The Portable
Skeletal X-Ray
Library

The Portable
Skeletal X-Ray
Library

Marshall N. Deltoff, DC, BSc, DACBR, FCCR(C)

Director, Images Radiology Consultants
Toronto, Ontario, Canada

Former Assistant Professor, Radiology Residency Coordinator and Chairman
Department of Radiology, Canadian Memorial Chiropractic College
Toronto, Ontario, Canada

Ancien coordonnateur, instructeur et consultant en radiologie
Département de chimie-biologie, Programme de doctorat en chiropratique
Université du Québec à Trois-Rivières
Trois-Rivières, Québec, Canada

Peter L. Kogon, DC, DACBR, FCCR(C), FICC

Professeur, radiologie clinique
Département de chimie-biologie, Programme de doctorat en chiropratique
Clinique universitaire de chiropratique
Université du Québec à Trois-Rivières
Trois-Rivières, Québec, Canada

Former Associate Clinical Professor
Department of Radiology,
Canadian Memorial Chiropractic College
Toronto, Ontario, Canada

Former Director, Chiropractic X-Ray Services
Toronto, Ontario, Canada

Immediate Past President
Chiropractic College of Radiologists (Canada)

with 948 illustrations

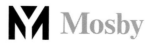 Mosby

St. Louis Baltimore Boston Carlsbad Chicago Naples New York Philadelphia Portland
London Madrid Mexico City Singapore Sydney Tokyo Toronto Wiesbaden

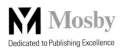

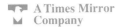

Publisher and Vice President: Don Ladig
Executive Editor: Martha Sasser
Developmental Editor: Kellie F. White
Project Manager: Linda McKinley
Production Editor: Paul Stoecklein
Composition Specialist: Wendy Bellm
Designer: Elizabeth Young
Manufacturing Supervisor: Don Carlisle

Printed in the United States of America

Composition by Mosby Electronic Production—St. Louis
Lithography by Top Graphics
Printing/binding by Maple Vail Book Manufacturing Group

Mosby–Year Book, Inc.
11830 Westline Industrial Drive
St. Louis, Missouri 63146

Library of Congress Cataloging in Publication Data

Deltoff, Marshall N.
   The portable skeletal X-ray library/Marshall N. Deltoff, Peter L. Kogon.
     p. cm.
   Includes bibliographical references and index.
   ISBN 0-8151-2244-6
   1. Bones—Radiography—Atlases.   I. Kogon, Peter L. II. Title.
   [DNLM: 1. Bone Diseases—radiography—atlases. 2. Bone Diseases-
-radiography—handbooks.   WE 17 D366p 1998]
   RC930.4.D45   1998
   616.7' 107572—dc21
   DNLM/DLC
   for Library of Congress

97 98 99 00 01 / 9 8 7 6 5 4 3 2 1

Preface

So much information has been generated about clinical radiology that students and clinicians alike find it difficult, if not impossible, to remain aware of all the material available. There are comprehensive texts with exacting, detailed descriptions of the etiology, pathogenesis, and radiodiagnostic features of a diverse number of radiologic entities. Although comprehensive, these large volumes are impractical for the physician who needs a fast reference or for the student looking for a quick review. Many attempts have been made to create radiologic synopses, and these have succeeded in centralizing and compacting significant volumes of subject matter. For the most part, however, these synopses have taken on a scope that was too broad; consequently, they have dealt with too many conditions that assume little prominence in everyday general chiropractic practice.

Our goal in creating The Portable Skeletal X-Ray Library is to bridge the gap between comprehensive, voluminous texts and synopses that focus on rare disorders. This textbook provides a contemporary pictorial appreciation of pathologic lesions that can and do present in daily practice. This quick and concise reference provides information about conditions affecting bone that is vital to the appreciation and management of such disorders. We have not detailed every radiodiagnostic entity; instead, we have placed emphasis on common presenting phenomena. Because our text is created to resemble an atlas format, we have reserved our bibliographic notations for the end of our work. Readers desiring or requiring more detailed information on a particular topic are invited to review those references.

Each condition presented in this book is described briefly and includes, where appropriate, age, incidence, gender distribution, pathogenesis, radiologic description, laboratory assessment, and differential diagnosis. We have included over 900 radiographs and line drawings depicting examples of common radiographic features. The abundance of x-rays films and line drawings, as well as the emphasis on key radiographic descriptions, allows this "portable library" to be used at the desk or viewbox as a quick reference for the busy clinician or as a study aid for the intern or student.

We have added many features to this book to ensure its ease of use as a quick reference. The chapters of the book are organized according to the mnemonic device CATBITESS (*C*, congenital, *A*, arthritides, *T*, tumors, *B*, blood, *I*, infection, *T*, trauma, *E*, endocrine, *S*, soft tissue, *S*, scoliosis). Thumbprints are provided for each chapter so that the reader can easily flip the book open to the information needed. Every chapter begins with an outline containing page number references. Also, an expanded table of contents is located at the front of the book. These features, along with a heavily detailed index, should make searching for specific conditions easy.

It is our sincere hope and intent that the reader, whether a clinician, student, board candidate, or teacher, will enjoy and use the contents of these pages.

Marshall N. Deltoff
Peter L. Kogon

Acknowledgments

"Only the lesson which is enjoyed can be learned well."

—Talmud

This volume is the culmination of 6 years of persistence and hard work. Completing this book has been one of my life's dreams. I was able to draw from a myriad of valuable human resources, whom I would now like to thank most humbly and sincerely.

I have been truly blessed with exceptional parents. Freda and Bert Deltoff have always been my greatest teachers. My mother continues to encourage and teach me with her strength, courage, and love, and my father will forever inspire me. When I began lecturing as a radiology resident at Los Angeles College of Chiropractic, he told me, "Remember, Marshall, you're not a drill sergeant, you're a teacher!"

To my incredible bride, Joyce, I cannot adequately verbalize my love and appreciation. Thank you for understanding me and motivating me, for being patient and supportive, and for tolerating the hundreds of x-rays, photos, and manuscript sheets constantly strewn and restrewn all over our living room floor. You are a loving source of constant encouragement.

My brother and partner, Arnie B. Deltoff, DC, is deserving of abundant gratitude for his exceptional and extraordinary enthusiasm and assistance throughout this project and for always going above and beyond the call of duty. His extensive literacy with computer operation saved many hours of toil. His behind-the-scenes commitment to this book through his smooth, efficient daily operation of our practice during manuscript development and preparation has been exemplary. He is a pleasure to work with and a source of great professional pride as a teacher and doctor.

I thank my sister, Michele Nitkin, RN, for her continuous interest and support of this venture, and her children Brenna, Avery, and Terrah for their eager enthusiasm for "Uncle Marshall," the book author.

I am forever indebted to my radiology professors, mentors, colleagues, and friends. I thank Drs. Joseph W. Howe, Terry R. Yochum, and Lindsay J. Rowe for the many hours they each spent at the viewbox with me, for all the educational and professional opportunities they initiated, and for the love of teaching chiropractic radiology that they cultivated in me.

I must thank my colleagues and friends who were also radiology residents during my residency training at Los Angeles College of Chiropractic, most notably, Drs. Larry H. Wyatt Jr., Gary D. Schultz, Margaret A. Seron, Anita L. Manne, and Gary L. Bustin, for providing an enjoyable, fun, learning atmosphere.

To all my students over the past 13 years throughout North America and particularly at Los Angeles College of Chiropractic, Canadian Memorial Chiropractic College, and the Université du Québec à Trois Rivières, I would like to express my gratitude for the privilege of sharing the classroom with you. Through your questions and positive feedback, you have provided me with inspiration and numerous ideas for this text.

A special thank you is conveyed to my practice partners, Robert J. Bacon, DC, and Lisette A. Logan, MRT, for their interest and support in this project and for supplying several cases. Sincere thanks also goes to my chiropractic assistant Bibi Hameed, CHA, for her creative scheduling of patients when the numerous and various publishing deadlines approached.

I must also thank all the doctors who generously shared so many wonderful cases. I appreciate that you are my friends and colleagues.

I express much gratitude to our editorial staff members, Martha Sasser, Kellie F. White, Paul Stoecklein, and their entire team at Mosby, for displaying confidence and trust in us, showing their genuine enthusiasm for this project, and providing the vehicle by which a dream became a reality. To Jeanne Robertson, thank you for enhancing this volume with your exceptional artistic talent.

Finally, to my coauthor, Peter L. Kogon, DC, FCCR(C), DACBR, FICC, I extend my perpetual thanks for his intelligence, wit, fortitude, motivating skills, patience, tolerance, and most of all, friendship. To say that the writing of this book with him has been a most satisfying odyssey would be a great understatement. Enjoy!

Marshall N. Deltoff

After reflecting on this text and the work that has gone into its production, I find myself unable to resist the opportunity to acknowledge those people who have provided me with so much love and support. Certainly, I must mention members of my family, including my parents Ben and Matilda, my sister Debbie, and my children Risa and Evan. Their support and guidance has assisted me through each word of this text. Also, I cannot forget all those dear friends and colleagues who were in my corner at every moment; to them, I remain sincerely indebted.

I would like to thank the doctors who contributed so many interesting studies, which have been included in this text and will benefit all of us. We have collected these cases over many years and are pleased to now have this opportunity to share them.

My deepest appreciation is extended to all my teachers, especially those who inspired my radiographic senses. I was fortunate to learn from a cadre of undergraduate and postgraduate professors who somehow managed to make radiology an interesting, exciting, and challenging endeavor. Without their gifted insight and wonderful esprit, it is difficult to imagine how this text could have become a reality.

I am grateful in particular for two influential people in my life and career. Every person at one point embraces a mentor, and I have mine. I have been privileged to study radiology under Dr. Thomas Goodrich. His brilliant academic prowess is superceded only by his compassionate humanitarianism. I am grateful also to my coauthor, Dr. Marshall Deltoff. He is a young, energetic, talented radiologist with whom I have had the pleasure of being a close friend and colleague. This special man and I have continued to remain friends in spite of a few differences of opinion in the preparation of our manuscript. Somehow, we have managed to work through our disagreements with laughter and mutual respect.

I thank the staff members at Mosby as well as our artist, Jeanne Robertson, for their extreme patience and tolerance through the course of this project.

Lastly, I would like to say thanks to you, our readers, for having selected our text for your study and pleasure. If it were not for all of you, our efforts would go largely unnoticed.

Peter L. Kogon

Contents

The Portable

Skeletal X-Ray

Library

Congenital Anomalies and Normal Variants

OUTLINE

Congenital anomalies, dysplasias, and normal skeletal roentgen variants may be of particular concern to those who possess an interest in diagnostic imaging. Comprising perhaps the most frequently encountered conditions, anomalies, dysplasias, and roentgen variants may assume a multitude of radiographic presentations. These conditions may frequently simulate a wide variety of disease states. Not uncommonly, a normal skeletal variant is overdiagnosed as a destructive bone lesion or even a fracture. Distinguishing normal from abnormal states, thus, becomes a critical issue when contemplating case management. Only after careful consideration can an accurate radiodiagnostic impression be rendered, the benefits of which can then be extended to patients.

The following pages present some of the more common skeletal variants and dysplasias. One must always recognize this potential presence and include normal variants in the differential diagnosis.

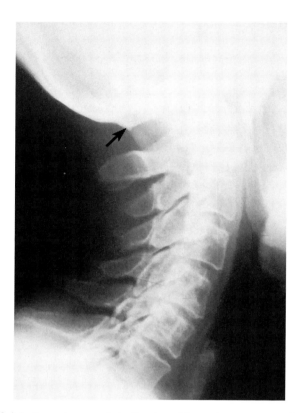

FIG. 1-1 Complete occipitalization. Note the remnant of posterior arch of atlas (*arrow*), which is fused to the occiput.

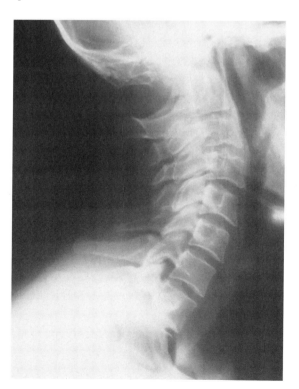

FIG. 1-2 Occipitalization. Posterior elements of atlas are absent.

OCCIPITOCERVICAL FUSION

- Extremely common skeletal malformation
- Usually consists of a total or partial fusion of the atlas to the rim of the foramen magnum (Figs. 1-1 and 1-2)
- Often associated with malformation of the foramen magnum, consisting of irregular shape, decreased size, and platybasia
- Usually accompanied by a low hairline, torticollis, shortness of the neck, and limitation of movement
- Possible increase of pain with coughing or neck movements
- Associated with fusion of C2 to C3 in 70% of patients (Fig. 1-3)

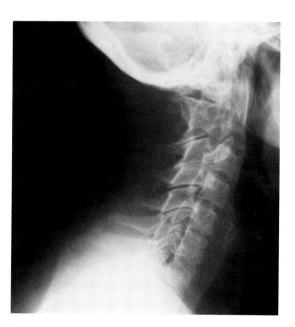

FIG. 1-3 Occipitalization. Note the concurrent congenital block vertebra at C2-C3 in this 41-year-old woman.

PARAMASTOID PROCESS

- ◆ An accessory osseous process originating at the jugular process on the occiput
- ◆ Projects caudad toward the ipsilateral atlas transverse process (Fig. 1-4)
- ◆ Possible formation of an accessory articulation with the transverse process of the atlas

AGENESIS/HYPOPLASIA

- ◆ Common condition in varying degrees
- ◆ Can be encountered at any spinal segment but most frequently at transitional sites (Figs. 1-5, 1-6, 1-7, 1-8, 1-9, and 1-10)

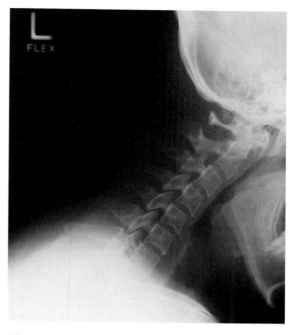

FIG. 1-5 This 29-year-old woman demonstrates a narrow, hypoplastic posterior arch of atlas.

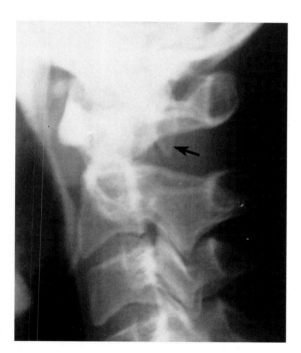

FIG. 1-4 Paramastoid process (*arrow*).

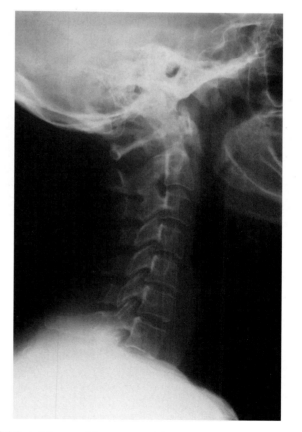

FIG. 1-6 A 56-year-old woman with a narrow posterior C1 arch.

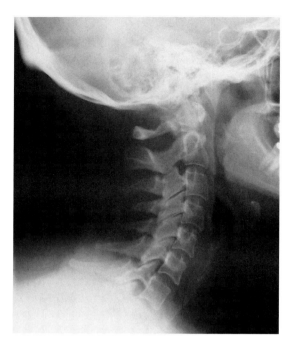

FIG. 1-7 Hypoplastic posterior arch of atlas in a 46-year-old woman.

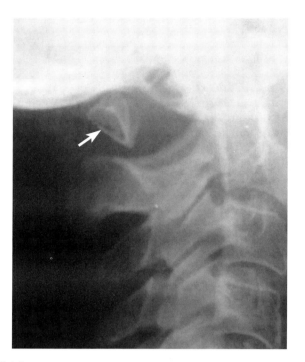

FIG. 1-8 Hypoplasia of atlas. Observe the posterior tubercle (*arrow*), with absent ossification of the remaining posterior arch.

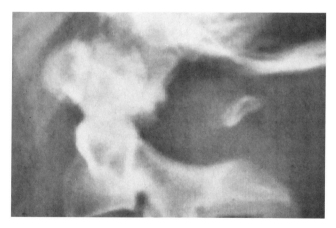

FIG. 1-9 Atlas posterior arch hypoplasia.

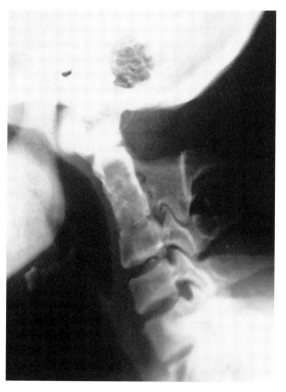

FIG. 1-10 Agenesis of posterior arch of atlas, demonstrating complete absence of posterior elements. Note the accompanying C2-C3-C4 block vertebrae.

POSTERIOR PONTICLE

- Observed in approximately 10% of all cervical spines
- Formed by the ossification of the oblique membrane of the atlanto-occipital ligament (Fig. 1-11)
- May demonstrate partial (Figs. 1-12, 1-13, and 1-14) or complete ossification
- When totally ossified, forms the arcuate foramen through which passes the suboccipital nerve and the vertebral artery (Figs. 1-15, 1-16, and 1-17)

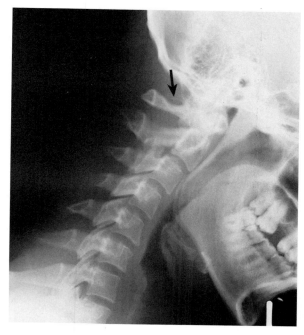

FIG. 1-12 Posterior ponticle. Partial ossification of the oblique membrane (*arrow*) is observed in this 28-year-old man. (Courtesy Ladislav Horak, MD, Toronto, Ontario.)

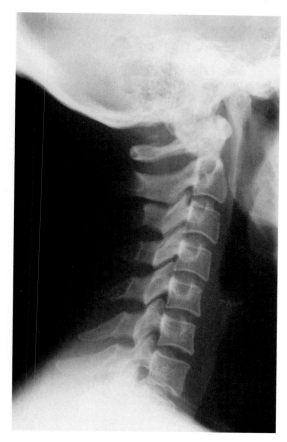

FIG. 1-11 Posterior ponticle. This 37-year-old woman demonstrates partial ossification of the oblique membrane. (Courtesy Ladislav Horak, MD, Toronto, Ontario.)

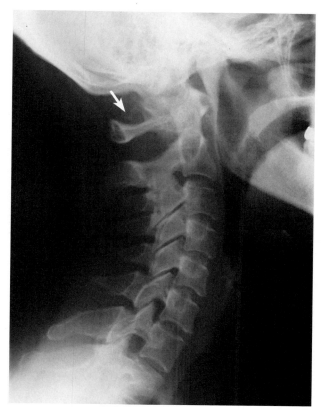

FIG. 1-13 Posterior ponticle. This 51-year-old woman demonstrates a near-complete arcuate foramen (*arrow*). (Courtesy Paul Anderson, MD, Toronto, Ontario.)

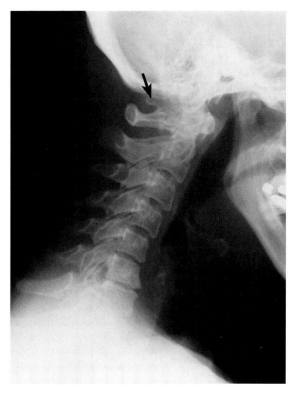

FIG. 1-14 Posterior ponticle. Partial pons posticus (*arrow*) in a 50-year-old woman.

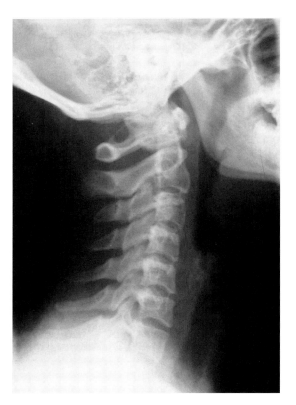

FIG. 1-15 Posterior ponticle. This 20-year-old woman demonstrates thin, almost total ossification of the oblique membrane.

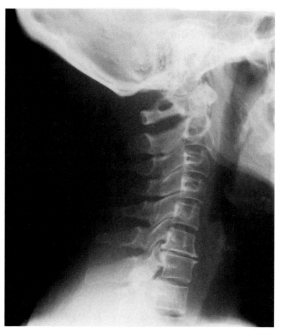

FIG. 1-16 Posterior ponticle. An arcuate foramen is formed in this 44-year-old woman as a result of complete ossification of the oblique membrane.

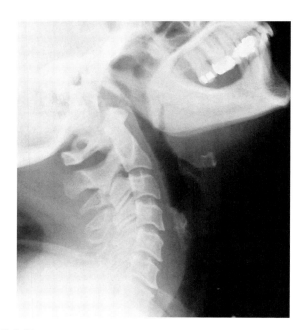

FIG. 1-17 Posterior ponticle. This 49-year-old man demonstrates an arcuate foramen. (Courtesy Lisette Logan, MRT, Brampton, Ontario.)

OS ODONTOIDEUM

- The apex and base of the dens fuse at approximately 9 years of age, but the base does not fuse to the body of C2 until adulthood. This situation is normal and must not be construed as an os odontoideum unless the odontoid is displaced.
- It is the most common anomaly of the odontoid process.
- It is characterized by a round ossicle of bone that may vary in size (Fig. 1-18).
- The ossicle is round or oval and roughly half the size of the normal odontoid (Fig. 1-19).
- A smooth, sclerotic border separates the os from the axis and is postulated to be a congenital nonunion (Figs. 1-20 and 1-21, *A* and *B*).

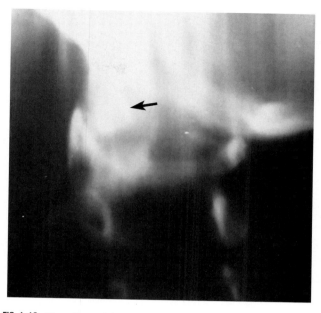

FIG. 1-19 Os odontoideum. This tomogram depicts the characteristic ossicle (*arrow*).

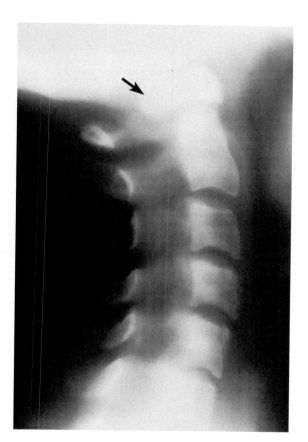

FIG. 1-18 Os odontoideum. Note the superior ossicle (*arrow*) in this neutral projection.

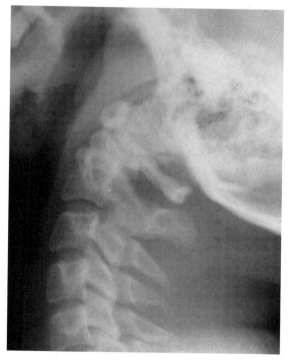

FIG. 1-20 This extension view demonstrates a posterior translation of atlas and the os odontoideum.

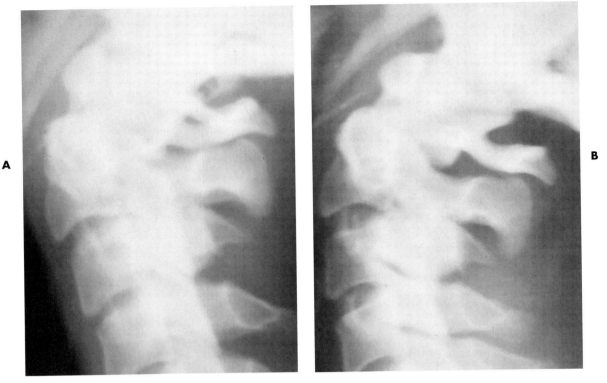

FIG. 1-21 Os odontoideum. **A,** Neutral. **B,** Extension. Note the posterior translation of atlas.

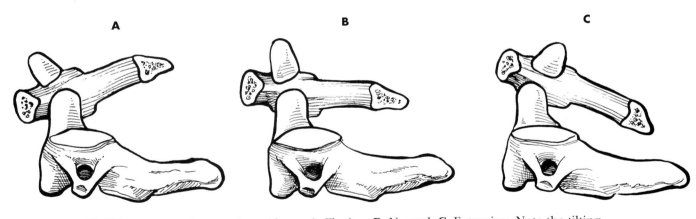

FIG. 1-22 Diagram of an os odontoideum. **A,** Flexion. **B,** Neutral. **C,** Extension. Note the tilting of the superior dens on movement.

- The patient is asymptomatic.
- Os odontoideum may be demonstrated on the anteroposterior open mouth (APOM) film, neutral lateral film and, when clinical indications permit, flexion and extension views (Figs. 1-22 and 1-23).
- Its radiologic appearance is often mistaken for a traumatic fracture.
- The gap is wide with smooth margins (Fig. 1-24, *A* and *B*).
- In an odontoid fracture the gap between the fragments is irregular and narrow.
- No marginal cortex adjacent to the fracture fragments is seen.
- Instability and complications resulting from relatively insignificant trauma pose a serious health risk.
- Prophylactic stabilization is still controversial in the asymptomatic patient.
- Surgical intervention is frequent in unstable cases or in the presence of severe neurologic manifestations.

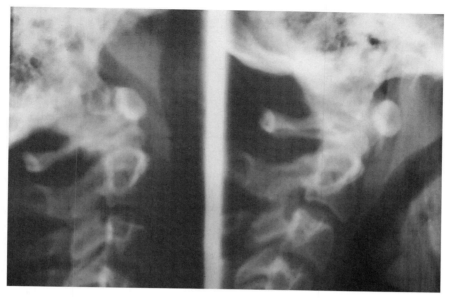

FIG. 1-23 Os odontoideum. Extension (left) and flexion views demonstrate the anterior movement of C1 on flexion.

A

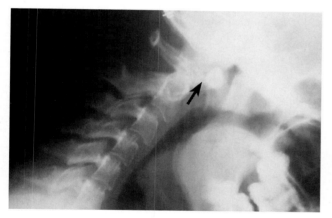

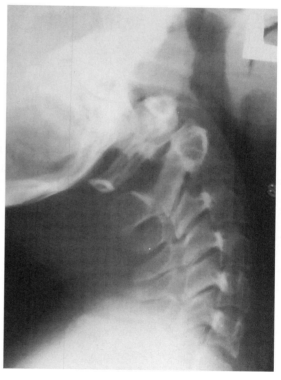

B

FIG. 1-24 Os odontoideum. **A,** Flexion. Note the increase in the atlantodental interspace (*arrow*). **B,** Extension. Note the posterior atlas migration.

OSSICULUM TERMINALE

- This condition occurs when the secondary ossification center on the apex of the dens fails to unite (Fig. 1-25, *A* and *B*).
- This small ossification center usually appears by age 3 and fuses to the dens by age 12.

- Ossiculum terminale persistens manifests as a V-shaped depression in the apex of the odontoid (Figs. 1-26, 1-27, and 1-28).
- This condition is rarely of clinical significance.
- The ossiculum is usually secured to the remaining dens by fibrous tissue.

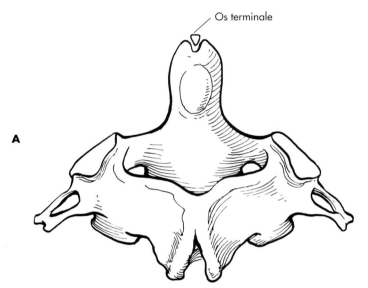

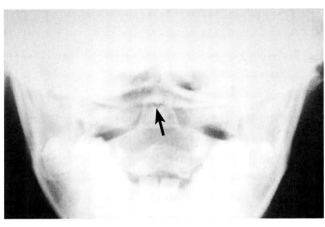

FIG. 1-26 Ossiculum terminale. Note the V-shaped depression (*arrow*).

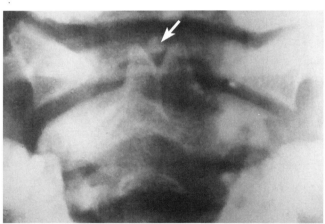

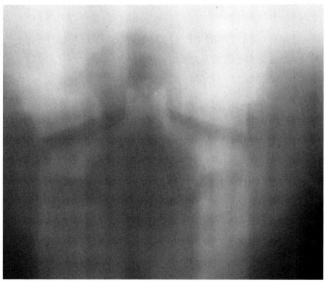

FIG. 1-25 Ossiculum terminale. **A,** Diagram. **B,** Radiograph. Observe the ununited apex of the dens (*arrow*).

FIG. 1-27 Ossiculum terminale. Tomogram depicts superior dens ossicle with V-shaped depression.

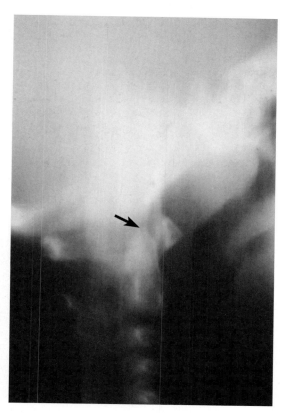

FIG. 1-28 Ossiculum terminale. Note the V-shaped depression (*arrow*) at the apex of the superior dens on this lateral cervical radiograph.

CONGENITAL APLASIA AND DYSPLASIA OF THE DENS

♦ Rare malformation
♦ Usually asymptomatic and discovered incidentally
♦ With severe trauma, may result in quadraplegia
♦ Appears radiographically as a flattened superior surface of C2 or a moundlike bulge in the region corresponding to the aplastic dens (Figs. 1-29 and 1-30)

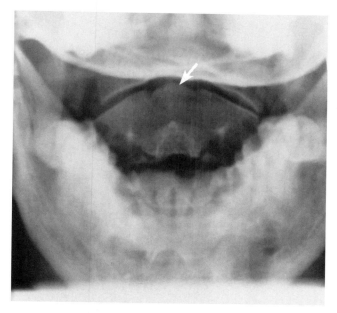

FIG. 1-29 Agenesis of the dens. The absence of the odontoid is noted with only a rudimentary "mound" of bone visualized (*arrow*).

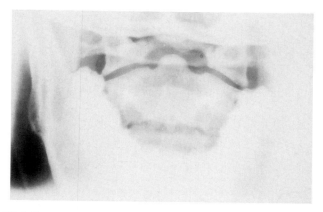

FIG. 1-30 Odontoid agenesis.

INTERCALARY BONE

◆ Small bony ossicle in the anterior vertebral interspace
◆ Usually in cervical spine (Fig. 1-31)

◆ Represents calcification in the anterior longitudinal ligament or outer annular disc fibers (Figs. 1-32, 1-33, 1-34, and 1-35)
◆ Of no clinical significance

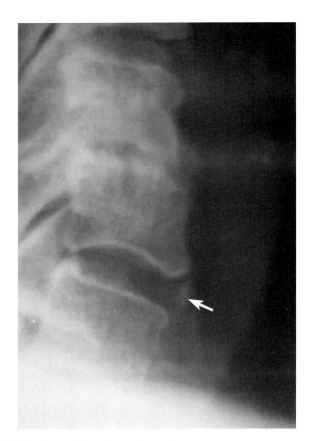

FIG. 1-31 Intercalary bone (*arrow*).

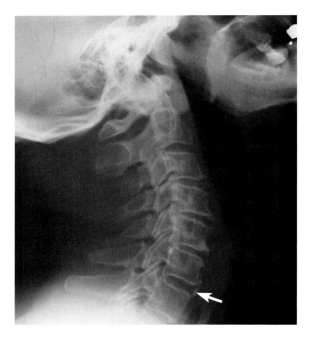

FIG. 1-32 Intercalary bone. Note the vertical ossicle at the anterior aspect of the C6-C7 disc space (*arrow*).

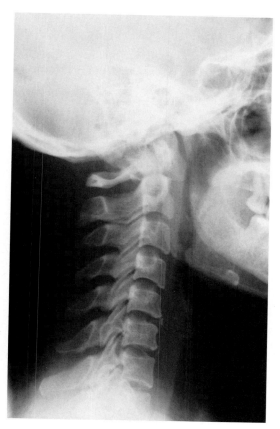

FIG. 1-33 Intercalary bones. C5-C6 and C6-C7 levels demonstrate intercalary bones.

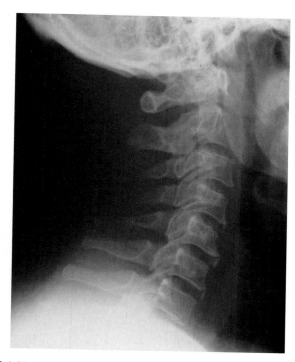

FIG. 1-34 Multiple intercalary bones. Levels C3-C4 through C6-C7 each demonstrate an intercalary bone. (Courtesy Pavit Kapoor, DC, Burlington, Ontario.)

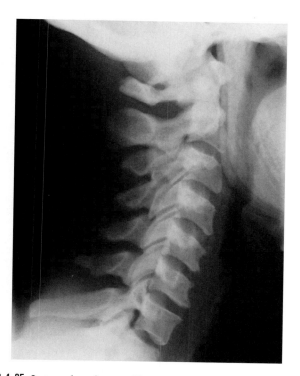

FIG. 1-35 Intercalary bones. Two are noted at the C4-C5 level.

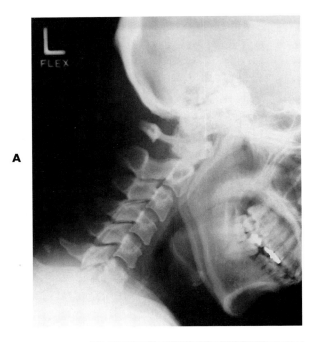

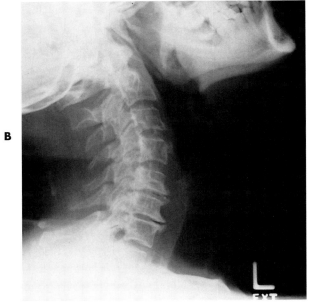

NUCHAL BONE

- Not uncommon
- Calcifications and ossifications in the nuchal ligament that vary in number, size, and shape (Fig. 1-36, *A-C*)
- Not clinically significant

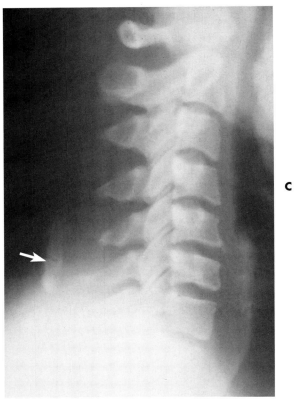

FIG. 1-36 Nuchal bones. **A,** A nuchal bone is noted between the tips of the C6 and C7 spinous processes in this 47-year-old woman. **B,** Small nuchal bone in a 69-year-old man. **C,** Extremely large nuchal bone (*arrow*).

STYLOHYOID LIGAMENT OSSIFICATION

- ◆ May observe partial or complete ossification
- ◆ Unilateral (Fig. 1-37) or bilateral (Fig. 1-38)
- ◆ Possible formation of pseudoarthroses along the length of the ossifying ligament (Fig. 1-39)
- ◆ May be symptomatic (Eagle syndrome)

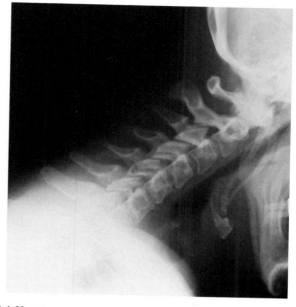

FIG. 1-38 This 43-year-old woman demonstrates marked bilateral stylohyoid ligament calcification.

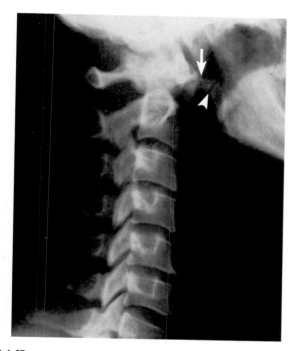

FIG. 1-37 This stylohyoid ligament ossification (*arrow*) demonstrates an accessory articulation (*arrowhead*).

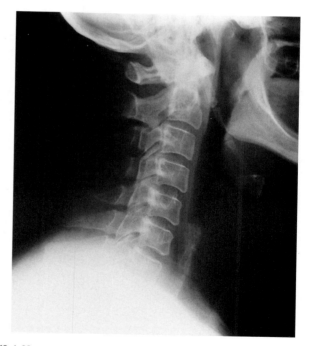

FIG. 1-39 Stylohyoid ligament calcification in a 37-year-old woman.

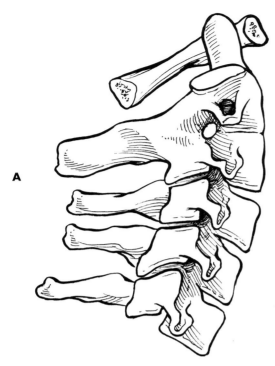

BLOCK VERTEBRAE

- Common
- Occurs when segmentation of somites is disturbed (Figs. 1-40, *A* and *B;* 1-41; and 1-42)
- Can occur at any level (Figs. 1-43; 1-44; 1-45, *A* and *B;* and 1-46)
- Often discovered incidentally
- May involve the body, arch, or entire segment
- May be multiple (Figs. 1-47, 1-48, 1-49, and 1-50)

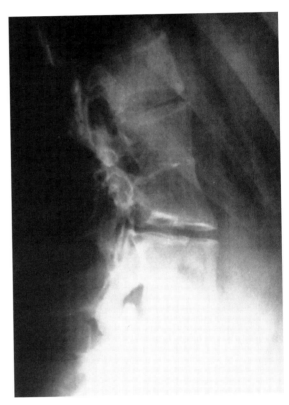

FIG. 1-41 Lateral lumbar view depicting congenital fusion at L3-L4.

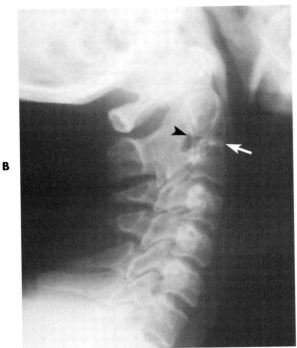

FIG. 1-40 Block vertebra at C2-C3. **A,** Diagram. **B,** Lateral cervical radiograph. Note the rudimentary disc (*arrow*), visualization of the intervertebral foramen (*arrowhead*), and facet fusion.

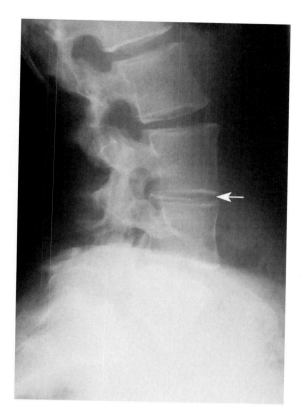

FIG. 1-42 Congenital block at L3-L4. Note the rudimentary disc (*arrow*).

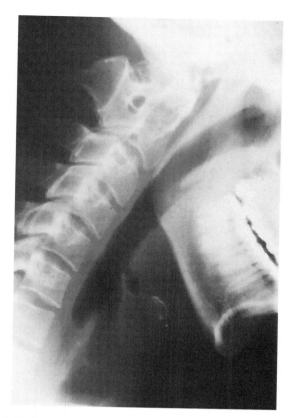

FIG. 1-43 Congenital block at atlas-axis in a 31-year-old man. (Courtesy Sheldon Hershkop, MD, Toronto, Ontario.)

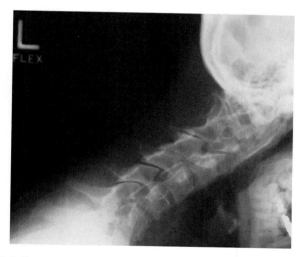

FIG. 1-44 Congenital block at C2-C3 with concurrent occipitalization in a 41-year-old woman.

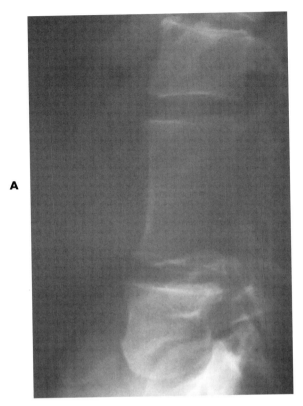

A

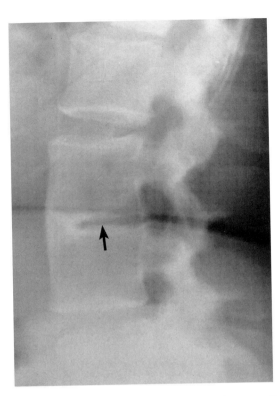

FIG. 1-46 L3-L4 congenital block demonstrating a rudimentary disc (*arrow*).

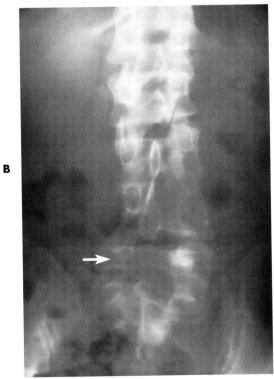

B

FIG. 1-45 L3-L4 congenital block. **A,** Lateral. **B,** Anteroposterior. Note the L5 hemivertebra (*arrow*), which accompanies the congenital fusion at L3-L4.

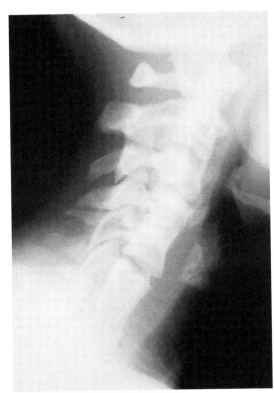

FIG. 1-47 Multiple-level block vertebrae. C4-C5 as well as C6-C7 demonstrate congenital fusion.

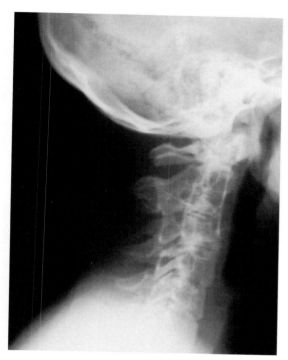

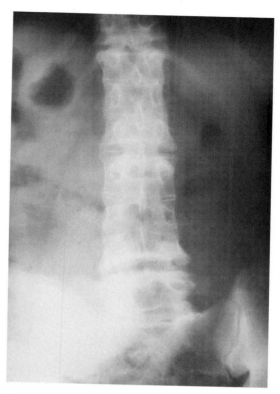

FIG. 1-48 Multiple-level congenital fusion from C2 through C5. (Courtesy Jacinthe Desmarais, DC, Brossard, Quebec.)

FIG. 1-49 Block vertebra. This anteroposterior view demonstrates a multiple-level congenital synostosis from L2 through L4.

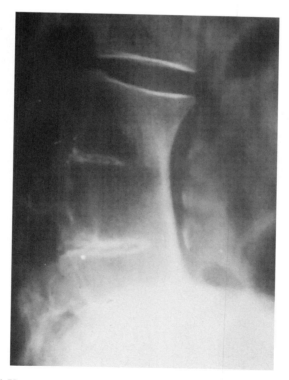

FIG. 1-50 Lateral projection of L2-L4 multilevel block.

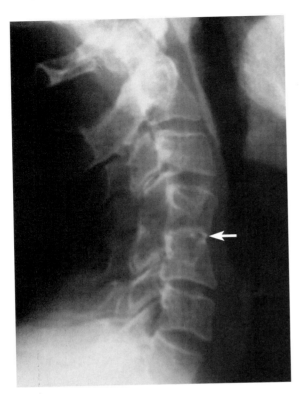

FIG. 1-51 Congenital block vertebra at C4-C5 demonstrates characteristic "wasp-waist" central concavity (*arrow*) at the site of the rudimentary disc.

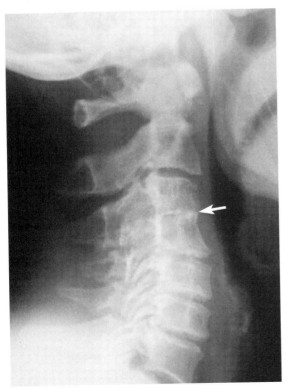

FIG. 1-52 Rudimentary disc (*arrow*) at C3-C4 block.

- Possible attributes of a congenital block segment:
  - "Wasp-waist" deformity: central anterior indentation at the site of the vestigeal disc (Fig. 1-51)
  - Rudimentary or absent disc (Figs. 1-52 and 1-53)
  - Fusion of posterior elements as well as adjacent vertebral bodies (Fig. 1-54)
  - Visualization of the intervertebral foraminae on a neutral lateral cervical view (Figs. 1-55 and 1-56)
  - Total height of a congenital block vertebra often equaling the height of the two separate segments plus the intervening disc space

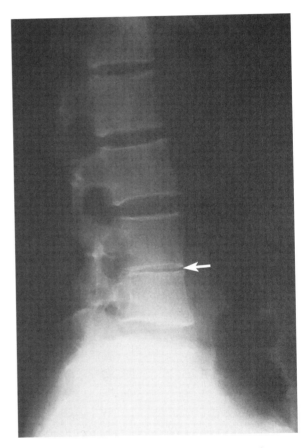

FIG. 1-53 Rudimentary disc (*arrow*) at L3-L4 block.

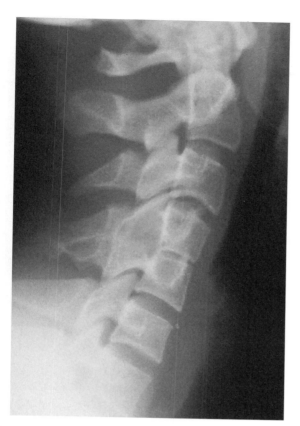

FIG. 1-54 Note the facet fusion at C4-C5.

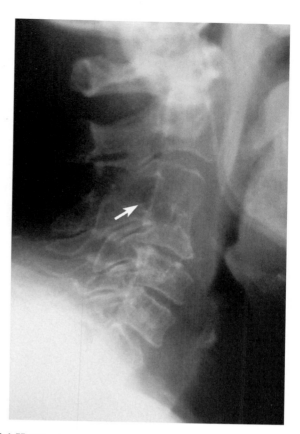

FIG. 1-55 The intervertebral foramen (*arrow*) is visualized on this lateral projection of a C3-C4 congenital block.

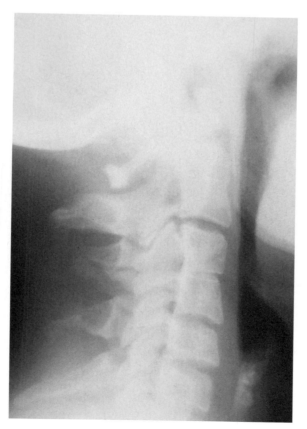

FIG. 1-56 Two sets of block vertebrae are observed in this patient; C2-C3 and C4-C5 each demonstrate congenital synostosis.

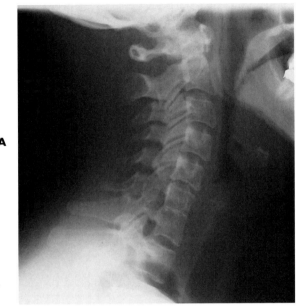

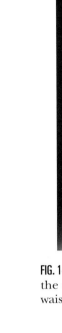

FIG. 1-58 Surgical arthrodesis from C5 through C7. Note the absence of rudimentary discs, facet fusion, and "wasp waist" deformities.

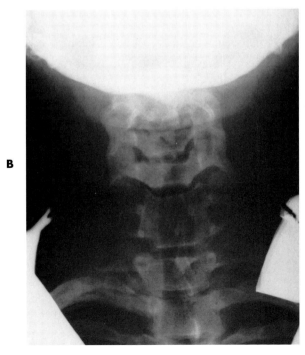

FIG. 1-57 A, Congenital fusion at C6-C7 in a 37-year-old woman. **B,** C6-C7 congenital block in an 18-year-old woman.

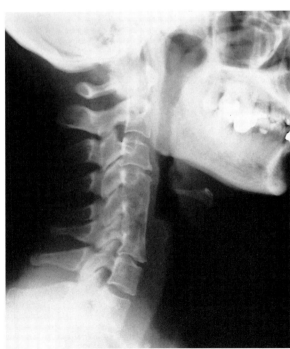

FIG. 1-59 C4 through C6 demonstrates surgical fusion.

- Necessary to differentiate congenital block (Fig. 1-57, *A* and *B*) from acquired fusion caused by infection, arthritic involvement, trauma, or surgical arthrodesis (Figs. 1-58 and 1-59)

KLIPPEL-FEIL SYNDROME

- A combination of congenital malformations involving the lower cervical spine
- Extensive fusions, marked shortening of the neck, and often a rounded back
- Exact etiology unknown
- Presence of three clinical signs required:
  - Short neck
  - Low posterior hairline
  - Limited range of motion

- Because of the involvement of the neural arches, the intervertebral foraminae are often smaller, smooth, and round or oval.
- Possible presence of hemivertebrae, spina bifida occulta, and disc aplasia or hypoplasia (Fig. 1-60)
- Scoliosis of 20 degrees or greater in more than half the cases
- Presence of Sprengel's deformity in more than one fifth of the cases (Fig. 1-61)
- Genitourinary tract anomalies found in over two thirds of the cases (e.g., unilateral renal agenesis, kidney malrotation, renal ectopia, and duplex collecting systems)

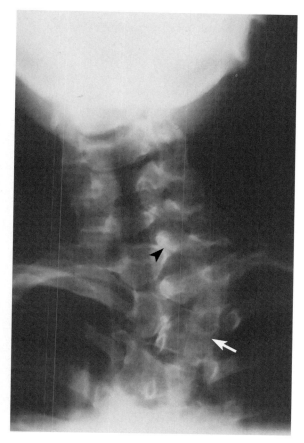

FIG. 1-60 Klippel-Feil syndrome. Multiple anomalies are noted, including hemivertebra (*arrow*) and spina bifida (*arrowhead*). (Courtesy Jacinthe Desmarais, DC, Brossard, Quebec.)

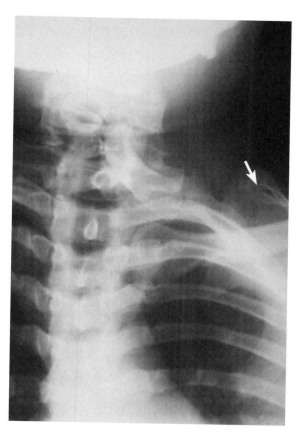

FIG. 1-61 Klippel-Feil syndrome. Multiple cervical anomalies and Sprengel's deformity (*arrow*).

SPRENGEL'S DEFORMITY

- A congenital anomaly in which the scapula fails to descend normally
- Scapula positioned so that the superior angle lies on a plane higher than the neck of the first rib (Figs. 1-62 and 1-63)
- Usually unilateral
- Seen in association with Klippel-Feil syndrome in 25% to 30% of cases
- In approximately 30% to 40% of cases, presence of a connection between the elevated scapula and one of the vertebra, usually C5 or C6; connection sometimes osseous, seen on plain film, and termed the *omovertebral bone*

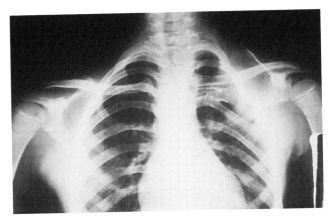

FIG. 1-62 Sprengel's deformity in a teenager. Note the nondescent of the left scapula.

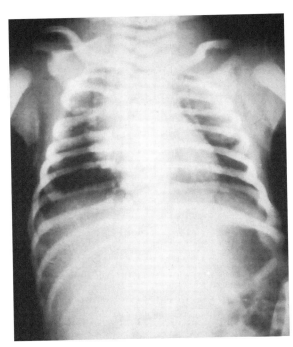

FIG. 1-63 Pediatric Sprengel's deformity of the right scapula.

SPINA BIFIDA

- ◆ Abnormal development of neural arch caused by failure of neural tube to close completely

Spina Bifida Occulta

- ◆ Most common and least severe neural arch deformity
  - · Etiology: failure of complete development of neural arch ossification centers
- ◆ Localized fusion defect of the halves of the vertebral arch with no neurologic deficit (Fig 1-64)
- ◆ Most commonly involves incomplete fusion of a single spinous process (Figs. 1-65 and 1-66)
- ◆ Asymptomatic; does not predispose a patient to back pain

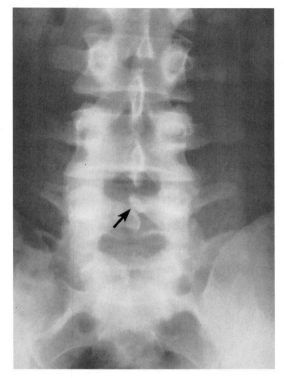

FIG. 1-65 L5 spina bifida. Note the central posterior arch defect (*arrow*).

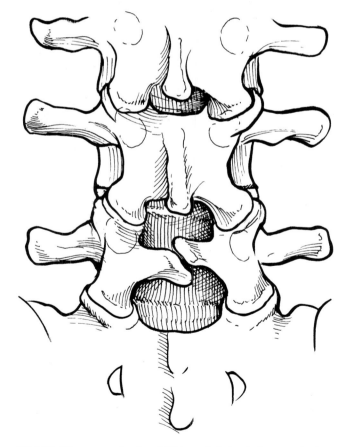

FIG. 1-64 Diagram of spina bifida at L5 depicting central nonfusion of the posterior arch.

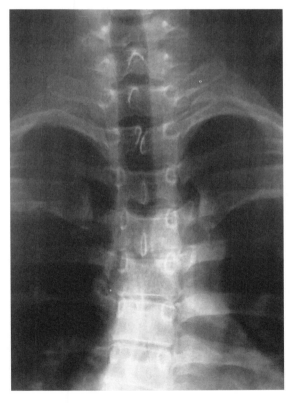

FIG. 1-66 T2 demonstrates spina bifida.

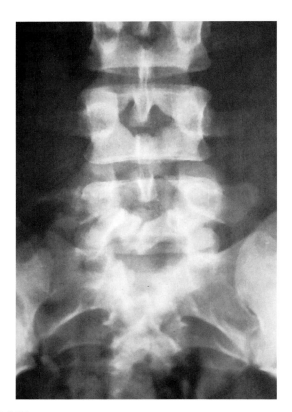

FIG. 1-67 Spina bifida at L5 and S1.

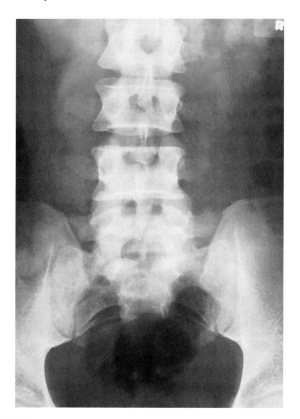

FIG. 1-68 L5 and S1 each demonstrate spina bifida.

- Lower lumbar and upper sacral segments most commonly affected (Figs. 1-67, 1-68, 1-69, 1-70, and 1-71)
- Nonunion of halves of the spinous process apparent on the A/P projection on radiographic examination
- May vary from a slight midline cleft defect to an absence of most of the vertebral neural arch (Fig. 1-72)
- Generally rare in the cervical spine

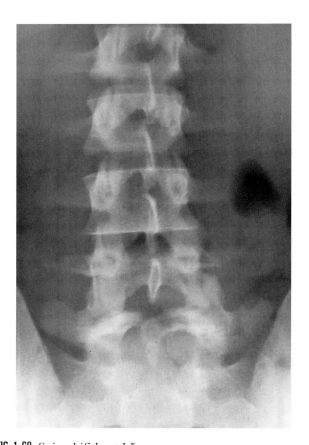

FIG. 1-69 Spina bifida at L5.

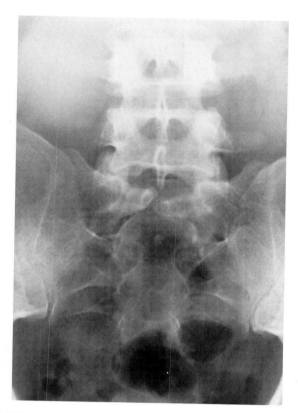

FIG. 1-70 Spina bifida at S1.

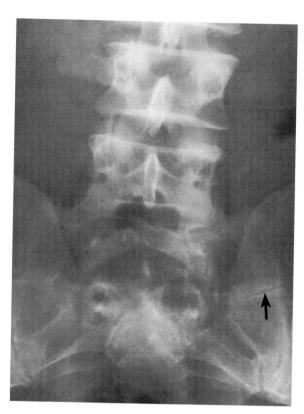

FIG. 1-71 Spina bifida at S1 transitional segment. Note the accessory articulation (*arrow*).

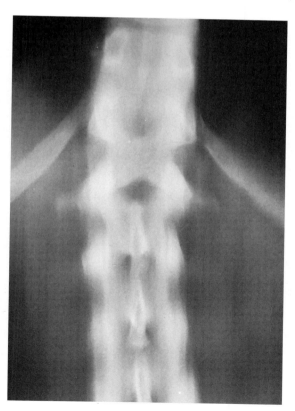

FIG. 1-72 Tomogram demonstrating an absent spinous process at T12.

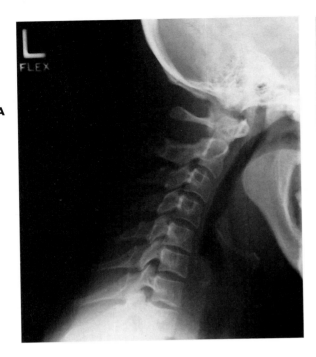

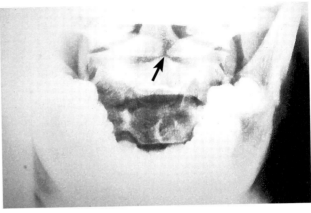

FIG. 1-73 Spina bifida of atlas. **A,** Lateral view demonstrating the absence of the spinolaminar junction line of atlas. **B,** Anteroposterior open-mouth view depicting a midline cleft (*arrow*) in the posterior arch. (Courtesy Arnie Deltoff, DC, Toronto, Ontario.)

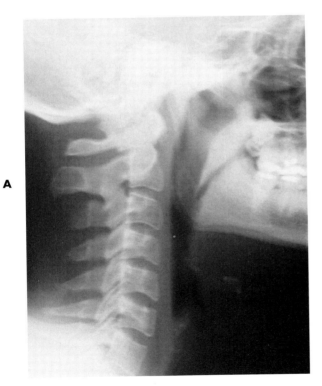

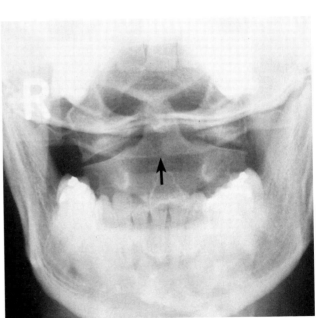

FIG. 1-74 Atlas spina bifida in a 21-year-old man. **A,** Lateral. Note the absence of the spinolaminar junction line. **B,** Anteroposterior open-mouth. Observe the midline defect (*arrow*).

- Lateral cervical: search for absence of the spino-laminar junction line (Figs. 1-73, *A* and *B*; and 1-74, *A* and *B*)
- C1 (Figs. 1-75 and 1-76, *A* and *B*), C2 (Figs. 1-77 and 1-78), and C7 (Fig. 1-79) most common cervical segments affected

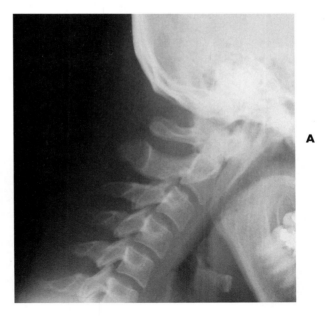

A

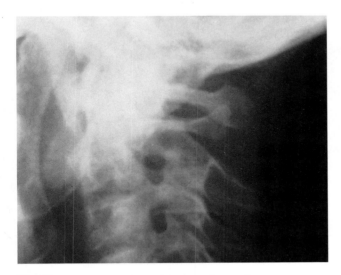

FIG. 1-75 Nonfusion of the C1 posterior arch.

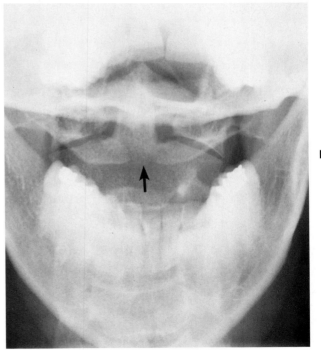

B

FIG. 1-76 A 33-year-old woman with nonfusion of the posterior arch of atlas. **A,** Lateral. **B,** Anteroposterior open mouth. Note the relatively wide defect (*arrow*).

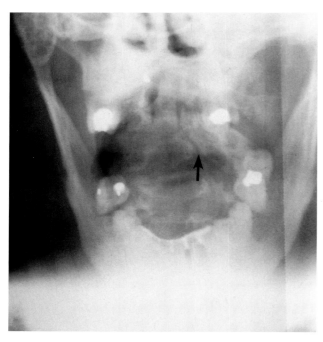

FIG. 1-77 Anteroposterior open-mouth projection demonstrating spina bifida of the axis (*arrow*). (Courtesy Kevin Dinsmore, DC, Belleville, Ontario.)

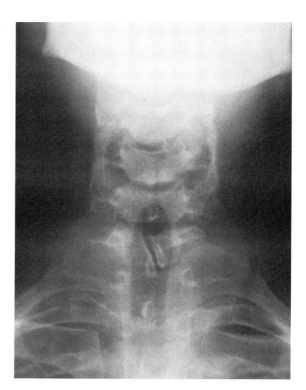

FIG. 1-79 C7 spina bifida is noted on this anteroposterior lower cervical film.

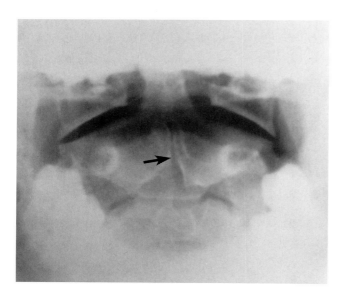

FIG. 1-78 Anteroposterior open-mouth view depicting spina bifida at C2 (*arrow*).

- Most common C1 malformation, occurring in approximately 3% of the population; occurs almost always without complications
- Lumbosacral spina bifida occurring in 5% to 10% of the population
- May occur at multiple levels (Figs. 1-80, 1-81, and 1-82) or in conjunction with other anomalies, such as block vertebrae (Fig. 1-83)

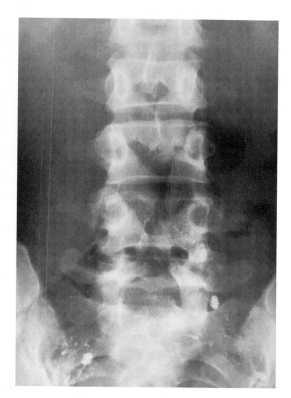

FIG. 1-80 Multiple-level spina bifida of the lumbar spine.

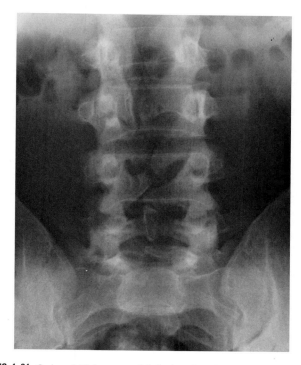

FIG. 1-81 Spina bifida at multiple lumbar levels.

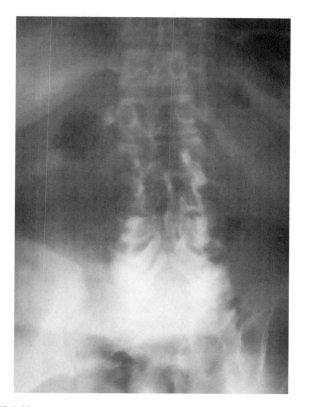

FIG. 1-82 Spina bifida at multiple lumbar levels.

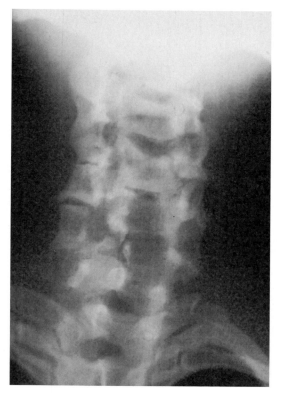

FIG. 1-83 This anteroposterior projection depicts spina bifida at C6 in conjunction with a block vertebra.

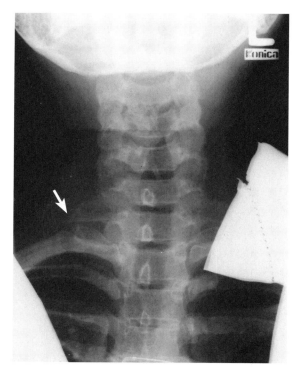

FIG. 1-84 The right C7 transverse process is hyperplastic (*arrow*) in this 34-year-old woman. (Courtesy James Clark, MD, Toronto, Ontario.)

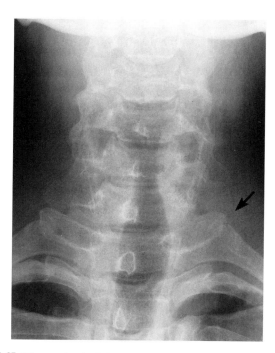

FIG. 1-85 Hyperplastic left transverse process of C7 in a 56-year-old man (*arrow*). (Courtesy Howard Jacobs, MD, Toronto, Ontario.)

CERVICAL RIBS

- Occur in 0.5% to 1% of the human population
- Requires the presence of an articulation for diagnosis; otherwise, referred to as a *hyperplastic transverse process* (Figs. 1-84, 1-85, 1-86, 1-87, and 1-88)
- May be unilateral or bilateral, with the majority of the latter asymmetrical (Figs. 1-89, 1-90, and 1-91)
- In females, 10% to 15% increased frequency
- Can be distinguished from a T1 rib because the orientation of the C7 transverse process is downward or horizontal, whereas the T1 transverse process has an upward projection (Figs. 1-92 and 1-93)
- Cervical ribs or fibrous bands usually asymptomatic (Fig. 1-94, *A* and *B*)
- Appearance of symptoms in fewer than 10% of patients and usually not until middle age

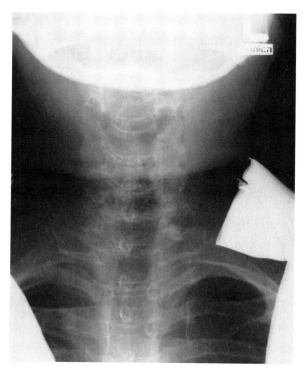

FIG. 1-86 This 74-year-old woman demonstrates a right hyperplastic C7 transverse process.

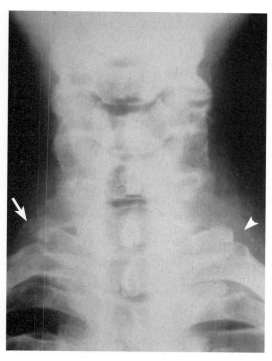

FIG. 1-87 Small right cervical rib at C7 (*arrow*) with a left hyperplastic transverse process (*arrowhead*).

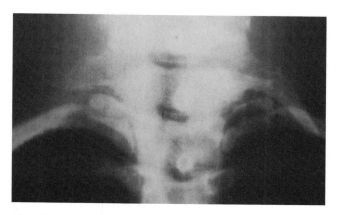

FIG. 1-88 A large, well-formed cervical rib at C7 is observed on the reading right. There is a contralateral hyperplastic transverse process.

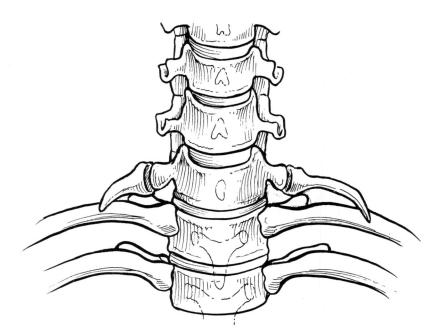

FIG. 1-89 Diagram depicting bilateral C7 cervical ribs. Note their typical asymmetry.

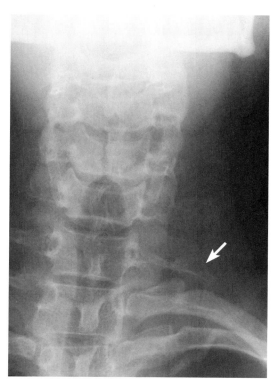

FIG. 1-90 A small left C7 cervical rib (*arrow*) is observed in this 30-year-old woman.

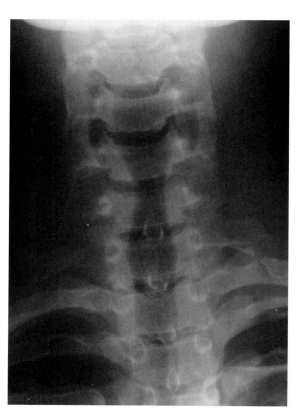

FIG. 1-91 A 29-year-old man demonstrates a complete articulation between the left C7 transverse process and its corresponding cervical rib. The right transverse process is moderately hyperplastic.

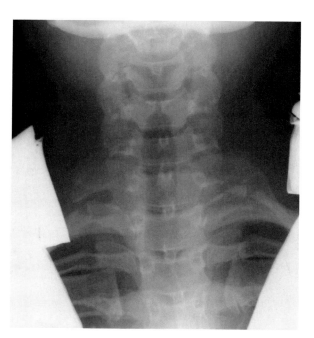

FIG. 1-92 This 32-year-old woman demonstrates a complete rib on the left at C7 with a hyperplastic transverse process on the right. (Courtesy Robert Bacon, DC, Toronto, Ontario.)

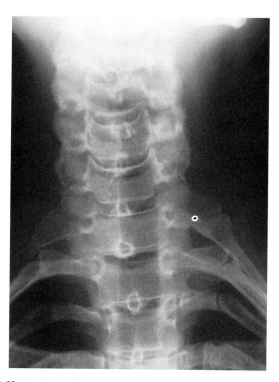

FIG. 1-93 Full left C7 rib with a mildly hyperplastic right transverse process in a 53-year-old woman.

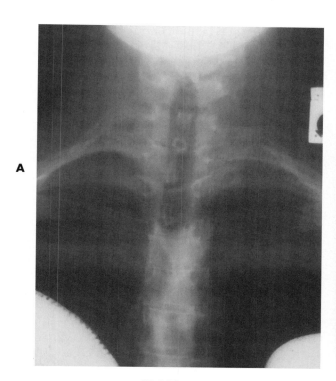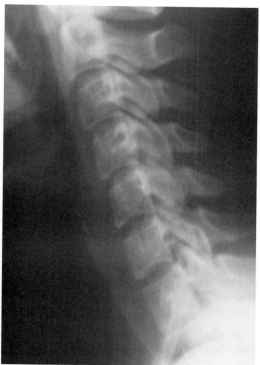

FIG. 1-94 Bilateral cervical ribs at C7. **A,** Anteroposterior. **B,** Lateral.

COSTAL CARTILAGE CALCIFICATION

♦ Present to some degree in most humans by the age of 25
  • Males: "railroad-track" appearance whereby the upper and lower margins of the cartilage become calcified initially (Fig. 1-95)

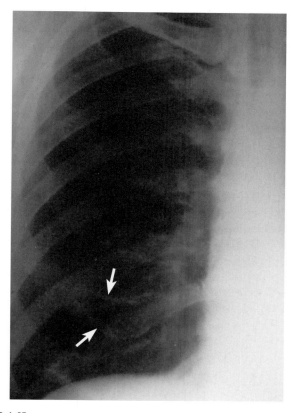

FIG. 1-95 Marginal "railroad track" costochondral calcification (*arrows*) in a male patient.

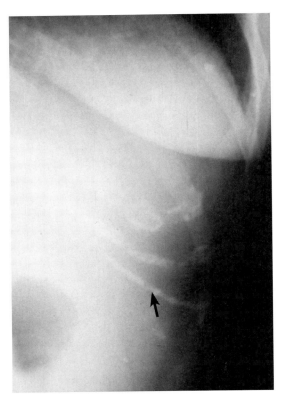

FIG. 1-96 Central "dagger" costochondral calcification (*arrow*) typically noted in women.

- • Females: "dagger" or "wagging-tongue" appearance whereby the central portion of the cartilage calcifies first (Fig. 1-96)
- ◆ No correlation to any disease

HAHN'S FISSURES

- ◆ Slitlike clefts that traverse the central portion of the vertebral body horizontally (Figs. 1-97 and 1-98)
- ◆ Represents an indurated vascular venous groove
- ◆ Of no clinical significance

KNIFE-CLASP DEFORMITY

- ◆ An elongated L5 spinous process in the presence of an S1 spina bifida occulta (Figs. 1-99, 1-100, 1-101, and 1-102)
- ◆ Occasionally associated with low back pain and radiculopathy, especially in the hyperextension posture

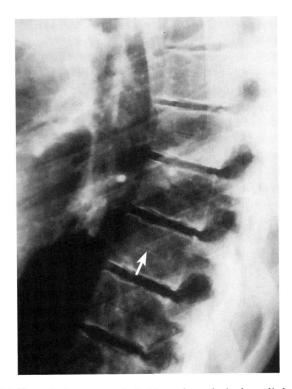

FIG. 1-97 Hahn's venous cleft. Note the relatively radiolucent "slit" (*arrow*) traversing the vertebral body.

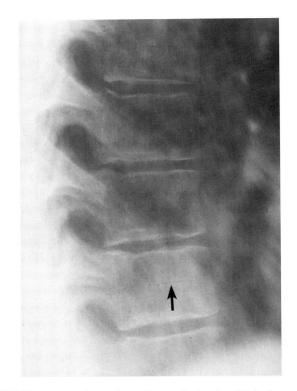

FIG. 1-98 Lateral thoracic radiograph depicts Hahn's venous fissure (*arrow*).

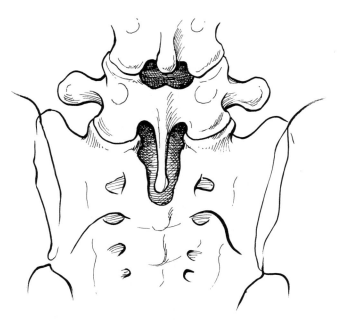

FIG. 1-99 Knife-clasp deformity diagram. Spina bifida at the S1 posterior arch is accompanied by an elongated L5 spinous process.

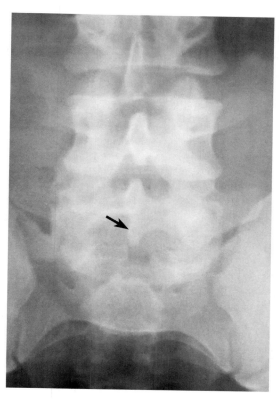

FIG. 1-100 Knife-clasp deformity. Note the slightly elongated spinous process at L5 (*arrow*).

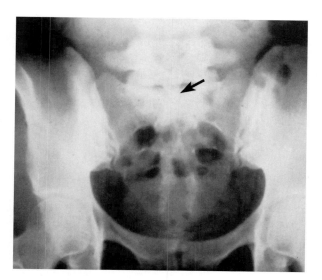

FIG. 1-101 Knife-clasp deformity (*arrow*).

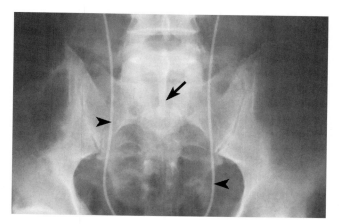

FIG. 1-102 Knife-clasp deformity (*arrow*). Of incidental note are ureterogram tubes (*arrowheads*).

- Symptoms a possible result of the L5 spinous process impinging on the fibrous membrane overlying the area of the spina bifida occulta and irritating neural tissue in the cauda equina (Figs. 1-103 and 1-104)
- May require surgical removal or shortening of the spinous process

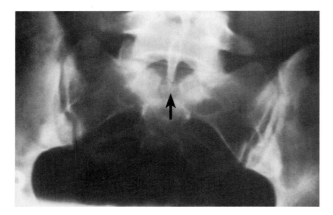

FIG. 1-103 Large L5 spinous process (*arrow*) forming a knife-clasp deformity.

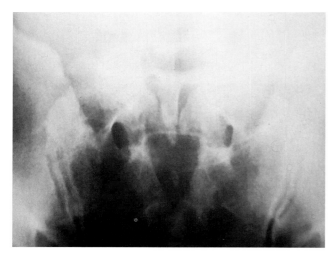

FIG. 1-104 Knife-clasp deformity.

TRANSITIONAL SEGMENTS

- Occur in approximately 20% of skeletons
- Vertebra assuming characteristics of both adjacent areas
- Most commonly lumbosacral or thoracolumbar (Figs. 1-105 and 1-106)
  - Accessory articulations: large L5 transverse processes possibly forming true joints with the sacral base (including cartilaginous surfaces and joint capsules) (Figs. 1-107, 1-108, 1-109, 1-110, 1-111, and 1-112)
  - Sacralization: Bertolotti's syndrome
  - Lumbarization (Fig. 1-113)

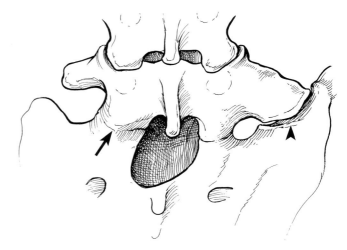

FIG. 1-105 Attempted sacralization of L5 is depicted in this diagram. Observe the fusion of L5 to the sacral base on the reading left (*arrow*) and the accessory articulation formed contralaterally (*arrowhead*) by the enlarged, spatulated transverse process.

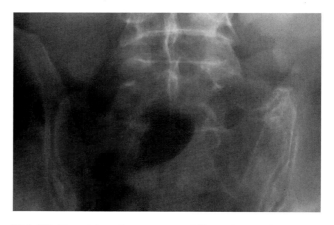

FIG. 1-106 Transitional segment at L5 on the reading right.

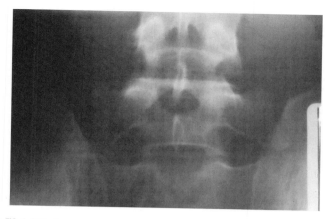

FIG. 1-107 Accessory articulation at the L5 transverse process on the reading left.

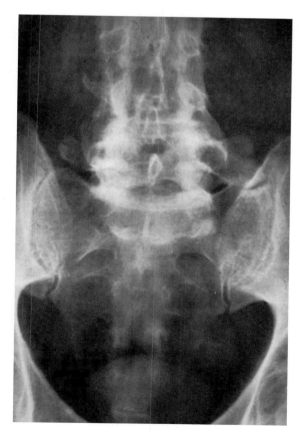

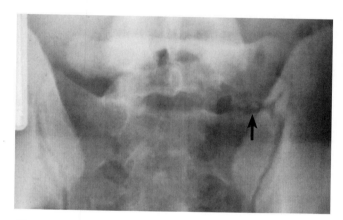

FIG. 1-109 Unilateral accessory articulation (*arrow*) demonstrating mild osteoarthritic changes.

FIG. 1-108 Mildly arthrotic accessory articulation on the reading right at L5.

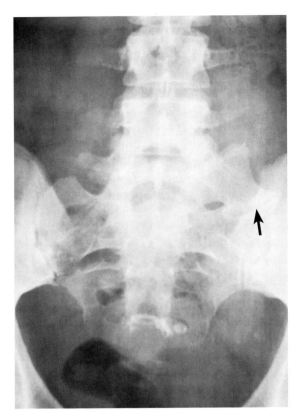

FIG. 1-110 Moderate degenerative changes in a unilateral accessory articulation (*arrow*).

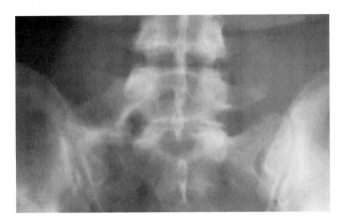

FIG. 1-111 Enlarged L5 transverse process has fused to the sacral base on the reading left.

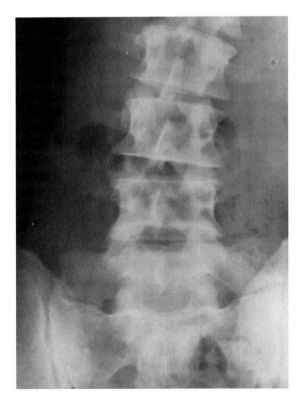

FIG. 1-112 Transitional segment. L5 demonstrates bilateral, enlarged, spatulated transverse processes that form accessory articulations bilaterally.

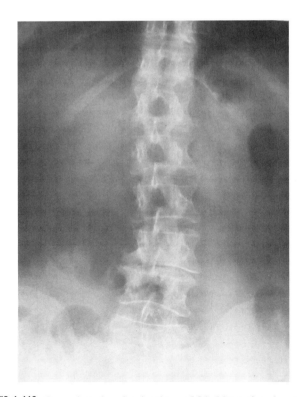

FIG. 1-113 Complete lumbarization of S1. Note the six vertebrae, which display lumbar characteristics.

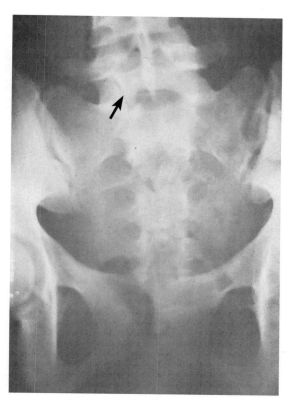

FIG. 1-126 Facet asymmetry at L5-S1. Note the primarily sagittal facet orientation on the reading left (*arrow*), whereas the contralateral side is primarily coronal.

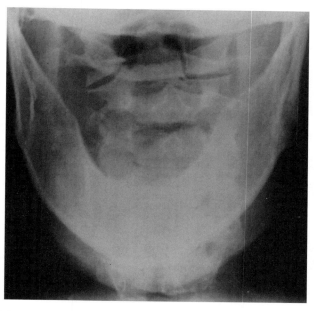

FIG. 1-127 Articular asymmetry at atlas-axis is demonstrated in this patient with a relatively right-angle facet orientation on the reading right.

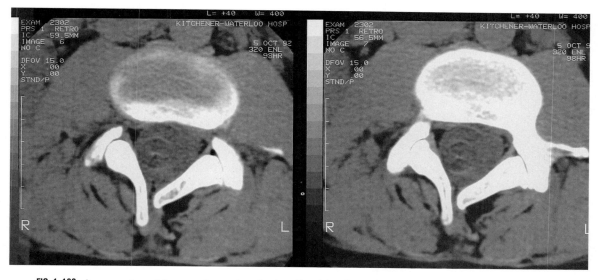

FIG. 1-128 Asymmetry of facet orientation is visualized in these sequential computed tomographic images of a lumbar vertebra.

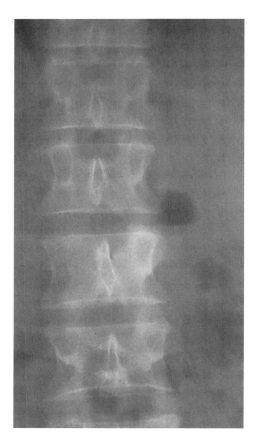

FIG. 1-129 Pedicle agenesis. Absence of the L2 pedicle on the reading left. Note the enlarged, sclerotic contralateral pedicle.

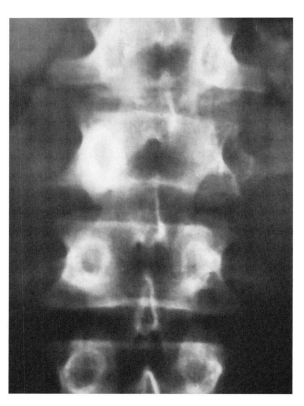

FIG. 1-131 Congenital pedicle agenesis with increased sclerosis contralaterally.

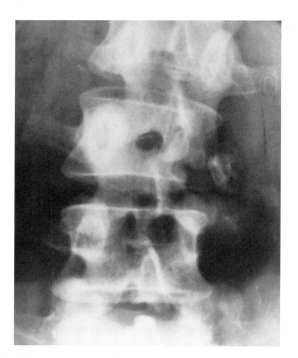

FIG. 1-130 L4 absent pedicle. Observe the hypertrophy of the contralateral pedicle.

ABSENT PEDICLE

- Due to failure of osseous formation (Fig. 1-129)
- Not clinically significant
- Must be differentiated from osteolytic metastasis or erosion caused by a neural tumor
- Characterized by increased sclerosis and hypertrophy of the contralateral pedicle; sclerosis caused by chronic asymmetric biomechanical stresses, suggesting congenital absence (Figs. 1-130 and 1-131)

LIMBUS BONE

- A small, fairly triangular bony ossicle often adjacent to the anterior aspect of the vertebral body (most often the anterosuperior corner) (Figs. 1-132 and 1-133)
- May represent marginal anterior herniation of discal material (a type of Schmorl's node) (Figs. 1-134 and 1-135)
- May be a persistent secondary ossification center
- Of no clinical significance

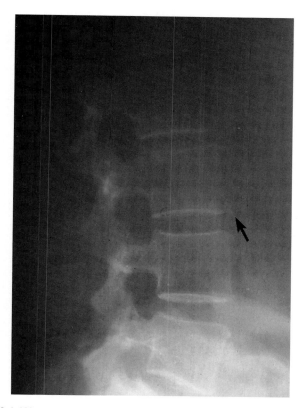

FIG. 1-132 Limbus bone. L3 demonstrates a small anteroinferior ossicle (*arrow*).

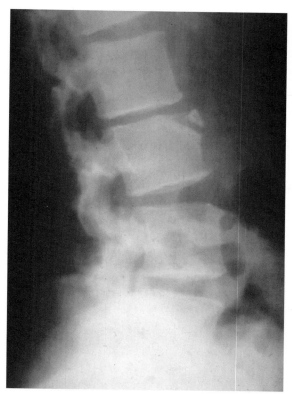

FIG. 1-133 Limbus bone at the anterosuperior corner of L3.

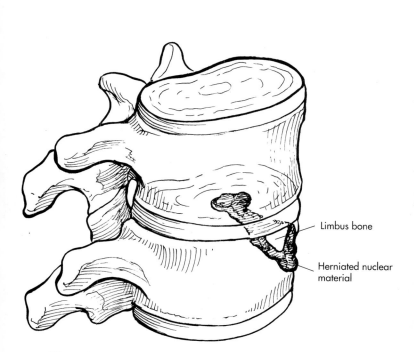

Limbus bone

Herniated nuclear material

FIG. 1-134 Diagram of a limbus bone depicting nuclear herniation (Schmorl's node) as the possible etiology.

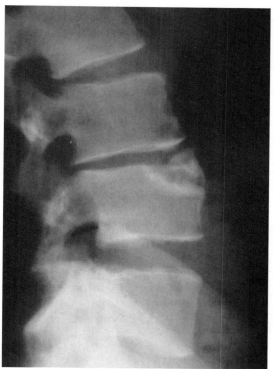

FIG. 1-135 Extremely large limbus bone at L4 with marked nuclear herniation. (Courtesy Arnie Deltoff, DC, Toronto, Ontario.)

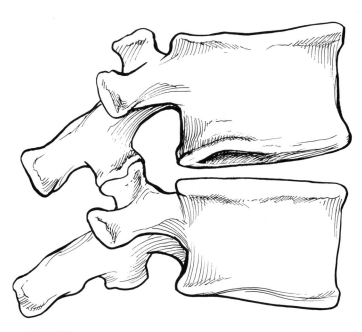

FIG. 1-136 Diagram of a nuclear impression. Note the smooth, undulating contour of the inferior end plate of the superior vertebral body.

NUCLEAR IMPRESSION

- End-plate depression or invagination secondary to notochordal remnant (Fig. 1-136)
- Must be differentiated from a Schmorl's node
  - Nuclear impressions:
    Broader
    Smoother
    More commonly posterior
    Tending to run the entire length of the vertebral end plate (Figs. 1-137, 1-138, and 1-139)
- Of no clinical significance

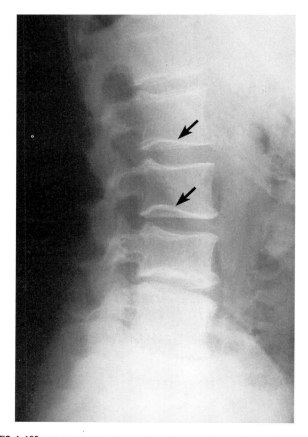

FIG. 1-138 Multiple-level nuclear impressions (*arrows*).

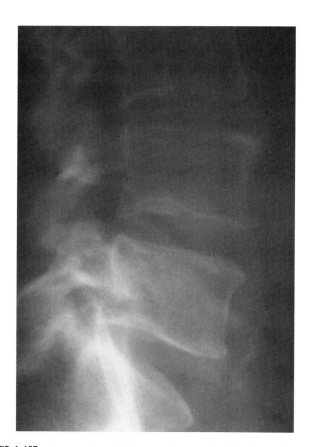

FIG. 1-137 A notochordal impression is visualized on the inferior surface of L5.

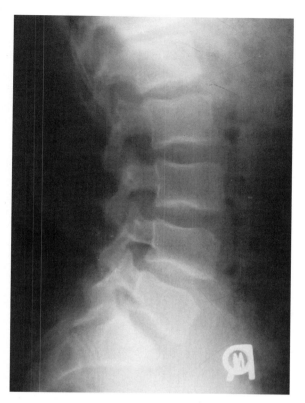

FIG. 1-139 This lumbar spine demonstrates nuclear impressions of the superior and inferior vertebral end plates of all visualized vertebrae.

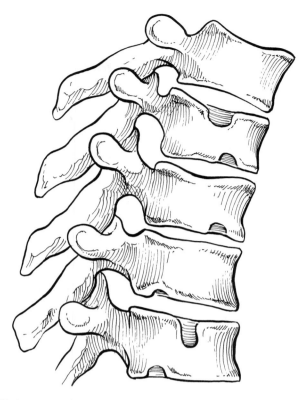

FIG. 1-140 In this diagram, multiple Schmorl's nodes are observed throughout the thoracic spine.

SCHMORL'S NODE

- Herniation of nucleus pulposus through vertebral end plate (Figs. 1-140, 1-141, 1-142, and 1-143)
- Etiologies: idiopathy, osteoporosis, posttrauma, Scheurmann's disease, and Paget's disease

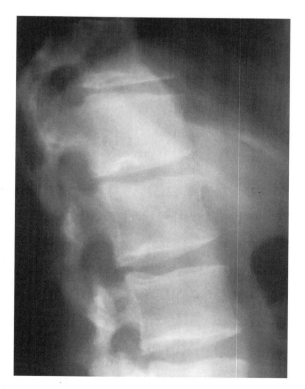

FIG. 1-141 Schmorl's nodes are noted on the inferior end plates of L1 and L2.

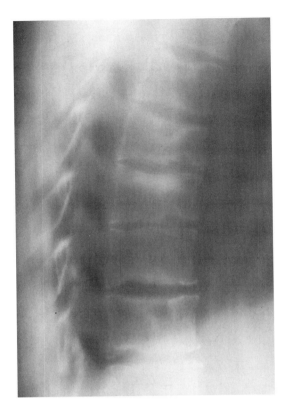

FIG. 1-142 Multiple-level Schmorl's nodes are observed in the thoracic spine.

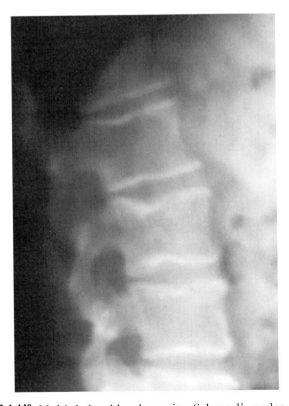

FIG. 1-143 Multiple-level lumbar spine Schmorl's nodes.

OS ACETABULUM

- ◆ Small accessory bone found at the superolateral aspect of the acetabulum (Figs. 1-144, 1-145, and 1-146)
- ◆ Of no clinical significance; discovered as an incidental finding

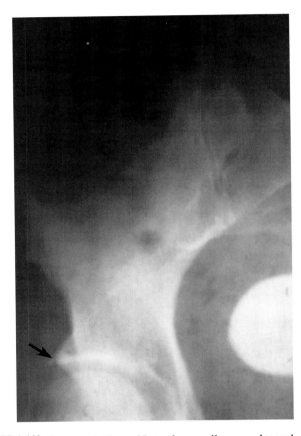

FIG. 1-144 Os acetabulum. Note the small superolateral acetabular ossicle (*arrow*).

FABELLA

- A common, normal variant sesamoid bone found in the lateral head of the gastrocnemius muscle tendon (Fig. 1-147)

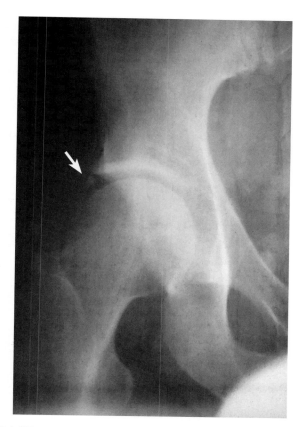

FIG. 1-145 Os acetabulum (*arrow*).

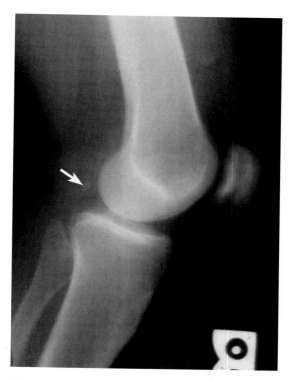

FIG. 1-147 Fabella. This accessory ossicle (*arrow*) is located in the tendon of the lateral head of the gastrocnemius.

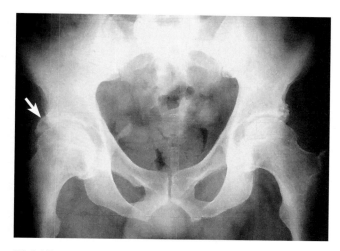

FIG. 1-146 Large os acetabulum (*arrow*).

BIPARTITE, TRIPARTITE, AND MULTIPARTITE PATELLA

- The patella is a sesamoid bone that usually develops from a single ossification center at 5 or 6 years of age.
- Occasionally, this ossification may be fragmented.
- Bipartite is the most common presentation (two pieces) (Figs. 1-148 and 1-149).

- The bipartite patella is bilateral in 80% of cases.
- These anomalies are present in 2% to 3% of the population and usually are clinically insignificant; however, they must be differentiated from a patellar fracture.
- The ununited segment is usually located adjacent to the superolateral aspect of the patella.
- The osseous margins are smooth and rounded, with no adjacent soft tissue edema (Fig. 1-150).

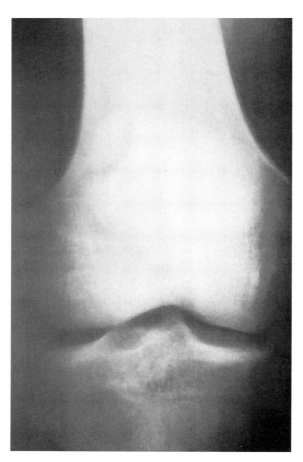

FIG. 1-148 Bipartite patella. Note the ununited segment of the patella.

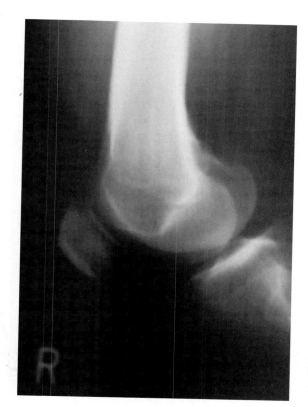

FIG. 1-149 Bipartite patella. This lateral projection demonstrates an ununited patellar segment.

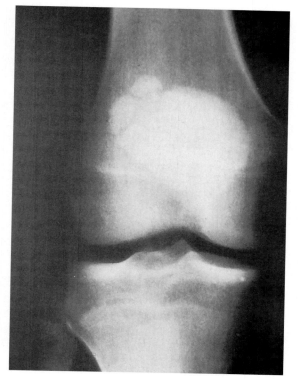

FIG. 1-150 Tripartite patella.

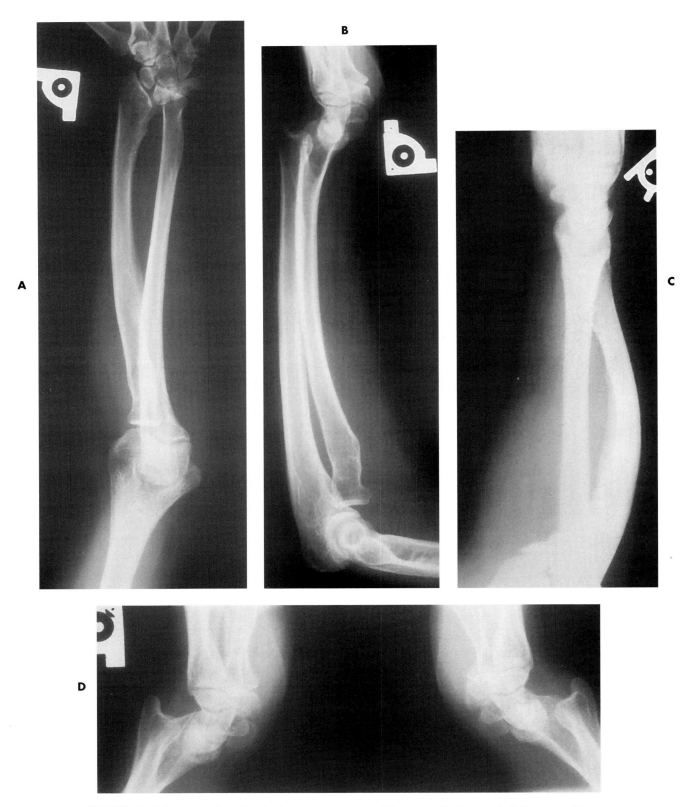

FIG. 1-151 Madelung's deformity. **A,** Anteroposterior left forearm. **B,** Lateral left forearm. Note the bowing of the radius (bayonet deformity). **C,** Lateral right forearm. In the bayonet deformity, observe marked radial bowing. **D,** Bilateral lateral wrists. Note the abnormal alignment.

MADELUNG'S DEFORMITY

- Fundamental abnormality arising as retarded growth of the medial portion of the distal radial epiphysis, resulting in asymmetric development of the distal radius and ulna
- Physical description is termed *bayonet deformity* (Fig. 1-151, *A-C*)
- More common in females
- Usually bilateral
- Associated wrist pain during periods of rapid growth, accounting for its frequent diagnosis in adolescence

Radiographic Features

- Ulnar deviation of the hand
- Dorsal prominence of ulnar styloid process caused by posterior ulnar subluxation (Fig. 1-151, *D*)
- Characteristic V-shaped deformity on ulnar side of distal radius apparent on P/A
- Widening of the radioulnar articulation

FIBROUS DYSPLASIA

- One of the great imitators of bone disease (along with Paget's disease)
- Developmental condition of unknown etiology that may involve any bone in the skeleton
- May have neoplastic or inflammatory origins
- Fundamental lesion that of a fibrous-based matrix with scattered bony spicules intermixed; renders an increase in radiopacity to the existing radiolucent lesion called the *ground glass appearance*
- Difficult to ascertain incidence because most lesions are asymptomatic
- May be monostotic or polyostotic

Clinical Presentation

- The usual age of presentation is from 8 to 14 years, but it can affect patients between 4 months and 70 years.
- Sex predilection is equal, except for McCune-Albright syndrome, which is almost exclusively found in females.
- Most lesions are asymptomatic.
- Bowing deformities, leg length discrepancies, and pathologic fractures are the most common causes of symptoms.
- Café au lait spots (Coast-of-Maine pattern) are chestnut-pigmented, nonelevated macules present in 30% to 35% of patients with polyostotic fibrous dysplasia. These macules have irregular, rough margins and are few (differentiate from smooth margins of the Coast-of-California pattern of multiple café au lait spots found in neurofibromatosis).
- The pigmentation is dark, with serrated margins, and is located in the lumbosacral area or buttocks.
- Café au lait spots are not seen in the monostotic form of fibrous dysplasia.
  - The monostotic form is most common in the ribs, proximal femur, anterior tibia, and skull.
  - The polyostotic form is most common in the femur, skull, tibia, humerus, ribs, fibula, radius, and ulna.
- The deformity is more commonly linked to the polyostotic form and is often unilateral.
- Vertebral involvement is quite rare.
- Malignant transformation to fibrosarcoma or osteosarcoma is rare (0.5%).
  - McCune-Albright syndrome features polyostotic fibrous dysplasia associated with skin pigmentation, precocious puberty, and endocrine disturbances.

Laboratory Findings

- Serum alkaline phosphatase may be elevated.

Radiographic Features

- Skeletal lesions are not present at birth. They occur several years before puberty.
- Most lesions are radiolucent, loculated, and primarily diaphyseal (Fig. 1-152).
- They often appear as eccentric, well-defined, cystic defects with an intact cortex (Fig. 1-153).
- Localized widening of the medullary canal occurs, with no periosteal response (Fig. 1-154).
- A ground glass or smoky appearance of the radiolucent lesion is typical. A cancellous matrix of bone is replaced by fibrous tissue that contains disseminated, irregular, extremely small spicules of bone. These spicules are poorly ossified and provide a gritty consistency to the lesion, which can be likened to sand in putty.
- The lesion is usually fairly lytic but can calcify. At this time it appears as a sclerotic lesion.
- Most lesions demonstrate an encapsulated sclerotic border (Fig. 1-155) around the geographic lesion ("rind" of sclerosis).
- Weight-bearing forces on the softened abnormal femur can produce a bowing deformity resembling the staff of a shepherd ("shepherd's crook" deformity) (Fig. 1-156).
- Bowing may be markedly progressive, leading to severe deformity (Fig. 1-157).
- Expansile ribs can create an extrapleural sign.
- Pseudoarthrosis infrequently occurs as a complication of pathologic fracture and nonunion.
- The lower extremity is most often affected.
- Pelvic involvement has been noted (Fig. 1-158).

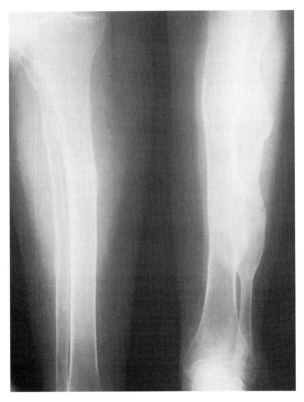

FIG. 1-152 Fibrous dysplasia of the fibula. Note the radiolucent diaphyseal lesion with an irregular undulating contour.

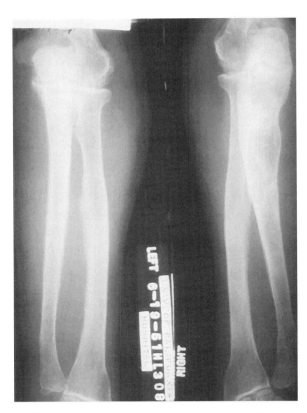

FIG. 1-153 Fibrous dysplasia of the proximal ulna. The thin, expanded cortex imparts a cystic appearance to the lesion.

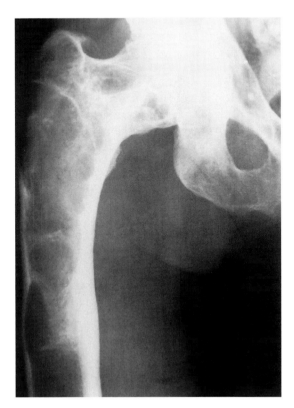

FIG. 1-154 Fibrous dysplasia of the proximal femur. The radiolucent lesion manifests with a widened medullary cavity, endosteal scalloping, and a thinned, intact lateral cortex.

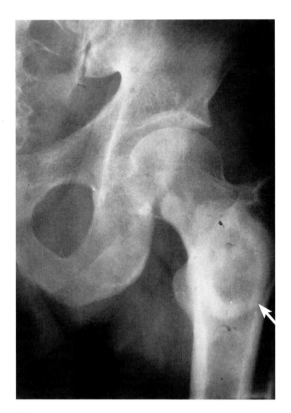

FIG. 1-155 Fibrous dysplasia of the proximal femur. Note the thick, geographic, sclerotic rind (*arrow*) in the intertrochanteric region.

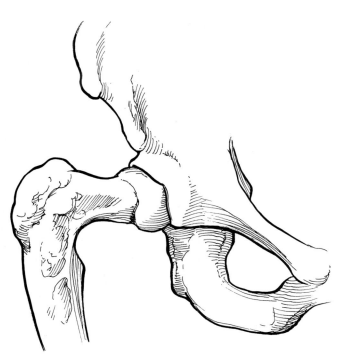

FIG. 1-156 Diagram of fibrous dysplasia. The abnormal angulation at the junction of the femoral neck and diaphysis is due to bone softening (Shepherd's crook deformity).

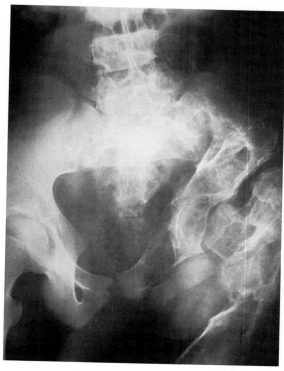

FIG. 1-158 Fibrous dysplasia of the hemipelvis and ipsilateral femur. Severe osseous deformity is observed.

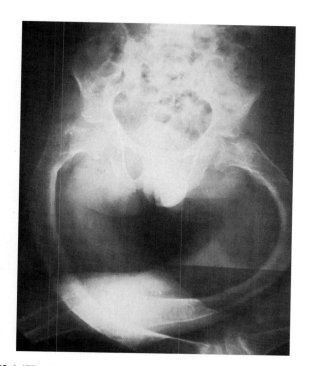

FIG. 1-157 Fibrous dysplasia; bilateral femora. Marked bowing deformity testifies to the bone-softening effect of the disease seen in this unusually advanced case.

- If calvarium is involved, lesions must be differentiated from Paget's disease. In fibrous dysplasia, an expansion of diploic space may be seen. However, the cortex is not uniformly thickened; it is usually thinned.
- Cherubism involves fibrous dysplasia of the jaws. The name relates to the physical appearance of the affected child, wherein puffed–out cheeks produce an angelic look. These jaw lesions regress in adulthood.
- Leontiasis ossea (lion facies) occurs if fibrous dysplasia affects the skull base or paranasal sinuses. Osseous expansion then occurs, with obliteration of the sinuses.
- The disease usually progresses throughout the patient's life but tends to stabilize in adulthood. Patients who experience early symptoms and extensive skeletal involvement usually demonstrate fractures and deformity.

Differential Diagnosis

- Paget's disease
- Neurofibromatosis
- Unicameral bone cyst
- Early aneurysmal bone cyst
- Brodie's abscess (osteomyelitis)
- Brown tumor (hyperparathyroidism)

Arthritides

The arthritides are a collation of disorders that produce an inflammatory response in a joint. Each condition is unique in its etiology, clinical presentation, and radiographic features. Arthritides may be categorized under four general headings: (1) degenerative joint disease, (2) inflammatory rheumatoid and rheumatoid-like arthritides, (3) infectious arthritis, and (4) metabolic arthritis.

DEGENERATIVE JOINT DISEASE

- Osteoarthritis
- Diffuse idiopathic skeletal hyperostosis (DISH)

INFLAMMATORY RHEUMATOID AND RHEUMATOID-LIKE ARTHRITIDES

- Rheumatoid arthritis
- Juvenile rheumatoid arthritis
- Ankylosing spondylitis
- Psoriatic arthritis
- Reiter's syndrome
- Enteropathic arthritis

INFECTIOUS ARTHRITIS

See Chapter 5.
- Tuberculosis
- Pyogenic arthritis

METABOLIC ARTHRITIS

- Gout
- Calcium pyrophosphate dihydrate crystal deposition disease (CPPD)

DEGENERATIVE ARTHROPATHIES

Osteoarthritis

- A progressive, degenerative disorder that affects amphiarthrodial and diarthrodial joints
- Characterized by a deterioration of articular cartilage and periarticular hypertrophic new bone formation
- The most common arthritide, affecting 70% to 80% of the adult population over 50 years of age

Pathophysiology

- The disease initially affects articular hyaline cartilage, which becomes softened as a result of the loss of chondroitin sulfate from the matrix.
- The cartilage becomes roughened by shearing forces that produce flaking and vertical splitting (fibrillation).
- The loss of supportive matrix weakens the collagen fibers in the cartilage.
- Cartilaginous atrophy exposes subchondral bone with resultant stress-related subchondral bone formation (eburnation) and marginal lipping.
- The disease is caused by trauma, either from a solitary episode or an accumulation of microtraumas over a period of years.

SECONDARY OSTEOARTHRITIS (MOST COMMON FORM)

- Not gender or age related; usually caused by trauma, but obesity, postinflammatory joint disease, articular deformity, and metabolic deposition diseases also identified with the development of this condition
- May affect any articulation
- The large, weight-bearing joints (such as the knee, hip, and articulations of the spine) most frequently involved in classic osteoarthritis
- Possible involvement of the distal interphalangeal (DIP) joints of the hands, first metatarsophalangeal joint, first carpometacarpal joint, temporomandibular joints, sacroiliac joints, and sternoclavicular joints; no joint immune

Clinical Presentation

- Stiffness, immobility, or "gelling" caused by capsular contraction and fibrosis typically appear in the morning and are short-lived.
- Joint swelling, due to a low-grade synovitis and effusion, produces a decreased range of joint motion.
- Joint locking and crepitis caused by joint cartilage irregularity are common.

Laboratory Analysis

- No tests are of specific diagnostic significance.

Radiographic Features

- A classic radiographic triad composed of nonuniform (asymmetric) joint-space narrowing, subarticular sclerosis, and osteophytosis is usually identified.
- Another process that can occasionally be observed is a subchondral pseudocyst, or geode.
- Presumably, pseudocysts result from synovial fluid being forced into the subchondral bone, producing a cystic accumulation of joint fluid.

Hip

- Changes in the hip typically follow a unilateral course of involvement.
- Joint-space narrowing occurs in the area of greatest weight bearing (superior joint compartment), producing a nonuniform loss of joint space (Figs. 2-1 and 2-2).
- Marginal spurs and subchondral sclerosis caused by excessive wear form circumferentially at the junction of the femoral head and neck.
- Spurring also arises along the lateral and medial aspects of the femoral head and adjacent acetabular margins (Fig. 2-3).

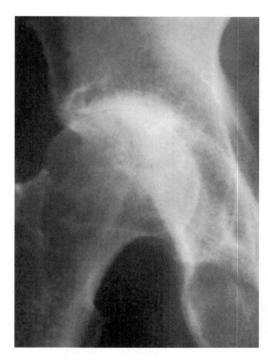

FIG. 2-1 Moderately advanced osteoarthritis of the hip. Note the acetabular and femoral head subchondral sclerosis with a severe decrease in superior joint space. The medial joint space is preserved.

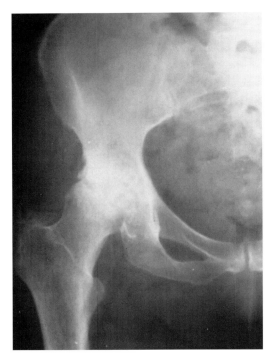

FIG. 2-2 Mild to moderate osteoarthritis of the hip. Observe the periarticular sclerosis, subchondral pseudocysts, and joint-space diminution.

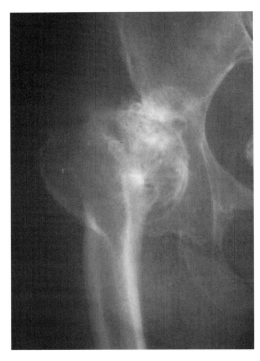

FIG. 2-4 Hip osteoarthritis. This is an advanced case demonstrating coxa vara angulation of the femur.

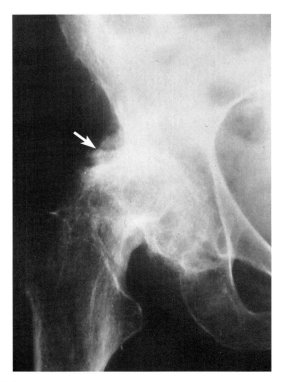

FIG. 2-3 Advanced degenerative disease of the hip. Marked sclerosis is evident, with significant spurring (*arrow*) and loss of joint space.

- Synovial fluid, being forced under compression into the subchondral spongiosa, can produce well-marginated pseudocysts (geodes), which may frequently communicate with the joint cavity.
- Joint compression may produce subchondral cystic collapse, resulting in deformity of the femoral head.
- Excessive muscular contracture and osseous deformity can predispose to a superolateral migration of the femoral head within the acetabulum.
- Progressive joint alterations may give rise to coxa vara deformities (Fig. 2-4).
- Advanced, long-standing osteoarthritis of the hip has been linked to avascular necrosis of the femoral head.
- Extreme degenerative hip-joint alterations in older individuals have been termed *malum coxa senilis* (Fig. 2-5).

Knee
- Unilateral involvement of the knee initially favors the medial joint compartment (Figs. 2-6, 2-7, 2-8, and 2-9).

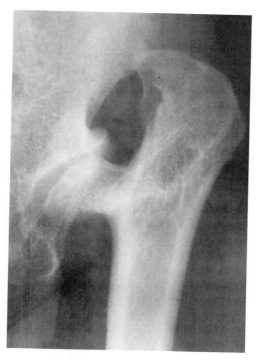

FIG. 2-5 Osteoarthritis of the hip. Note the marked resorption of the femoral head resulting from a long-standing degenerative process.

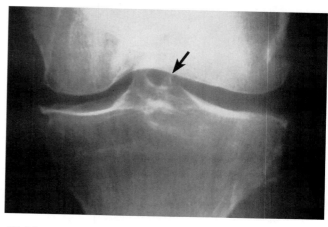

FIG. 2-6 Early osteoarthritis of the knee. Observe the tibial eminence spiking (*arrow*), one of the first radiographic indications of degenerative disease in the knee.

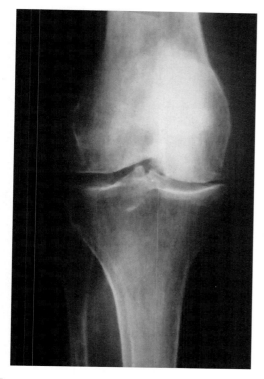

FIG. 2-7 Mild to moderate osteoarthritis demonstrated by a selective decrease in the medial joint-space compartment.

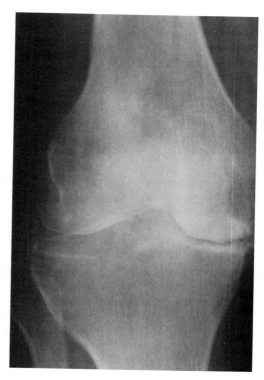

FIG. 2-8 Moderately advanced decrease in the medial joint space of the knee, with subarticular sclerosis.

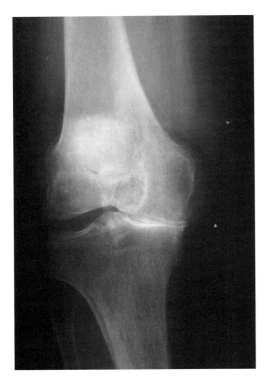

FIG. 2-9 Marked degenerative disease manifests as complete obliteration of the medial joint space compartment and articular surface roughening, with maintenance of the lateral compartment, resulting in a genu varum posture.

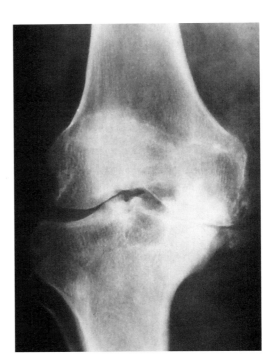

FIG. 2-10 Advanced medial compartment decrease, with subchondral sclerosis, medial spurring, and medial femoral shifting.

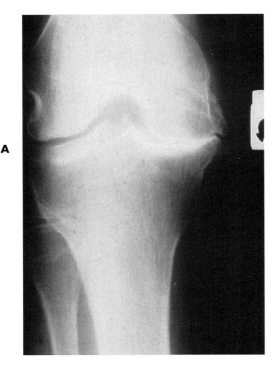

A

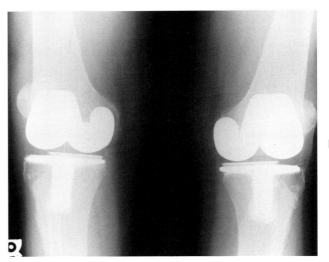

B

FIG. 2-11 A, Tunnel projection demonstrating tibial eminence blunting with advanced medial compartment osteoarthritic changes. **B,** Bilateral prosthetic articular surface replacement as a sequela of advanced osteoarthritis of the knees. (Courtesy Henry Clark, DC, Toronto, Ontario.)

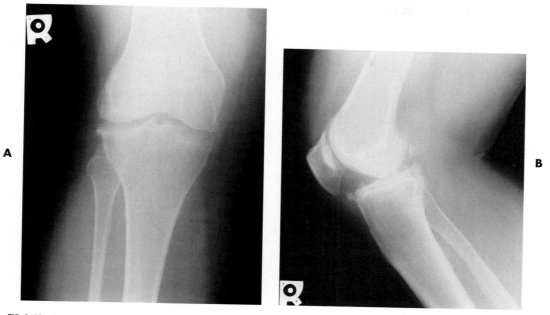

FIG. 2-12 Osteoarthritis of the knee. **A,** Anteroposterior. Tibial eminence blunting is observed. **B,** Lateral. Note the superior patellar spurring, with posterior femoral and anterior tibial spur formation. (Courtesy James Clark, MD, Toronto, Ontario.)

- This may be associated with medial shifting of the distal femur on the tibial plateau (Fig. 2-10).
- Subchondral sclerosis and pseudocystic formation are common, as is marginal articular spurring.
- Spurring may also arise from the superior and inferior poles of the patella, as well as the tibial intercondylar eminences (Figs. 2-11, *A* and *B;* 2-12, *A* and *B;* and 2-13).
- Lateral compartment involvement occurs in advanced, progressive states.

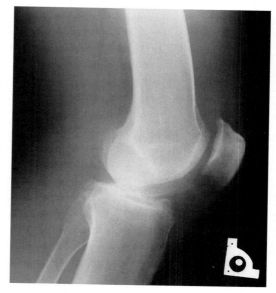

FIG. 2-13 Patellofemoral osteoarthritis. Note the moderate posterior patellar roughening and mild spurring.

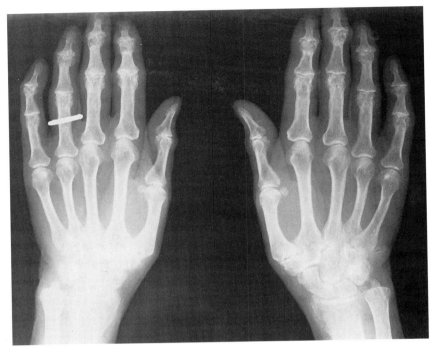

FIG. 2-14 Osteoarthritis of the hands; bilateral, asymmetric distribution. Note the proximal inter-phalangeal articular involvement with sparing of the metacarpophalangeal joints.

A

B

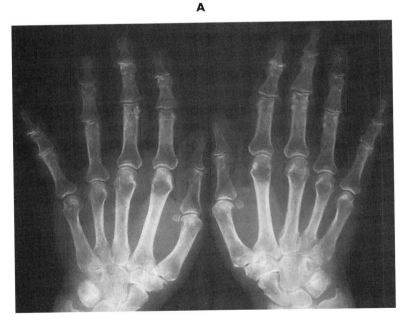

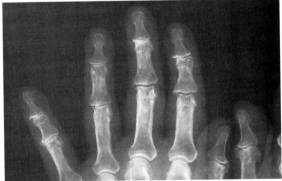

FIG. 2-15 Osteoarthritis of the hand. **A,** Observe the involvement of the first carpometacarpal joints and distal interphalangeal articulations. **B,** Close-up of distal interphalangeal joints. Note the characteristic nonsymmetric decrease in joint space and mild spurring.

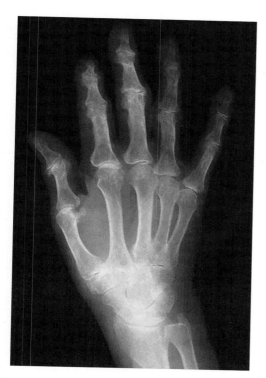

FIG. 2-16 Marked involvement of the distal and proximal interphalangeal joints, with complete sparing of the metacarpophalangeal joints. Moderately advanced degenerative changes in the wrist are also present.

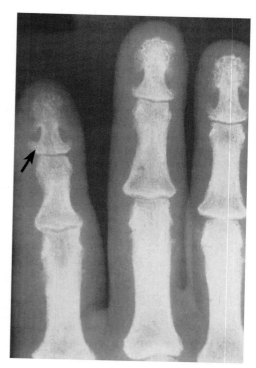

FIG. 2-17 Marked spurring of the distal phalanx (*arrow*).

Hands

- Distribution is asymmetric (Fig. 2-14).
- Degenerative changes may be evident in any joint of the hand, but the DIP, first carpometacarpal, and radiocarpal joints appear to be favored (Figs. 2-15, *A* and *B;* 2-16; and 2-17).
- Soft tissue edema, nonuniform joint-space narrowing, subchondral sclerosis, and pseudocystic production are common findings in the scaphoid, trapezium, first metacarpal base, and distal radius.
- Osseous excrescences on the dorsal aspects of the distal and proximal interphalangeal (PIP) joints represent Heberden's and Bouchard's nodes, respectively.
- Exuberant spurring occurring at joint margins of adjacent phalanges, combined with joint-space narrowing, produces the "seagull" sign.
- Heberden's and Bouchard's nodes are frequently observed (Figs. 2-18 and 2-19).

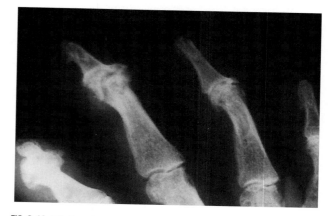

FIG. 2-18 Heberden's nodes of varying severity with marked osteophytic formation. These become clinically visible as knuckle enlargement and deformity.

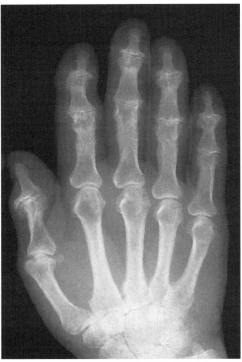

FIG. 2-19 Marked involvement of the distal interphalangeal joints (Heberden's nodes) and proximal interphalangeal joints (Bouchard's nodes). Note the complete sparing of the metacarpophalangeal joints.

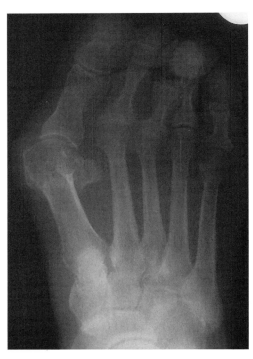

FIG. 2-21 Hallux valgus. Marked lateral deviation of the first digit, with lateral subluxation of the first proximal phalanx on the metatarsal head.

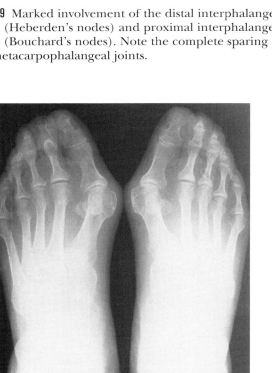

FIG. 2-20 Bilateral hallux valgus with osteoarthritis of the first metatarsophalangeal and interphalangeal joints.

Feet
- The first metatarsophalangeal (MTP) joint is most commonly affected.
- Uneven joint-space narrowing results in the typical hallux valgus deformity, with marginal spurring, subchondral sclerosis, and pseudocystic formation being the most common features (Figs. 2-20, 2-21, and 2-22).
- Advanced osteoarthritis of the first MTP joint may result in the classic bunion-type deformity of bone, with associated adjacent periarticular soft tissue thickening.

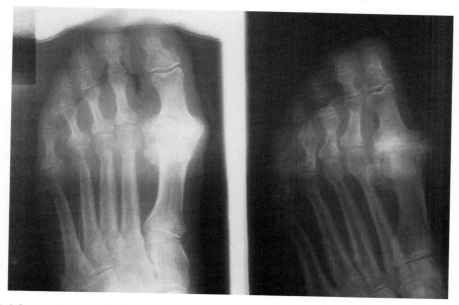

FIG. 2-22 Advanced osteoarthritis of the first metatarsophalangeal joint, with significant spurring, sclerosis, and loss of joint space.

Spine

- Apophyseal joint involvement is termed *osteoarthrosis.*
- A similar change noted within the discovertebral joints or intervertebral discs is generally termed *discogenic spondylosis.*
- Degeneration of the intervertebral discs causes bulging of the annular fibers, producing abnormal amounts of tensile stresses at their fibrous insertions.
- Calcium deposition in the annular insertions, combined with continued degeneration of the annulus, produces bone spurs or spondylophytes (Figs. 2-23, 2-24, and 2-25).

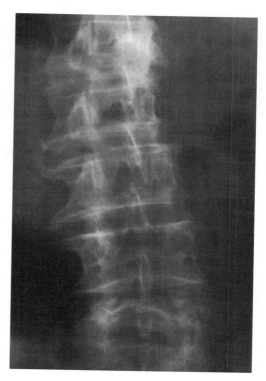

FIG. 2-23 Lumbar osteoarthritis: osteophytosis. Note the proliferative spurring at multiple levels on the reading left. Marked sclerosis is also observed at L1-L2.

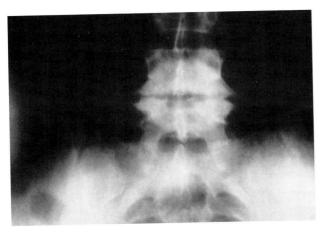

FIG. 2-24 Advanced degenerative disc disease at L4-L5 demonstrates a significant decrease in disc height, sclerosis, and spur formation.

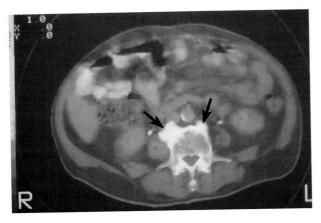

FIG. 2-25 Lumbar osteoarthritis. This computed tomographic image depicts large anterolateral osteophytes (*arrows*), suggesting advanced disease.

- Spondylophytes arise from the anterior and lateral margins of the vertebral bodies and invariably involve a horizontal component in their orientation (Figs. 2-26 and 2-27).
- Spondylophytes typically have a wide base and extend from the vertebral margins, exhibiting a contiguous cortex with their host bone (Figs. 2-28 and 2-29).

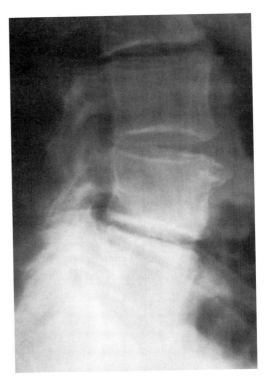

FIG. 2-26 Note the relatively horizontal orientation of the spurs at the anterosuperior corner of L3 and L4. Advanced disc height diminution is observed at L4-L5.

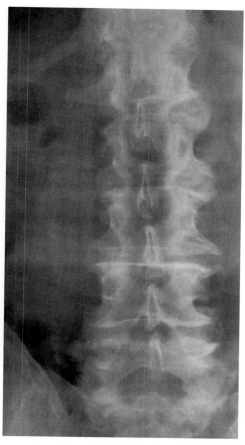

FIG. 2-27 Advanced to moderately advanced degenerative disc disease throughout the lumbar spine. The spur orientation tends to be predominantly horizontal.

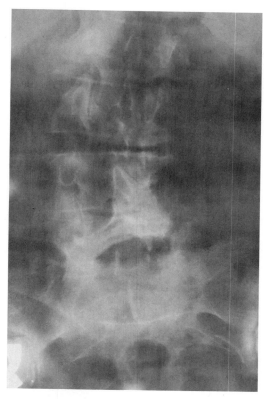

FIG. 2-28 Marked degenerative disc disease with convexity of the lower lumbar spine, demonstrating large, wide-based osteophytes on the concavity at L3-L4.

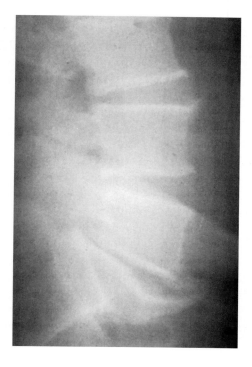

FIG. 2-29 Advanced osteoarthritis at L5-S1. A Grade 1 degenerative spondylolisthesis of L5 is evident. S1 demonstrates attempted buttressing with a large anterior spur.

◆ Radiographic features are characteristically located in the lower portions of the cervical, thoracic, and lumbar regions and consist of roughening, sclerosis, and osseous hypertrophy of the joint margins (Figs. 2-30, 2-31, 2-32, 2-33, 2-34, 2-35, and 2-36).

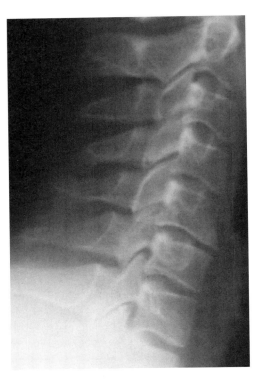

FIG. 2-31 Early osteoarthritis demonstrated by mild C5-C6 spurring.

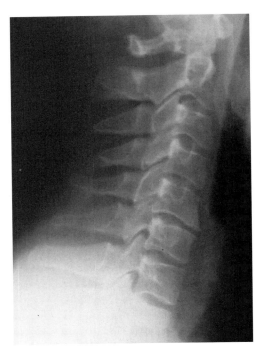

FIG. 2-30 Osteoarthritis of the cervical spine. This alordotic spine demonstrates early degenerative change at C5-C6, with mild spurring.

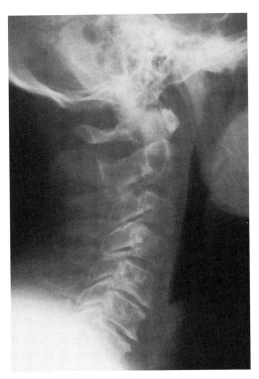

FIG. 2-32 Mild to moderate degenerative disc disease at C5-C6 and C6-C7, with some evident decrease in disc height accompanied by anterior spondylophyte formation.

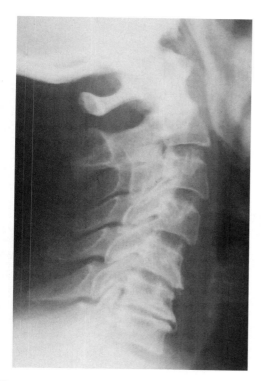

FIG. 2-33 Advanced osteoarthritis at C6-C7, with roughened end plates, decreased disc height, subarticular sclerosis, and spondylophytosis. Moderate changes are noted at C5-C6.

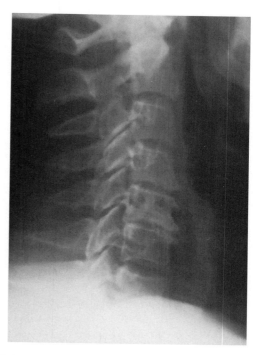

FIG. 2-34 Marked classic degenerative changes at C5-C6, with moderate C4-C5 osteoarthritis in an alordotic cervical spine.

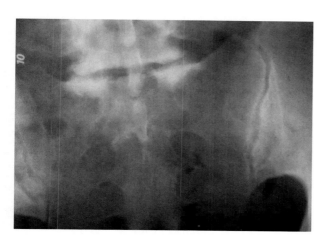

FIG. 2-35 L5-S1 degenerative disc disease displaying prominent subarticular sclerosis.

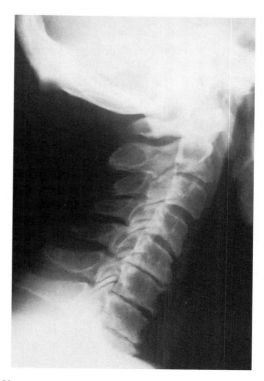

FIG. 2-36 Alordotic cervical spine demonstrating advanced degenerative disc disease from C5-C6 through C7-T1. Early spurring has begun at C4-C5.

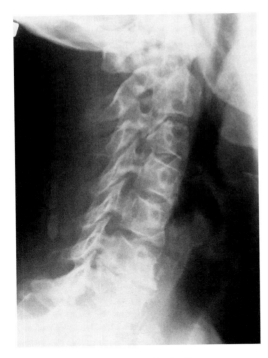

FIG. 2-37 Oblique cervical spine depicting uncinate process spurring encroaching into the intervertebral foramen at C6-C7. Observe the accompanying advanced degenerative disc disease. Of incidental note is a large nuchal bone.

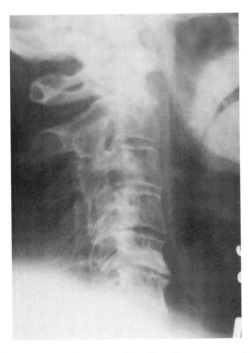

FIG. 2-38 Advanced degenerative disc disease at multiple levels. Anterior and posterior osteophytosis (C5-C6) is evident. Multilevel facet arthrosis is also present. (Courtesy Arnie Deltoff, DC, Toronto, Ontario.)

♦ In the cervical spine, degenerative arthritis may produce posteriorly oriented spondylophytes, which may compromise the integrity of the spinal canal (Figs. 2-37, 2-38, and 2-39).

♦ Degenerative arthrosis of the uncovertebral joints of Luschka or the posterior zygopophyseal articulations, featuring hypertrophy, asymmetry, and spurring, may also give rise to intervertebral foraminal encroachment (Figs. 2-40, *A;* 2-40, *B;* 2-41, *A* and *B;* 2-42; 2-43, *A* and *B;* and 2-44).

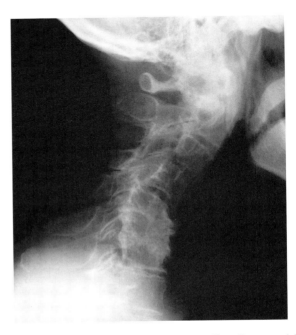

FIG. 2-39 Advanced C5-C6 degenerative disc disease with anterior and posterior spurring. Note the striking kyphosis and absence of lower cervical disc spaces.

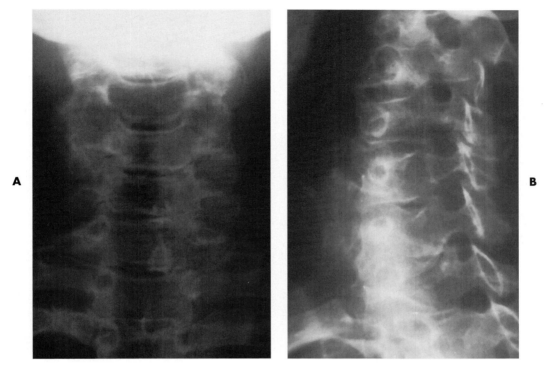

FIG. 2-40 Uncinate arthrosis. **A,** Anteroposterior lower cervical view. Observe the blunting and roughening of the uncinate processes at C5-C6 on the reading left and at C6-C7 bilaterally. **B,** Oblique view. Note the osseous compromise of the intervertebral foramen at C6-C7.

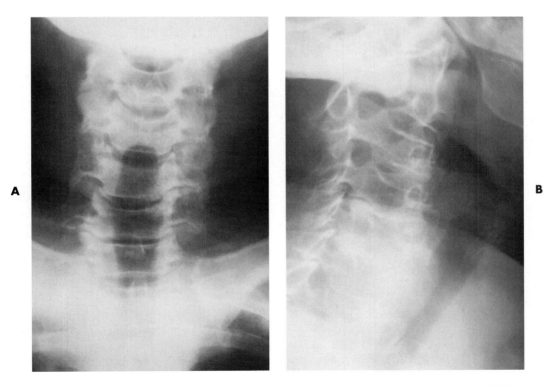

FIG. 2-41 Uncinate arthrosis. **A,** Anteroposterior lower cervical view. Observe the marked blunting and spurring of the C6 uncinate process on the reading right and at C7 on the reading left. **B,** Oblique view. Note the intervertebral foraminal encroachment at C5-C6 and C6-C7, resulting in an "hourglass" countour of these foramina.

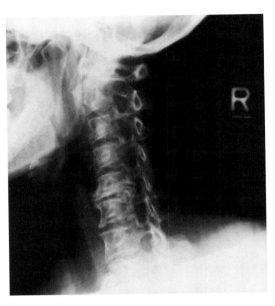

FIG. 2-42 Right anterior oblique view demonstrating advanced degenerative disc disease at C5-C6 and uncinate arthrosis. Note the intervertebral foraminal encroachment at this level. (Courtesy Paul Anderson, MD, Toronto, Ontario.)

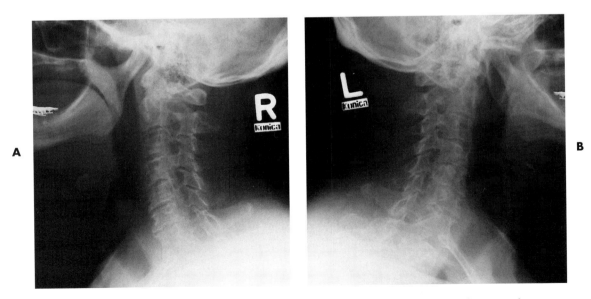

FIG. 2-43 A 71-year-old man with uncinate arthrosis and intervertebral foraminal encroachment at multiple levels. **A,** Right anterior oblique view. **B,** Left anterior oblique view. (Courtesy Arnie Deltoff, DC, Toronto, Ontario.)

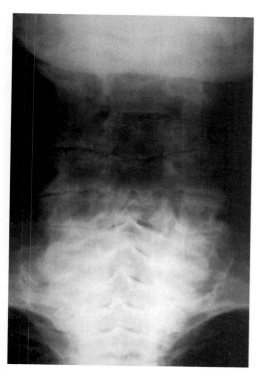

FIG. 2-44 Advanced facet arthrosis with sclerosis, spurring, and nonuniform decreased joint spaces at multiple levels is demonstrated on this bilateral pillar projection.

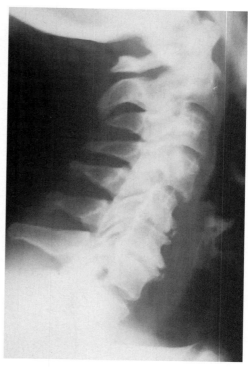

FIG. 2-45 Marked spondylophytosis at C6-C7. This may cause dysphagia, along with advanced changes at C5-C6, and a Grade 1 degenerative anterolisthesis at C4 caused by facet arthrosis at C4-C5.

◆ Large anterior spondylophytes, especially at the C5-C6 disc level, rarely impinge on the esophagus, thereby producing dysphagia (Figs. 2-45 and 2-46).

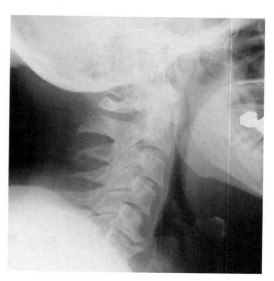

FIG. 2-46 A 68-year-old man with dysphagia. Note the marked anterior spondylophytosis at C5-C6. Milder changes are observed at C3-C4 and C4-C5. (Courtesy Sheldon Hershkop, MD, Toronto, Ontario.)

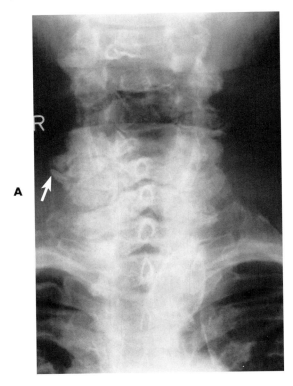

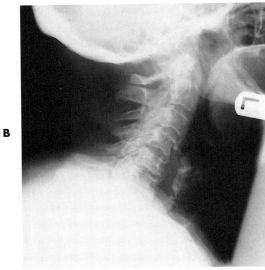

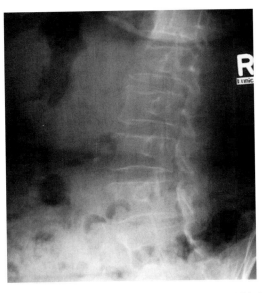

FIG. 2-48 A 62-year-old woman demonstrating mild left facet arthrosis at L3-L4, L4-L5, and L5-S1 on a right anterior oblique study. (Courtesy John Tyl, MD, Toronto, Ontario.)

FIG. 2-47 Facet arthrosis. **A,** Anteroposterior lower cervical. Marked prolific osteophytosis of the facet joints at multiple levels is demonstrated, most prominently at C5-C6 on the right (*arrow*). **B,** Lateral. The advanced facet degeneration is accompanied by significant degenerative disc disease at C5-C6 and C6-C7, with milder changes at C4-C5. C3 and C4 each demonstrate a degenerative Grade 1 anterolisthesis. (Courtesy Kathy Wickens, DC, Perth, Ontario.)

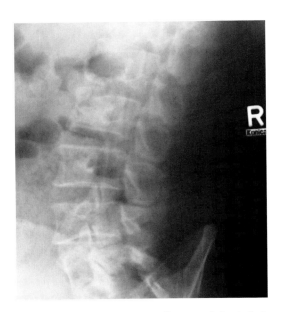

FIG. 2-49 Advanced degenerative disease of the left facet joint is observed at L5-S1 on this right anterior oblique study of a 39-year-old man. Note the marked subarticular sclerosis. (Courtesy John Tyl, MD, Toronto, Ontario.)

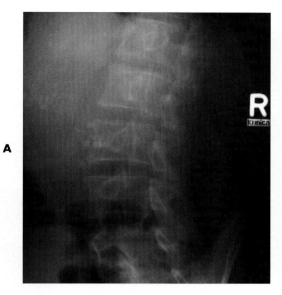
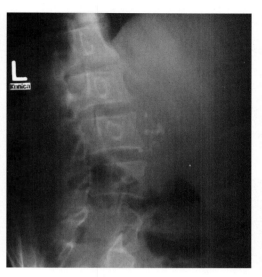

FIG. 2-50 A, Right anterior oblique. Apophyseal joint osteoarthritis in a 42-year-old man. Observe the sclerosis of the facets at L5-S1. **B,** Left anterior oblique. Note the multiple densities in the soft tissue, characteristic of the stippled pattern of pancreatic calcification. (Courtesy John Tyl, MD, Toronto, Ontario.)

◆ Advanced, degenerative arthrosis of the apophyseal joints (Figs. 2-47, *A* and *B;* 2-48; 2-49; 2-50, *A* and *B*) can result in subluxation and anterolisthesis (Fig. 2-51).

◆ In the lower thoracic spine, spondyloarthrosis typically produces increased kyphosis, paravertebral ligamentous calcification, and intervertebral disc thinning with calcification and spondylophytosis.

◆ Early changes may be seen as annular calcification producing intercalary bones.

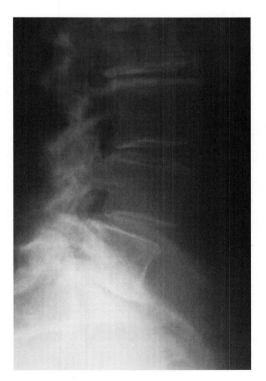

FIG. 2-51 The facet arthrosis at L4-L5 has resulted in a degenerative Grade 1 anterolisthesis of L4. Also, note the advanced disc degeneration at L2-L3 and L5-S1.

- Spondylophytosis may be more prominent on the right side because of aortic pulsations on the left, but this finding is not consistent (Fig. 2-52).
- In the lumbar spine, degenerative changes of the intervertebral discs and apophyseal joints can resemble each other in severity, but often one precedes and predisposes to the other (Figs. 2-53, 2-54, and 2-55).

- Advanced spinal degenerative changes generally produce disc narrowing, vacuum phenomena (Figs. 2-56 and 2-57), spondylophytosis, and apophyseal joint arthrosis (Figs. 2-58, 2-59, and 2-60).

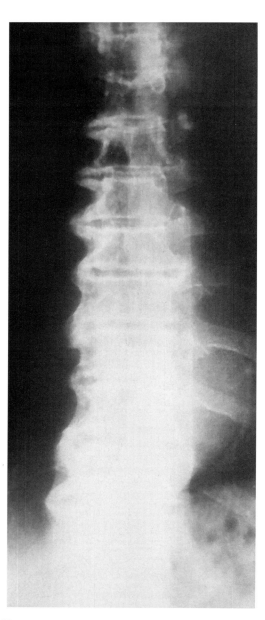

FIG. 2-52 Osteophytes at multiple thoracic levels are present on the patient's right side and absent on the left side of the spine. Aortic pulsations prevent their development on the left.

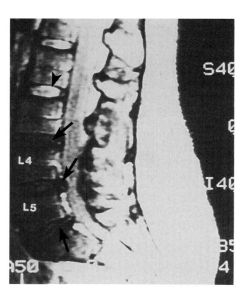

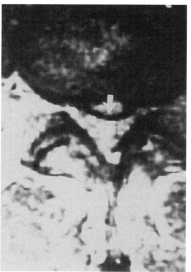

FIG. 2-53 Lumbar degenerative disc disease: magnetic resonance imaging. Note the normal bright signal of a healthy, hydrated disc (*arrowhead*) compared with those at L3-L4, L4-L5, and L5-S1, which are uniformly dark (*black arrows*). In addition, L4-L5 and L5-S1 demonstrate some degree of posterior bulging into the spinal canal (*white arrow*).

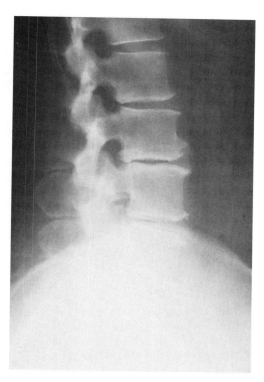

FIG. 2-54 Advanced degenerative disc disease at multiple midlower lumbar levels.

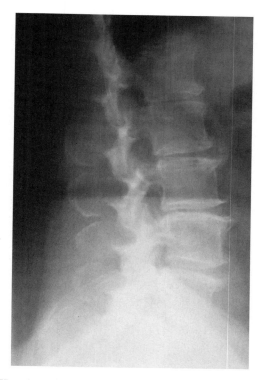

FIG. 2-55 Lumbar spine with marked multilevel degenerative changes involving facets and discs.

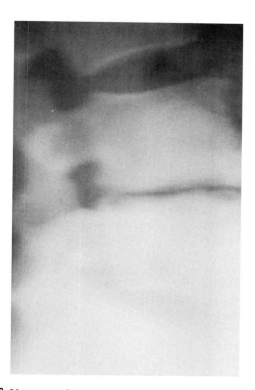

FIG. 2-56 Vacuum phenomenon of the lumbar spine. Observe the thin, radiolucent linear density in the markedly narrowed L4-L5 disc space, indicative of nitrogen gas formation from nuclear degeneration.

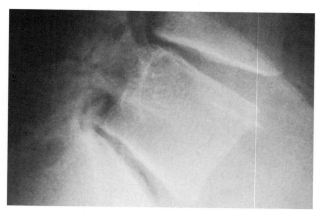

FIG. 2-57 Vacuum phenomenon. The L5-S1 disc space demonstrates a thin, central gas density.

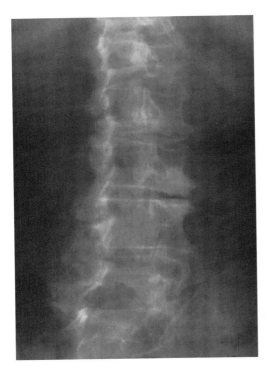

FIG. 2-58 Facet arthrosis is observed at multiple levels, accompanied by disc involvement.

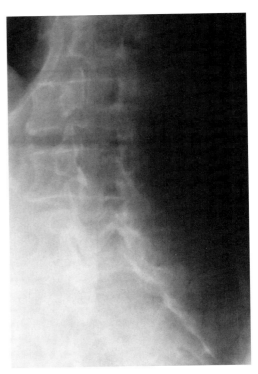

FIG. 2-59 Marked facet arthrosis at L4-L5 and L5-S1 has resulted in entrapment of the L5 pars interarticularis.

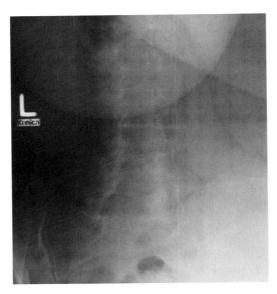

FIG. 2-60 Advanced facet arthrosis in an 81-year-old woman. Note the significant subarticular sclerosis and joint-space diminution at L4-L5 and L5-S1. (Courtesy Paul Anderson, MD, Toronto, Ontario.)

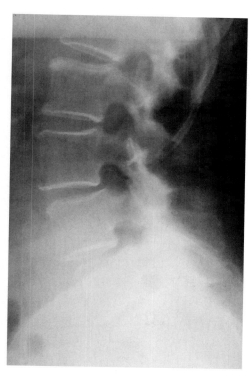

FIG. 2-61 Baastrup's disease. Note the approximation and articulation of the spinous processes at L2-L3, L3-L4, and L4-L5. In addition, L4 demonstrates a degenerative Grade 1 anterolisthesis due to L4-L5 facet arthrosis.

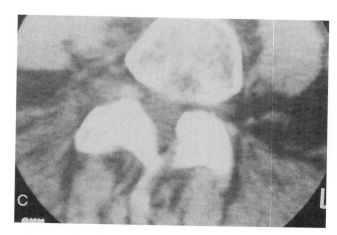

FIG. 2-62 Facet arthrosis: computed tomography. Both facet articulations exhibit marked degenerative spur formation. Note the intervertebral foraminal compromise on the reading right.

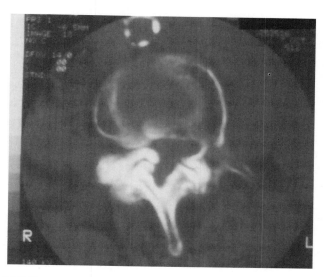

FIG. 2-63 Facet arthrosis: computed tomography. Observe the advanced bilateral hypertrophic spurring, severe on the right, resulting in significant spinal canal distortion and stenosis.

- Advanced, protracted osteoarthritis of the lumbar spine (spondylosis deformans) may lead to joint instability, Baastrup's phenomena (spinous process articulation, "kissing" spinouses) (Fig. 2-61), intervertebral foraminal encroachment (Fig. 2-62), spinal stenosis (Fig. 2-63), anterolisthesis, retrolisthesis, and laterolisthesis (Figs. 2-64 and 2-65).
- Although changes of osteoarthritis may be radiographically striking, they may be inconsistent with a correspondingly prominent clinical presentation.

Diffuse Idiopathic Skeletal Hyperostosis (DISH)

- A generalized degenerative articular disorder characterized by paraspinal and extraspinal ligamentous ossification
- Possesses a definite axial pattern of involvement focusing on the anterior and lateral paraspinal areas, including paraspinal ligamentous and tendinous attachments
- The only disorder that produces osteophytes in the absence of accompanying sclerosis or joint-space narrowing
- A common bone-forming disorder that initially resembles degenerative disc disease but with an absence of intervertebral disc joint-space narrowing
- Not considered to have a traumatic or weight-bearing etiology (as does degenerative disc disease)
- Characterized by paravertebral ligamentous calcification and ossification chiefly involving the anterior longitudinal ligament

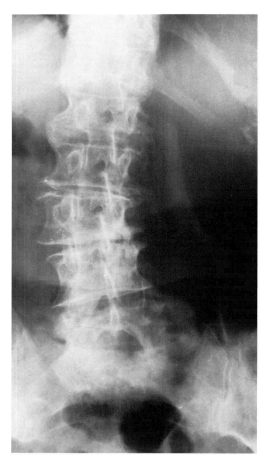

FIG. 2-64 A lumbar convexity accompanies advanced degenerative disc disease at multiple levels. L3 demonstrates a mild lateral migration to the reading left (laterolisthesis).

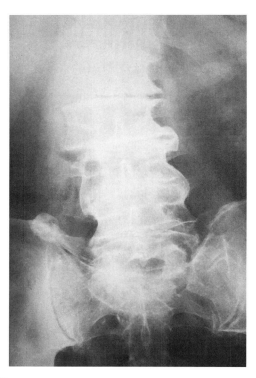

FIG. 2-65 Severely advanced degenerative disc disease throughout the lumbar spine. L2 demonstrates a laterolisthesis to the reading left.

◆ Possibly also involves the posterior longitudinal ligament (ossification of the posterior longitudinal ligament or OPLL)

◆ Represents the second most common etiology of vertebral body spurring

Clinical Presentation

◆ Patients are typically males over 50 years of age, but females are not immune.

◆ The most common symptom is a low-grade, aching pain with slow, progressive spinal stiffness, especially prevalent in the thoracolumbar junction.

◆ Peripheral musculoskeletal involvement occurs in up to 30% of patients.

◆ Palpable masses are the product of exuberant osseous proliferation common at the olecranon, calcanei, tibial tubercles, and patellar poles.

◆ Recurrent lateral epicondylitis and Achilles tendinitis are two conditions that are frequently noted.

◆ Diabetes mellitus is linked to approximately 25% to 30% of DISH cases.

Laboratory Features

◆ There are no tests of any specific diagnostic significance.

Radiographic Features

◆ Calcification of the anterior longitudinal ligament initially occurs adjacent to the midportion of the vertebral body.

◆ Long sections of the ligament appear to be involved, producing an anterolateral flowing ossified contour.

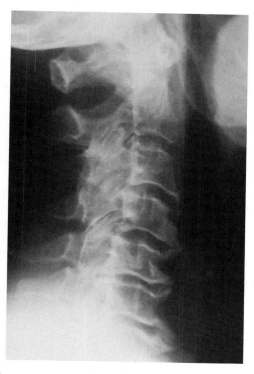

FIG. 2-66 Early diffuse idiopathic skeletal hyperostosis. Note the attempted anterior osseous vertebral bridging from C4-C5 caudad, with relative maintenance of the disc heights. Moderate facet arthrosis at multiple levels is also incidentally present.

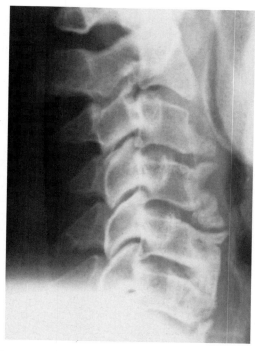

FIG. 2-67 Diffuse idiopathic skeletal hyperostosis. Prolific hyperostotic anterior bone formation is noted from C3-C4 caudad, with complete bridging of C5 and C6. Observe the normal disc spaces.

- Extensive involvement of anterior longitudinal ligamentous ossification in the spine usually incorporates a minimum of four contiguous vertebral segments.
- Because the intervertebral disc is usually not affected, normal disc integrity is relatively preserved.
- The posterior apophyseal joints and joints of Luschka are not involved.
- Normal bone density is expected.

Cervical spine

- Up to 80% of patients have cervical spinal involvement.
- OPLL occurs in 50% of patients, with subsequent production of spinal stenosis.
- Esophageal impingement by prominent anterior osseous protrusion can result in dysphagia (Figs. 2-66, 2-67, and 2-68).

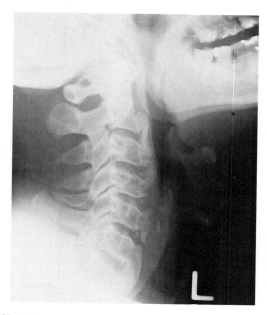

FIG. 2-68 Diffuse idiopathic skeletal hyperostosis. Marked anterior ossification is seen throughout the cervical spine, with bridging or attempted bridging at all levels. Discs are normal.

Thoracic spine

- The thoracic spine is the most common spinal area affected, with the thoracolumbar region appearing to be the site of greatest involvement (Fig. 2-69, *A* and *B*).
- Exuberant anterolateral ossification produces increased kyphosis and ankylosis, with a predominance on the right (Fig. 2-70).
- The left side is spared as a consequence of aortic pulsations.

Lumbar spine

- Favors the upper segments as ligamentous ossification ascends from the anterosuperior aspects of the upper lumbar vertebral bodies to involve the thoracolumbar junction (Fig. 2-71)

Pelvis

- Only the superior one third of the sacroiliac joint proper is affected because this area is ligamentous and nonsynovial.
- Ossification of the posterior sacroiliac ligaments produces the "star" sign, as observed in the oblique and anteroposterior projections.
- Bilateral involvement is not an uncommon occurrence.
- Ossification of the iliolumbar ligaments produces the "angel wing" sign.
- Prominent hyperostosis or "whiskering" frequently occurs at the ligamentous attachments of the iliac crests, anterosuperior iliac spine, ischial tuberosities, greater trochanters, and pubic symphysis, where frank osseous bridges may form.

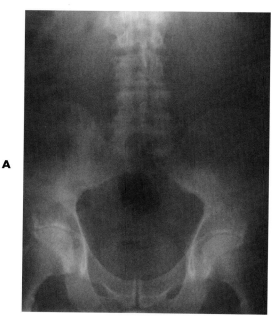
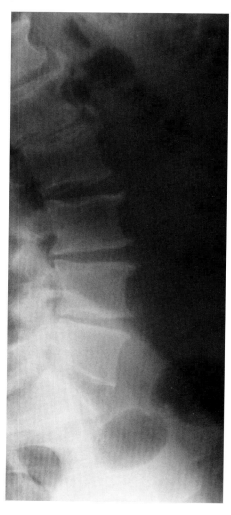

FIG. 2-69 A, Anteroposterior. Diffuse idiopathic skeletal hyperostosis of the thoracolumbar junction in a 68-year-old man. Note the mild unilateral hip osteoarthritis. **B,** Lateral. The thoracolumbar junction area demonstrates exuberant hyperostotic spurring. Mild degenerative disc disease is seen caudally. (Courtesy Sheldon Hershkop, MD, Toronto, Ontario.)

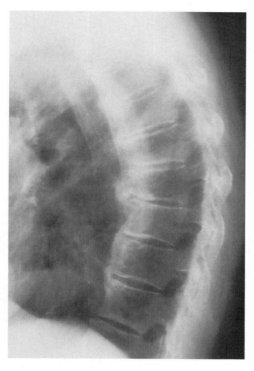

FIG. 2-70 Diffuse idiopathic skeletal hyperostosis. "Flowing" hyperostotic bone is observed along the anterior margin of virtually the entire thoracic spine, with accompanying increase in the kyphosis.

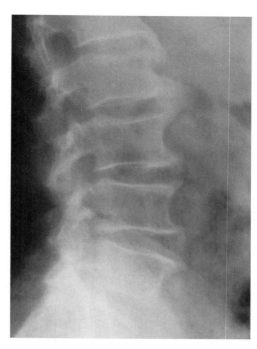

FIG. 2-71 Diffuse idiopathic skeletal hyperostosis. Marked involvement from L2-L3 cephalad is visualized.

Extremities

- Hyperostoses may also occur at the patellar poles, distal tibia, fibular interosseous membrane, calcaneus, tarsus, phalangeal tufts, distal radius, ulnar interosseous membrane, acromion, distal clavicle, and olecranon.

OSSIFIED POSTERIOR LONGITUDINAL LIGAMENT (OPLL) SYNDROME

- This syndrome may result in compression myelopathy of the spinal cord.
- The most common site of occurrence is the cervical spine.

Clinical Presentation

- May be asymptomatic

Radiographic Features

- Signs are distinctive and best portrayed on the lateral radiograph.

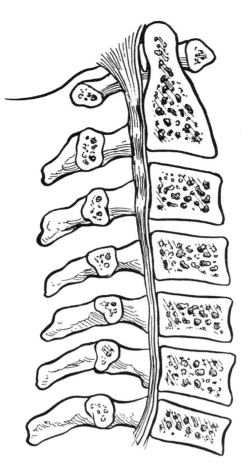

FIG. 2-72 Diagram of the posterior longitudinal ligament.

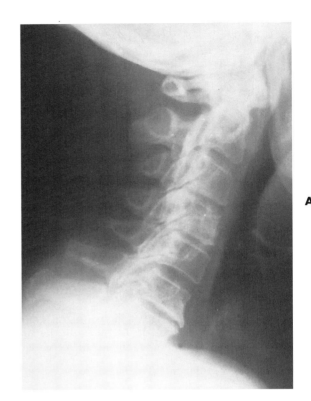

A

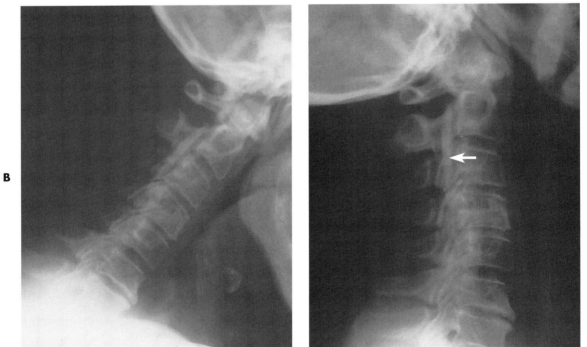

B

C

FIG. 2-73 Ossification of the posterior longitudinal ligament. **A,** Neutral. **B,** Flexion. **C,** Extension. Observe the thick osseous bar immediately posterior to the C2 and C3 bodies (*arrow*), corresponding to ossification of the posterior longitudinal ligament.

- The most reliable diagnostic sign is the characteristic, dense, linear radiopaque osseous bar, 1 to 5 mm thick, paralleling the posterior vertebral body margins (Figs. 2-72 and 2-73, *A-C*).
- A radiolucent zone is commonly interspaced between the ossified ligament and vertebral body, corresponding to the unossified deeper ligamentous layers.
- The length of this ossification may comprise only one vertebral body height or traverse a number of contiguous segments.
- Usually the adjacent intervertebral discs and apophyseal joints remain normal.
- OPLL is reported to occur in 50% of patients with DISH.
- Subsequent studies using conventional and computerized tomography as well as myelography are necessary to delineate the degree of suspected cord compromise present.

INFLAMMATORY ARTHROPATHIES
Rheumatoid Arthritis
Pathophysiology

- Rheumatoid arthritis is defined as a disorder of connective tissue that affects extraarticular and intraarticular structures.
- Its etiology is not yet fully understood, but various causes, such as infection, auto-immunity, and heredity, have been postulated.
- In the early stage of the disease the synovium becomes hyperemic and thickened.
- The synovium proliferates to form villi, which fill the joint space; at this point, the hypertrophied synovium is known as *pannus.*
- The pannus extends over the articular cartilage and bone at the articular margins where granulation tissue forms, resulting in cartilaginous destruction and bony erosions.
- Later, joint destruction can lead to subluxation, deformity, and ankylosis.
- The juxtaarticular bone becomes osteopenic as a result of inflammatory hyperemia and pannus development. (This can be intensified late in the disease because of steroid therapy and disuse atrophy.)
- Pannus erodes into bone at joint margins, where inflamed synovium is in direct contact with bone that is unprotected by articular cartilage (marginal erosions).
- Cartilage breaks down because of the catabolic effect of pannus enzymes and impedance of

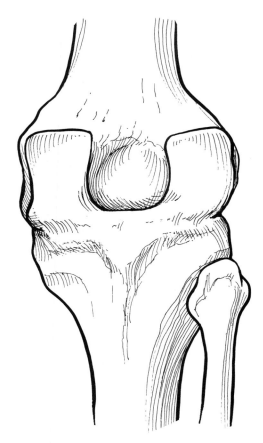

FIG. 2-74 In this diagram fibrous ankylosis has fused the femorotibial articulation in end-stage rheumatoid arthritis.

nutritional supply, resulting in a uniform loss of joint space.
- Eventual fibrous and bony ankylosis across the joint space may ensue (Fig. 2-74).

Clinical Presentation

- The disease typically afflicts middle-aged women, but people of any age and gender may be involved.
- The typical onset of the disease is the gradual development of symmetrical polyarthritis, involving the small joints of the hands and feet.
- Other joints are less commonly affected.
- The disease may strike those between 20 and 60 years of age, with peak incidence at 40 to 50 years of age.
- The ratio of women to men with the disease is 3:1 in the 20 to 40 age group and 1:1 after age 40.
- When patients are under age 16, the condition is termed *juvenile rheumatoid arthritis.*

- The most common signs and symptoms are painful, swollen, stiff joints.
- Morning stiffness, muscle wasting, and later, deformity, may also be evident.
- Subcutaneous nodules, evident in up to 30% of patients, are especially prominent on the extensor surfaces of the forearms and olecranon processes.
- The presence of the nodules denotes generalized systemic involvement and carries a poor prognosis.
- Constitutional symptoms such as fever, malaise, and weight loss are common during the active phase of the disease.
- The course and prognosis of the disease are unpredictable.
- Usually, the disease involves periods of remission and exacerbation, with gradual progression of deformity and disability.

Laboratory Analysis

- A complete blood count (CBC) may demonstrate normochromic or hypochromic anemia.
- The erythrocytic sedimentation rate (ESR) may be elevated during the active phase of the disease.
- Serology is as follows:
  - The latex-fixation rheumatoid factor (RF) test is positive in 80% of adults who have established rheumatoid arthritis but may be negative for several years.

Radiographic Features

- Areas of the skeleton most commonly affected are the metacarpophalangeal (MCP) and PIP joints of the hands and the MTP joints.
- Axially, only the cervical spine is affected.
- The following are early alterations, classically bilaterally symmetric:
  - Soft tissue edema and intraarticular effusion
  - Juxtaarticular osteoporosis
  - Uniform loss of joint space
  - Marginal joint erosions
  - Subarticular pseudocysts, which can be large and contain a combination of synovial fluid and intraosseous pannus extension
- The following are later alterations:
  - Deformities, such as subluxations, dislocations, and osseous misalignments, caused by joint destruction, ligamentous laxity, and altered muscular action resulting from tendinous rupture
  - Marked articular bony destruction
  - Fusion

Hands

- The earliest changes are seen in the second and third MCP and PIP joints.

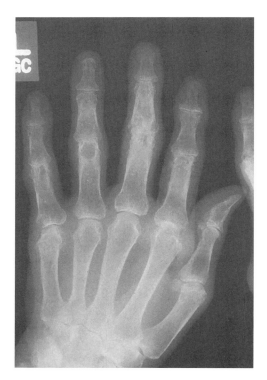

FIG. 2-75 Rheumatoid arthritis. Note the universal involvement of the proximal interphalangeal joints with adjacent soft tissue swelling, and sparing of the distal interphalangeal joints.

- The absence of DIP joint involvement assists in distinguishing rheumatoid arthritis from osteoarthritis (Fig. 2-75).
- Fusiform soft tissue edema produces the "spindle digit" sign (Figs. 2-76 and 2-77).
- Haygarth nodes are subcutaneous nodules located at the MCP joints.
- Joint-space widening is temporarily produced early on by intraarticular edema.
- Periarticular osteoporosis is due to hyperemia and disuse.
- Uniform joint-space narrowing is due to uniform destruction of articular cartilage by pannus (Fig. 2-78).
- Marginal erosions are produced by inflammatory pannus hypertrophy at capsular ligamentous insertions. This condition is termed *rat-bite erosions* (Fig. 2-79).
- Early rat-bite erosions are best visualized with a specialized Norgaard (ball catcher's) projection.

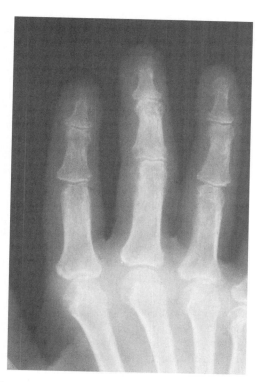

FIG. 2-76 Spindle digits. Mild soft tissue swelling surrounding the proximal interphalangeal joints is an early radiographic indication of rheumatoid arthritis.

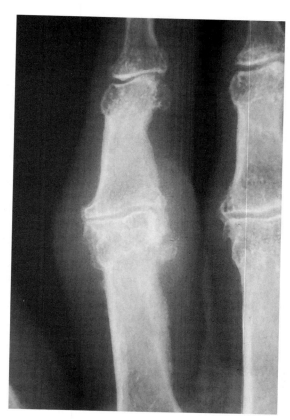

FIG. 2-77 Periarticular soft tissue swelling is evident at the proximal interphalangeal joint, accompanying the osseous alterations.

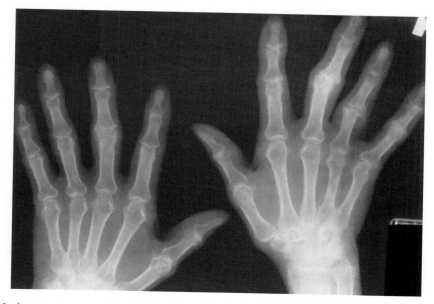

FIG. 2-78 Moderate rheumatoid arthritis. Note the periarticular osteopenia at the proximal interphalangeal and metacarpophalangeal joints, with uniform joint-space narrowing, subluxations, soft tissue swelling at the proximal interphalangeal joints, and ulnar deviation of the fingers. Advanced inflammatory arthritis of the wrists is noted.

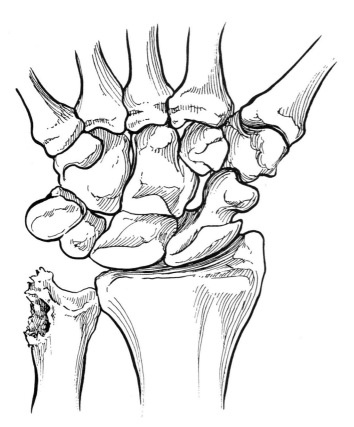

- Advanced erosions, interspaced by intact articular cortex, produce the characteristic "dot-dash" appearance of the subarticular cortex.
- Marginal erosions are most commonly located on the radial aspects of the metacarpal heads.
- Pseudocysts may be produced by synovial fluid and granulation tissue forced through weakened subarticular cortex into osteoporotic, subcortical spongiosa.
- Pseudocysts may be large.
- Compressive erosions, a later manifestation of the disease, are the result of muscular forces acting on the joint that collapse weakened articular cortex and subarticular osteoporotic bone.
- As the disease progresses, the periarticular osteoporosis advances to generalized, regional osteoporosis as a result of chronic inflammation and disuse.
- Advanced compressive erosions can produce a "ball-and-socket" configuration at the MCP and PIP joints.
- Another late manifestation of the disease is "telescoping fingers," in which the extensive destruction of bone ends, combined with muscular pull, produces collapse of the subarticular and metaphyseal regions of the short tubular bones of the hands (Fig. 2-80).

FIG. 2-79 Rheumatoid arthritis: rat-bite erosion. This diagram depicts erosion at the ulnar styloid as a result of hypertrophic inflammatory pannus.

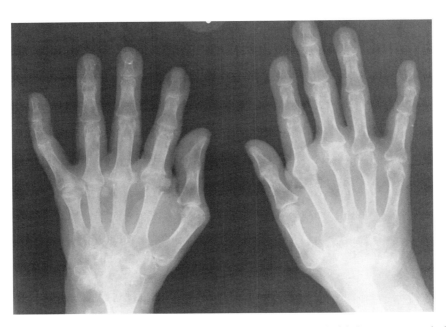

FIG. 2-80 Silastic hinge implants have been used at the second and third left metacarpophalangeal joints after the collapse of weakened articular cortex in advanced rheumatoid arthritis. Telescoping at the right second metacarpophalangeal joint is noted. Extensive wrist involvement with bilateral carpal coalition is also observed.

- Migration of granulation tissue from marginal erosions into the subarticular cortex, with resultant contact with articular pannus, may yield fibrous or osseous ankylosis of the joints of the hands.
- Interphalangeal bony ankylosis is rare in the hand.
- Muscular spasm produces ulnar deviation of the MCP joints; ligamentous laxity and bony erosions are seen in 50% of patients.
- The "boutonniere" deformity is usually a later manifestation of the disease and involves flexion of the PIP joint and extension of the DIP joint (Fig. 2-81).
- The "swan-neck" deformity is formed by extension of the PIP joint and flexion of the DIP joint (Figs. 2-82 and 2-83).
- The thumb may exhibit the Z-deformity (also known as *hitchhiker's thumb*), which involves flexion of the MCP joint with dorsal subluxation and hyperextension of the interphalangeal joint (Fig. 2-84).

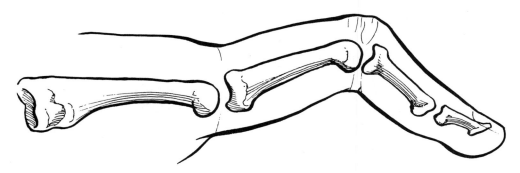

FIG. 2-81 Diagram showing a boutonniére deformity. Note the flexion at the proximal interphalangeal joint, with extension at the distal interphalangeal joint.

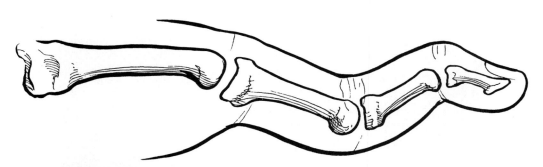

FIG. 2-82 Diagram showing a swan-neck deformity. Observe the extension at the proximal interphalangeal joint, with flexion at the distal interphalangeal joint.

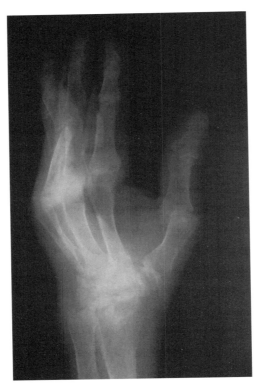

FIG. 2-83 Swan-neck deformity is observed in the fourth finger. A "hitchhiker's" deformity of the thumb is also present.

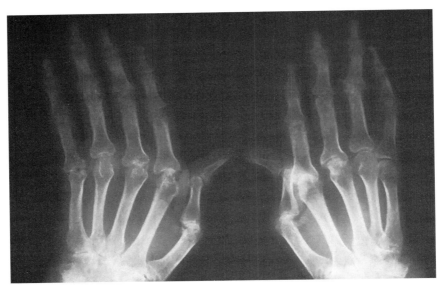

FIG. 2-84 "Hitchhiker's" thumb. Observe the bilateral marked flexion subluxations of the first metacarpophalangeal joints, with hyperextension subluxations of the first interphalangeal joints.

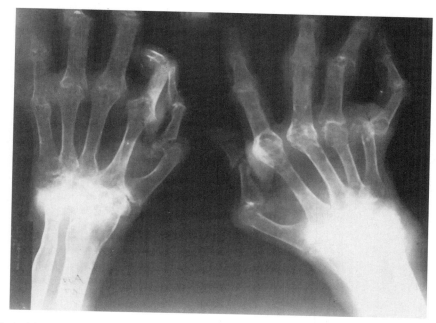

FIG. 2-85 Arthritis mutilans. Advanced end-stage rheumatoid arthritis demonstrates total carpal fusion, metacarpal head destruction with MCP joint subluxations and luxations, as well as severe interphalangeal joint involvement with deformities throughout.

- The DIP joints are less commonly affected in rheumatoid arthritis.
- *Arthritis mutilans* is defined as the end stage of severe rheumatoid arthritis in the extremities, characterized by gross deformity and joint subluxation (Fig. 2-85).

Wrist
- Soft tissue edema is the earliest manifestation, especially opposite the medial aspect of the distal ulna.
- Osteoporosis is common and regional.
- Rat-bite erosions commonly affect the ulnar styloid.
- Erosions may involve any bone of the wrist, producing the "spotty" carpal sign.
- As the disease progresses, the carpal bones become disorganized, and radial rotation often results.
- Intercarpal joint widening may also occur.
- Late changes of the disease may produce deformity.
- Uniform pancompartmental joint-space narrowing occurs.
- Fibrous ankylosis of the carpus may result, followed by bony ankylosis (Fig. 2-86).
- Radiocarpal fusion is rare.

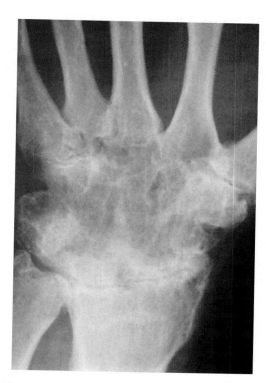

FIG. 2-86 Wrist coalition: complete carpal fusion with carpometacarpal fusion in advanced end-stage rheumatoid arthritis.

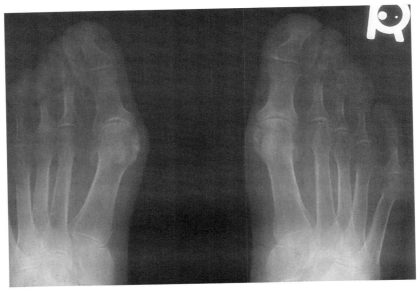

FIG. 2-87 Rheumatoid arthritis of the feet. Observe the marked bilaterally symmetric osteopenia of the metatarsal heads and periarticular aspects of all phalanges.

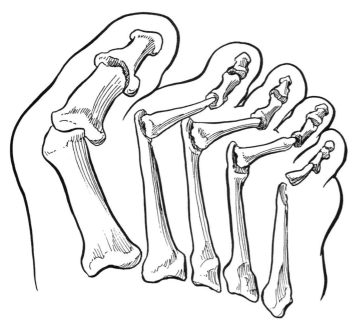

FIG. 2-88 Diagram showing Lanois deformity. Observe the metatarsal head resorption, with subluxations and fibular phalangeal deviation.

- Late rheumatoid arthritis of the hand and wrist produces severe marked destruction, deformity, and misalignment, with resultant fibrous and/or osseous ankylosis (arthritis mutilans).
- Treatment may include surgical ligation and prosthetic replacement of severely affected articulations.

Feet

- Feet are the initial site of disease in 15% of patients.
- Earliest changes are observed at the fourth and fifth MTP joints.
- Soft tissue edema may result in spreading of the metatarsal heads.
- Erosive changes are most commonly noted on the medial aspects of the metatarsal heads.
- Destructive changes resemble those found in the hands (Fig. 2-87).
- Calcaneal lesions at the attachments of the Achilles tendon and plantar aponeurosis produce well-defined spurs.
- Subluxation occurs later and usually affects the first MTP joint, producing a hallux valgus deformity.
- Plantar depression of the metatarsal heads combined with erosion and fibular deviation of the phalanges at the MTP joints and flexion of the interphalangeal joint produce the Lanois deformity (Fig. 2-88).

Cervical spine

- Atlantooccipital: erosions, sclerosis, and eventual fusion
- Osseous destruction sometimes facilitating vertical translocation of the dens, which can be fatal (Fig. 2-89)
- Pseudobasilar invagination
- Atlantoaxial articulations
- Frequent involvement

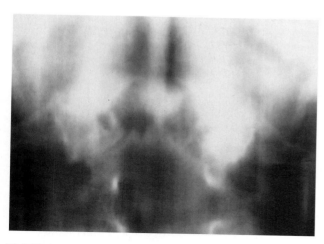

FIG. 2-89 Dens erosion. Note the considerable erosion of the midlower odontoid process.

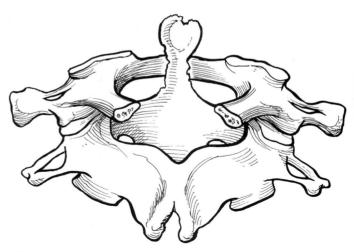

FIG. 2-90 Diagram showing erosion of the odontoid. The preferred sites for inflammatory erosion are depicted.

♦ Inflammatory rupture of the transverse ligament allowing an increased atlantodental interspace (especially in flexion) in excess of 3 mm in the adult (occurs in 25% to 50% of patients, depending on the severity of the disease)
♦ "Drumstick" deformity at the posterior base of the dens produced by erosions of the dens (Fig. 2-90)
♦ Loss of ligamentous integrity leading to atlas displacement
♦ Necessary to perform flexion and extension studies with caution
♦ Atlantodental interspace: adults (3 mm maximum); children (5 mm maximum)
♦ Surgical stabilization sometimes required
♦ Subaxial articulations
  • Generalized osteoporosis
  • Apophyseal joints: erosions, loss of joint space, instability, and possible ankylosis
  • Subluxations, especially at C2-C4 caused by ligamentous laxity and apophyseal joint involvement
  • "Stair-stepping": multilevel spondylolistheses (Fig. 2-91)
  • "Pencil-sharpened" spinouses: tapered because of nuchal bursal inflammation

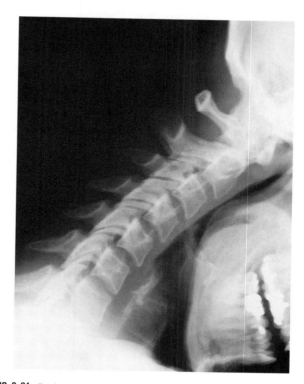

FIG. 2-91 Stair-stepping. Cervical flexion in this 35-year-old woman with rheumatoid arthritis demonstrates multilevel anterolistheses caused by ligamentous laxity. (Courtesy Doug Penrose, DC, Toronto, Ontario.)

Knee

- Rheumatoid arthritis is uncommon in the knee.
- Joint effusion, followed by marginal erosions, is most commonly seen at the medial tibial condyle (Fig. 2-92).
- Subchondral pseudocysts may form later.

- Uniform loss of joint space, regional osteoporosis, and Baker's cysts are characteristic findings (Fig. 2-93).
- Genu valgum and flexion deformities are late manifestations. Surgical intervention may be indicated (Fig. 2-94).

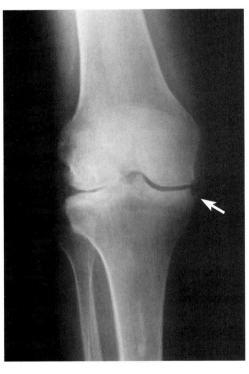

FIG. 2-92 Rheumatoid arthritis of the knee. Concentric medial and lateral compartment involvement contrasts rheumatoid arthritis with osteoarthritis, which selectively affects the medial compartment. Note the medial tibial erosion (*arrow*).

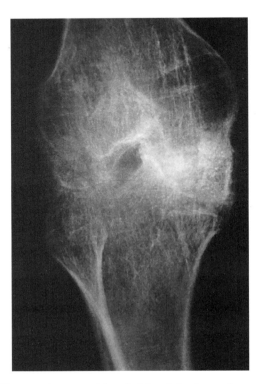

FIG. 2-93 Late rheumatoid arthritis of the knee demonstrates complete uniform joint-space loss, with marked regional osteoporosis. Superimposed osteoarthritis accounts for the medial compartment sclerosis.

Elbow

- Involvement, which occurs in a bilateral, symmetrical manner, is uncommon.
- Early changes include joint-space edema, which displaces the posterior and anterior fat pads and enables them to be clearly visualized in the lateral projection.
- The olecranon bursa is often involved and is visualized as a soft tissue mass overlying the olecranon.
- Periarticular osteoporosis, pathologic fracture, subluxation, and bony ankylosis are late changes (Fig. 2-95, *A* and *B*).
- Rheumatoid nodules may be formed in 20% to 30% of patients on the extensor surfaces of the forearms, just distal to the olecranon.

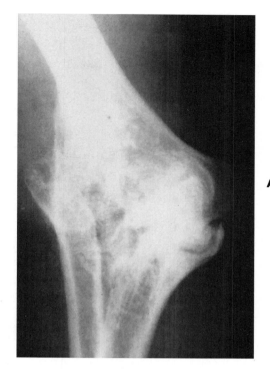

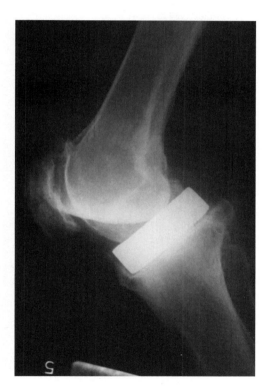

FIG. 2-94 Rheumatoid arthritis. A tibial plateau prosthesis was required in this patient after inflammatory destruction and deformity of the superior tibia. Note the marked degenerative changes of the patellofemoral joint.

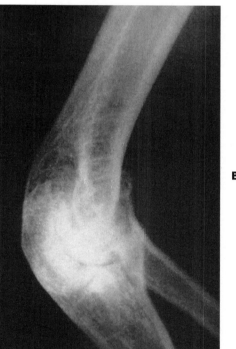

FIG. 2-95 Rheumatoid arthritis of the elbow.
A, Anteroposterior. **B,** Lateral. Advanced end-stage disease manifests as obliteration of the articular spaces, with accompanying deformity, luxation, and synostosis.

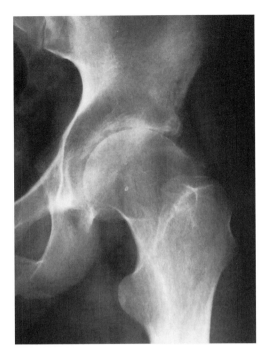

FIG. 2-96 Rheumatoid arthritis of the hip. Note the characteristic uniform loss of joint space.

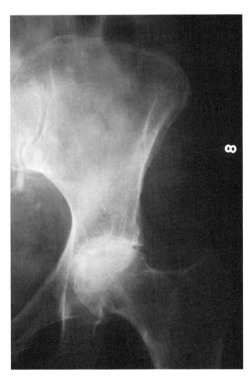

FIG. 2-97 Rheumatoid arthritis of the hip. Marked uniform loss of joint space is accompanied by periarticular erosion of the femoral head.

Hip

- This is an uncommon location but possible in longstanding, severe rheumatoid arthritis.
- Hip involvement is characterized by uniform loss of acetabular joint space and osteoporosis (Fig. 2-96).
- Erosions and subchondral pseudocysts in the femoral head and acetabulum are common, resulting in superior and medial migration of the

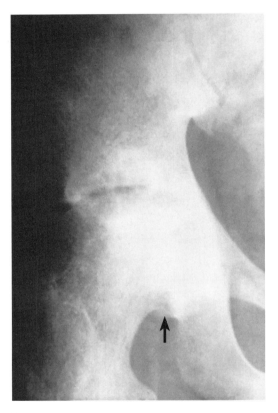

FIG. 2-98 Rheumatoid arthritis of the hip. Note the inflammatory erosion (*arrow*) with uniform joint-space diminution.

femoral head, along the axis of the femoral neck; this is referred to as *axial migration* (Figs. 2-97, 2-98, 2-99, and 2-100).

- Bilateral involvement is the rule (Fig. 2-101).
- Monoarticular rheumatoid arthritis is a rare condition.
- In protrusio acetabuli (arthrokatadysis), acetabular floor is displaced medially as a result of weight-bearing.

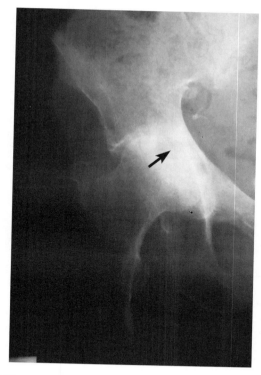

FIG. 2-100 Uniformly diminished joint space is noted along with subchondral pseudocyst (*arrow*) in progressing rheumatoid arthritis.

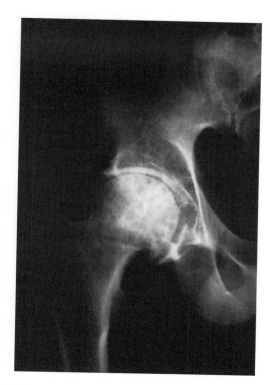

FIG. 2-99 Rheumatoid arthritis of the hip. Pseudocystic formations in the femoral head are noted with inferior erosion at the femoral head-neck junction.

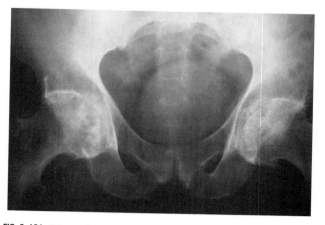

FIG. 2-101 Rheumatoid arthritis of the hips. Note the typical bilaterally symmetric involvement.

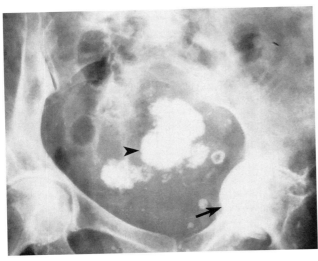

FIG. 2-102 Rheumatoid arthritis: protrusio acetabulum. Note the marked deformity of the pelvic basin caused by medial acetabular displacement with weight-bearing (*arrow*). Uterine fibroids are incidentally observed in the pelvis (*arrowhead*).

- Rheumatoid arthritis is the most common cause of bilateral protrusio acetabuli (Figs. 2-102 and 2-103).
- A possible end stage is fibrous ankylosis (Fig. 2-104).
- With time, overlying secondary osteoarthritis can form circumferentially around the femoral heads, including subchondral sclerosis, pseudo-cysts, and osteophytes.

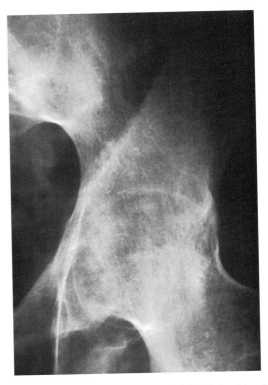

FIG. 2-104 End-stage rheumatoid arthritis of the hip depicts fibrous ankylosis, with nonvisualization of the femoral head cortex and negligible residual joint space.

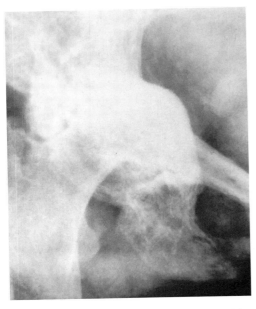

FIG. 2-103 Advanced rheumatoid arthritis of the hip demonstrates significant deformity of the femoral head and neck, with protrusio acetabulum.

- Later changes noted are generalized loss of lordosis and symmetric, bridging syndesmophytes, which produce the "bamboo-spine" appearance (Fig. 2-119).
- Ossification of apophyseal joint capsules results in fusion of facet surfaces.
- Ossification of the interspinous and supraspinous ligaments produces the "dagger sign" when visualized on the anteroposterior projection.
- Advanced paraspinal soft tissue ossification involving the annulus, joint capsule, and interspinous and supraspinous ligaments creates a "trolley-track" appearance of the lumbar spine on the anteroposterior projection (Fig. 2-120).
- Osteoporosis is usually mild to moderate.

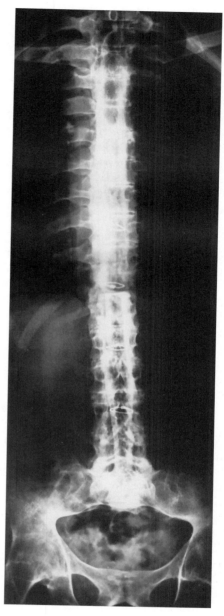

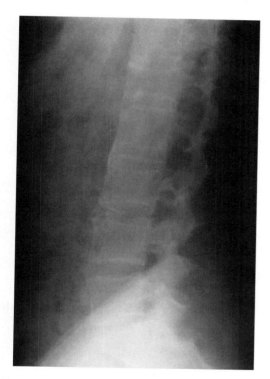

FIG. 2-119 Ankylosing spondylitis of the lumbar spine. Note the multilevel syndesmophytic fusion, referred to as a *bamboo spine*. The normal lordotic curve has been lost.

FIG. 2-120 Ankylosing spondylitis; anteroposterior full spine projection. The "trolley-track" sign manifests as ossification of the lumbar facet joint capsules on either side of ossified interspinous and supraspinous ligaments. Also note the bilateral sacroiliac joint fusion.

Pelvis

- Localized periostitis at ligamentous insertion sites produces the classical enthesopathy, or "whiskering."
- Enthesopathy commonly parallels inflammatory changes at the sacroiliac joint and arises from the iliac crests, ischial tuberosities, and greater trochanters.
- The symphysis pubis demonstrates changes similar and parallel to those that occur in the sacroiliac joints.
- With rhizomelic distribution the hips and shoulders are involved in ankylosing spondylitis in up to 50% of patients, with features quite similar to rheumatoid arthritis.

Hip

- Changes are usually bilateral and symmetric, with uniform loss of joint space and mild osteoporosis.
- Next, inflammatory osseous spurs may form at the articular margins of the femoral head and acetabular labrum, as well as between the head and neck of the femur.
- Later, protrusio acetabuli and osseous ankylosis may occur.

Shoulder

- Changes here are also bilateral and symmetric, with uniform loss of joint space, osteoporosis, and erosions occurring at the superolateral aspect of the humerus.
- "Whiskering" of the acromioclavicular joint and the insertion site of the coracoclavicular ligament may occur.
- Bony ankylosis occurs late.

Feet

- Changes center on the os calcis, where enthesopathy occurs most frequently.
- Erosions, reactive sclerosis, and "whiskering" occur at the insertion sites of the Achilles' tendon and plantar aponeurosis.
- Spurs may form but are commonly fluffy and irregular. This is an indication of their inflammatory nature.

Differential Diagnosis

- Clinically, osteoarthritis, tuberculosis, and disc lesions may simulate ankylosing spondylitis.
- Radiographically similar appearances can be produced by other seronegative spondyloarthropathies, rheumatoid arthritis, tuberculosis, osteoarthritis, and rarely, DISH.

ENTEROPATHIC ARTHRITIS

- Arthritis associated with ulcerative colitis and regional enteritis

Pathophysiology

- Its etiology is unknown, but it may be associated with a hypersensitivity reaction.

Clinical Presentation

- This disease is primarily seen in middle-aged men.
- Approximately 10% or fewer patients with ulcerative colitis and regional enteritis have associated arthritis.
- Conditions include a migratory arthralgia that is asymmetric in distribution and usually involves the hip and knee.

Laboratory Analysis

- Laboratory tests are nonspecific.
- Hematologic analysis reveals iron-deficiency anemia and leukocytosis.
- Stool examination may reveal the presence of steatorrhea.

Radiographic Features

- The areas most commonly affected are the sacroiliac joints, which demonstrate a symmetric involvement by sclerosis.
- In severe cases, erosions, joint-space widening (narrowing later), and ankylosis may occur.
- Spinal involvement may appear identical to ankylosing spondylitis, with marginal syndesmophytes and bony ankylosis of the facet joints.

Differential Diagnosis

- Ankylosing spondylitis, infectious arthropathy, and osteitis condensans illi should be considered.

PSORIATIC ARTHRITIS

- Patients with psoriasis may be predisposed to a specific type of arthropathy that involves peripheral joint destruction, sacroiliitis, and asymmetric, nonmarginal syndesmophyte formation.

Pathophysiology

- Articular symptoms may be acute or insidious.

Laboratory Analysis

- A minority (approximately 30%) of the patients may exhibit positive HLA B-27 tests and may have elevated serum uric acid.
- The ESR may be elevated.
- The RF is negative.

Radiographic Features

- ♦ The disease primarily affects the DIP joints of the hands and feet (Figs. 2-121 and 2-122).
- ♦ Tissue swelling over the entire digit gives the appearance of a "sausage digit."
- ♦ Soft tissue swelling appears first and progresses to marginal osseous erosions.

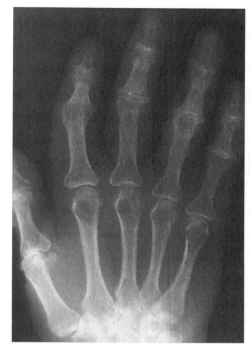

FIG. 2-121 Psoriatic arthritis of the hand. All interphalangeal articulations are affected, with inflammatory fusion noted at the second proximal interphalangeal joint.

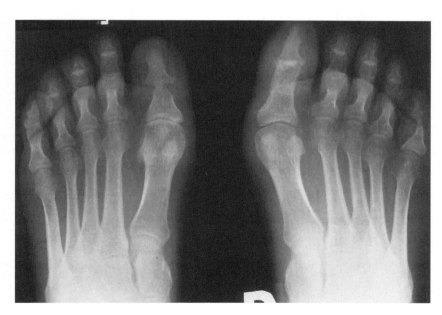

FIG. 2-122 Psoriatic arthritis of the feet. Observe the multiple site inflammatory osteopenia and erosive distal phalangeal whittling.

- In response, a prominent fluffy periostitis may be visualized (Fig. 2-123).
- Resorption of the terminal tufts of the distal phalanges results in a whittled appearance.
- In contrast to rheumatoid arthritis, involvement is asymmetric, and little or no hyperemic osteoporosis is detected.
- The joint-space width may increase because of the accumulation of intraarticular fibrous tissue, but progression of the disease results in osseous ankylosis.

- An "ivory phalanx" may appear and is due to osseous proliferation at the sites of erosion, subchondral sclerosis, and proliferation of the terminal ends of the distal phalanges.
- Telescoping of one bone into its neighbor (excess skin may be folded over involved joint) is known as *opera-glass hand*.
- In extreme conditions, resorption and erosion of the metacarpals or metatarsals result in a "pencil-in-a-cup" deformity, and if allowed to continue, develop into arthritis mutilans (Fig. 2-124).

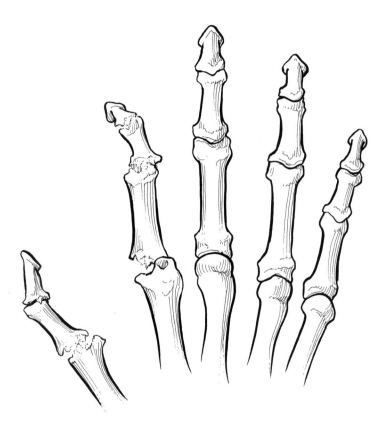

FIG. 2-123 Psoriatic arthritis of the hand. This diagram depicts characteristically "fluffy" periarticular periostitis in the first two digits. Also noted are inflammatory joint destruction and subluxation.

- Sacroiliac joint involvement is usually unilateral, with blurring of the subchondral margins, decrease in joint space, erosions, and reactive sclerosis that may eventually progress to bony ankylosis.
- In the spine, there is a pattern of asymmetric nonmarginal syndesmophyte (parasyndesmophyte) formation that skips areas of the spine and is most prevalent in the upper lumbar and lower thoracic regions.
- In contrast, the sydesmophytes of ankylosing spondylitis originate in the vertebral margins and not in the midvertebral body.
- Conditions seen in the cervical spine include atlantoaxial subluxation and dislocation, with blurring and irregularities at the apophyseal joint margins that rarely progress to ankylosis.

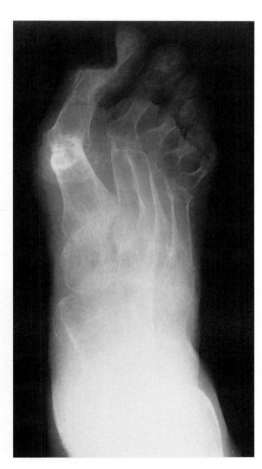

FIG. 2-124 Advanced psoriatic arthritis in the foot: arthritis mutilans. Note the complete inflammatory resorption of the metatarsal heads, severe phalangeal subluxation (Lanois deformity), and osseous fusion of the first metatarsophalangeal joint. Disuse osteoporosis of the digits is observed.

Differential Diagnosis

- Differential diagnosis of general radiographic features includes Reiter's syndrome and rheumatoid arthritis.

REITER'S SYNDROME

- Characterized by a classic triad consisting of urethritis, conjunctivitis, and polyarthritis, which may or may not arise concurrently

Pathophysiology

- Unknown etiology

Clinical Presentation

- The disease mainly affects young males and appears to be related to conditions of venereal disease and certain types of dysentery.
- The urethritis is mildly painful and produces a purulent discharge.
- The conjunctivitis is usually mild.
- The arthritic component is most commonly observed in the lower extremities and has an asymmetric distribution.

Articular signs and symptoms

- Asymmetric arthritis of lower extremity
- Initial involvement of knee and ankle, followed by the MTP joints and calcaneus
- Joint alterations of the upper extremity less frequent
- The sacroiliac joints, lumbar spine, symphysis pubis, and manubriosternal joint are involved.
- Arthritis is monoarticular during the early phase of the disease
- Common manifestations include heel pain and tenderness (also seen in psoriatic arthritis and ankylosing spondylitis, but not in rheumatoid arthritis).
- Heel pain may precede ocular and urethral findings.
- Joint aspiration reveals the presence of inflammatory synovial fluid.
- Ankylosing spondylitis may develop in approximately 25% of patients with recurrent Reiter's syndrome.

Laboratory Analysis

- The white blood cell count is usually at an elevated level.
- ESR is usually elevated.
- Hematuria may be seen.
- Approximately 80% of patients with Reiter's syndrome are HLA B-27 positive.

Radiographic Features

- Common areas of involvement include the feet, sacroiliac joints, and spine.
- Calcaneal involvement is characteristic.
- Initial changes include periarticular soft tissue swelling, which is followed by bony erosions and fluffy periostitis.
- Such features normally arise at the insertion of the plantar fascia and/or Achilles' tendon.
- Additional areas of involvement in the feet include the MTP and PIP joints.
- Periarticular osteoporosis may be seen, but it is visualized less frequently in this condition than in rheumatoid arthritis.
- In severe cases, arthritis mutilans may develop, producing a "Lanois" deformity, which is hallmarked by lateral deviation and dorsal dislocation of the toes.
- Sacroiliac joint involvement is normally unilateral and includes joint-space narrowing, bony erosions, and reactive sclerosis.
- Patterns of spinal involvement demonstrate coarse, nonmarginal, asymmetric syndesmophytes with discontinuous distribution (Fig. 2-125).

- The disease is most commonly seen in the lower thoracic and/or upper lumbar spine.

Differential Diagnosis

- Psoriatic arthritis, rheumatoid arthritis, and juvenile rheumatoid arthritis should be considered.
- Ankylosing spondylitis has a similar axial distribution (with marginal syndesmophytes instead of the nonmarginal variety) but demonstrates significantly less frequent peripheral articular changes.
- The resolving nature of the lesions is distinctive compared with the progressive and severe alterations in psoriatic arthritis.
- Sacroiliac and spinal joint changes are identical in Reiter's syndrome and psoriatic arthritis.

Osteitis Condensans Ilii

- In pregnancy, biomechanical changes occur that produce increased stress on pelvic articulations.
- Local tenderness and pain over the sacroiliac joints and symphysis pubis can be elicited.
- It involves the ilium adjacent to the sacroiliac joint.
- It is usually bilateral and has relatively symmetric involvement.
- It most often affects multiparous women.

Radiographic Features

- Well-defined triangular sclerosis on the iliac aspect of the sacroiliac joint (Figs. 2-126 and 2-127)
- Apex of the sclerosis extending into the auricular portion of the ilium

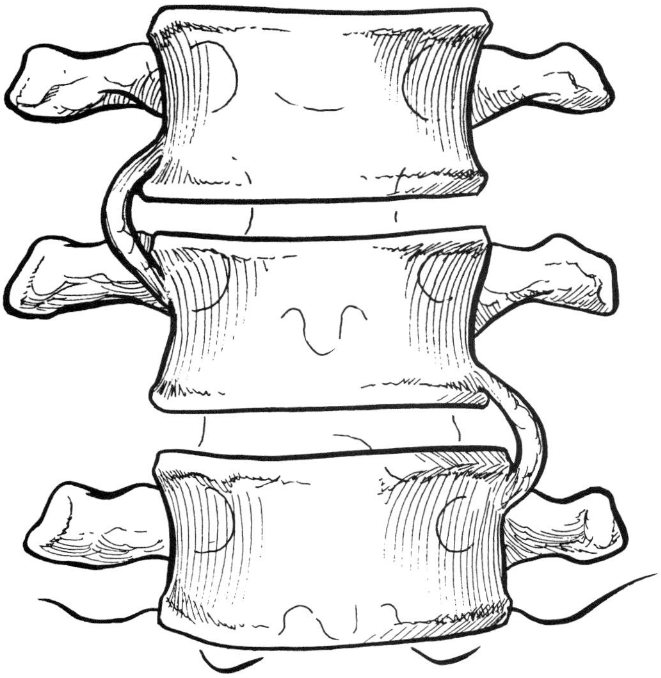

FIG. 2-125 Nonmarginal syndesmophytes. As seen in Reiter's syndrome and psoriatic arthritis, these osseous bridges are larger and bulkier than the marginal syndesmophytes of ankylosing spondylitis. They are also asymmetric in their distribution and are not strictly vertical in their orientation.

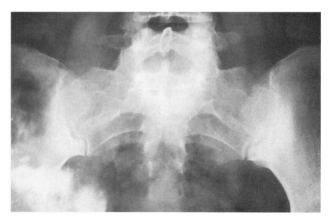

FIG. 2-126 Osteitis condensans ilii. Observe the marked bilateral triangular periarticular iliac sclerosis.

- Usually no significant joint-space narrowing or sacral involvement (Fig. 2-128)
- Size of lesion variable
- Possibility that condition resolves and disappears with time
- Unclear etiology
- According to predominant theory, condition secondary to mechanical stress across the sacroiliac joint, coupled with the hormone-induced pelvic ligamentous laxity

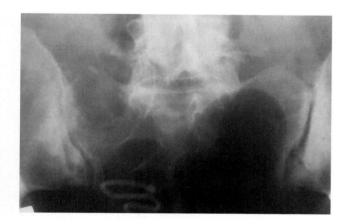

FIG. 2-127 Osteitis condensans ilii: bilateral sclerosis of the ilia immediately adjacent to the sacroiliac articulations. An intrauterine birth-control device is incidentally noted.

Osteitis Pubis

- May appear within a few months of child delivery or other pelvic operations
- In males, tends to follow prostatic or bladder surgery
- In females, tends to follow pregnancy
- In athletes, does not occur secondary to chronic stress across the articulation but is caused instead by acute avulsion at sites of attachment of adductor brevis, adductor longus, and gracilis

Clinical Presentation

- Local pain, tenderness, muscle spasm, and unstable gait

Radiographic Findings

- Widening of the symphysis, with bony erosion, resorption, and eburnation (Fig. 2-129)
- Usually involves both pubic bones symmetrically
- Eventually resolves by restoration of the normal osseous density, with disappearance of the sclerosis
- Possible persistence or fusion of irregular articular surfaces
- Differential diagnosis: trauma, infection, ankylosing spondylitis, and psoriatic arthritis

Metabolic Arthropathies

GOUT

- Gout is a condition of hyperuricemia, with deposition of sodium urate crystals in joints and soft tissues caused by a disorder of purine metabolism.

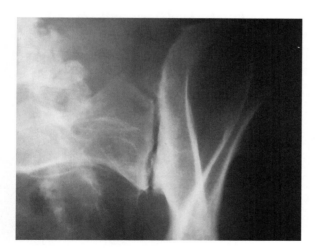

FIG. 2-128 Osteitis condensans ilii. No joint-space narrowing accompanies the subarticular iliac sclerosis.

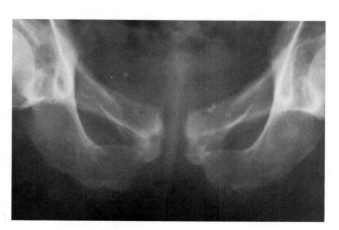

FIG. 2-129 Osteitis pubis. Widening of the symphysis pubis accompanies irregular periarticular osseous contour and sclerosis.

- As a consequence of overproduction or decreased excretion, high levels of uric acid precipitate out of the blood and are deposited into relatively avascular tissues, such as articular, periarticular, and subcutaneous tissue, as sodium urate crystals, or tophi.
- Tophi do not appear until about 10 to 12 years after the initial attack.
- Common sites of uric-acid crystal deposition include synovium, subchondral bone, ear cartilage, olecranon bursae, and infrapatellar bursae.
- With the deposition of crystals in the synovium the resultant irritation generates hyperplasia and the formation of granulation tissue known as *pannus.*
- Pannus formation causes cartilage destruction and marginal bony erosions.

Clinical Presentation

- The disease primarily affects males between 30 and 60 years of age.
- The primary disease may be transmitted as an autosomal dominant genetic characteristic.

- Polynesians, regular alcohol drinkers, and post-menopausal women on diuretics are predisposed to gouty attack.
- Usually monoarticular, the disease most frequently involves the first MTP joint (podagra).
- The joint appears red, hot, dry, and swollen and is exquisitely tender.
- Spinal involvement is rare.

Laboratory Features

- A serum uric acid level greater than 7 mg/100 ml constitutes hyperuricemia.
- Monosodium urate crystals are found in aspirated synovial fluid.

Radiographic Features

- The disease initially reveals the presence of asymmetric joint and bursal effusion predilected to the lower extremity.
- The arthropathy produced is radiographically characteristic, yet because it takes 4 to 7 years for gout to become radiographically evident and almost all patients are successfully treated long

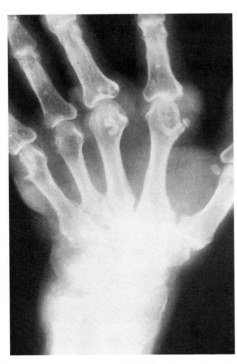

FIG. 2-130 Gout of the hand. Multiple sites of markedly increased soft tissue density are observed (tophi). Mild to moderate metacarpal head erosions are present.

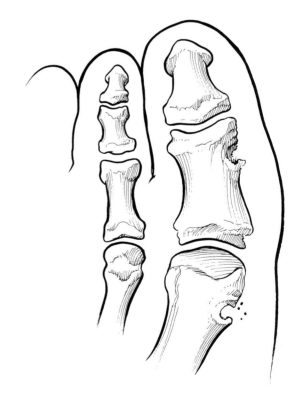

FIG. 2-131 Diagram showing "overhanging margin" signs. Observe the tophaceous subarticular erosion of the first metacarpal head and proximal phalanx, with a residual "overhanging" spicule of bone at each site.

before the destructive arthropathy occurs, it is seldom seen.

- As bone is destroyed, a periosteal response at the periphery of the tophus occurs, extending bone away from the erosion and producing an "overhanging edge" sign (Figs. 2-130 and 2-131).
- Symmetric joint-space narrowing usually occurs late in the disease.
- Secondary calcification within tophi may occur in the presence of renal failure.
- Long-standing subarticular erosions may ultimately lead to arthritis mutilans.
- Tophaceous softening of the transverse odontoid ligament can predispose to atlantoaxial subluxation.
- Unilateral sacroiliitis may develop.

Differential Diagnosis

- The following disorders may be considered radiographically in diagnosing gout: the rheumatoid variants, osteoarthritis, neuropathic arthropathy, and infectious arthropathy.

CALCIUM PYROPHOSPHATE DIHYDRATE (CPPD) DEPOSITION DISEASE

- Common synonyms for this disease include *pseudogout* and *chondrocalcinosis.*
- CPPD is defined as an inflammatory joint disease that results from the deposition of calcium pyrophosphate dihydrate into the synovial fluid, synovial membrane, joint capsule, and periarticular soft tissues.

Pathophysiology

- CPPD is a metabolic disturbance in which there is an impaired degradation or excessive production of pyrophosphate.
- CPPD crystals are deposited into cartilage lacunae, resulting in chondrocyte death and predisposing the articular cartilage to subsequent thinning and fissuring.

Clinical Presentation

- The condition may be acute, chronic, or asymptomatic.
- Symptomatic patients are usually over 60 years of age.

- The acute form of the disease is more prevalent in males, and the chronic form is more common in females.
- Acute attacks commonly affect the knees, wrists, MCP joints, shoulders, and elbows and cause the joints to become hot, swollen, and tender.
- The attack may last from 1 to 14 days.
- In chronic cases, clinical features include swelling, crepitus, and stiffness.
- Several associated diseases have been described, most frequently diabetes mellitus.

Laboratory Analysis

- CPPD crystals are present in the joint fluid aspirate.

Radiographic Features

- Features include articular cartilage calcification (chondrocalcinosis), periarticular calcification of synovia, capsule, tendon, bursa, or periarticular ligaments and soft tissues.
- The most common radiographic sign is articular cartilage calcification in which the knees and wrists (triangular cartilage) are most commonly affected; their involvement is virtually diagnostic of CPPD; symphysis pubis, elbows, hips, and intervertebral discs are most commonly affected.
- With hyaline articular cartilage involvement a fine radiopaque line appears parallel to the articular cortex.
- Fibrocartilage tissues demonstrate a characteristic punctate pattern of calcification.
- With knee involvement the menisci undergo chondrocalcinosis, and if the patellofemoral joint is affected, this diagnosis is strongly suggested.
- The joint destruction of arthropathy related to CPPD is virtually indistinguishable from that of degenerative joint disease.
- CPPD tends to affect the shoulder, elbow, radiocarpal joint, and patellofemoral joint.
- These areas are not normally affected by degenerative wear and tear.
- When degenerative joint disease is seen in the joints that CPPD tends to involve, a search for chondrocalcinosis should be undertaken.
- A joint aspiration for CPPD may be necessary to confirm the diagnosis.

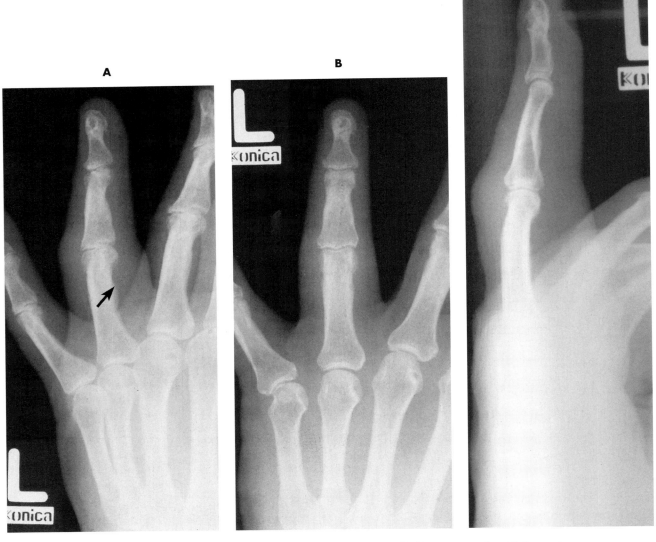

FIG. 2-132 Polyvillonodular synovitis of the finger. **A,** Oblique. **B,** Posteroanterior. **C,** Lateral. Observe the marked periarticular soft tissue swelling at the fourth proximal interphalangeal joint. Moderate fourth proximal phalanx erosion is noted (*arrow*). (Courtesy Cecil McQuoid, DC, Brighton, Ontario.)

Differential Diagnosis

◆ The radiographic differential diagnosis of chondrocalcinosis should include the following:
  - Cation disease
    Hyperparathyroidism
    Hemochromatosis
    Wilson's disease
  - Cartilage degeneration
    Degenerating and neuropathic joint disease
    Acromegaly
    Diabetes
  - Crystal deposition disease
    Gout
    Ochronosis (homogentisic acid)

Pigmented Villonodular Synovitis

◆ A chronic, inflammatory process of the synovium that causes synovial proliferation
◆ Etiology unknown
◆ Causes a swollen joint that has lobular masses of synovium, which leads to pain and joint destruction
◆ Primarily affects young adults
◆ Usually involves fingers and toes
◆ Originates in synovium of tendon sheaths
◆ Small soft tissue tumor that erodes bone from the outside (Figs. 2-132, *A-C*)

Tumor

Benign bone neoplasms comprise a wide variety of radiographic findings. Unfortunately, they may be misdiagnosed as their more sinister malignant counterparts. Although it frequently evokes symptoms, benign bone disease should not be confused with other categories of bone lesions. Many benign bone conditions are discovered only incidentally during examinations for other painful conditions. Still other benign states may worsen to produce significant osseous or soft tissue masses, which may result in adjacent neurovascular compromise. Other noteworthy considerations include the potential for malignant degeneration of previously benign lesions. In such instances, case management may extend from simple, periodic monitoring of the disease to more radical forms of surgical intervention. Practitioners are advised to familiarize themselves with this broad variety of disorders and their potential clinical consequences.

BENIGN TUMORS OF BONE

Fibrous Cortical Defect (FCD)

◆ A focal benign bone lesion of cellular fibrous tissue that replaces cortex

Clinical Presentation

◆ Asymptomatic
◆ Usually discovered incidentally in children

Radiographic Features

◆ FCD is most commonly observed in the posteromedial aspect of the distal end of the femur (Fig. 3-1).
◆ The proximal tibia (Fig. 3-2, *A* and *B*), humerus (Fig. 3-3, *A* and *B*), fibula, and femur (Fig. 3-4) are other common locations.

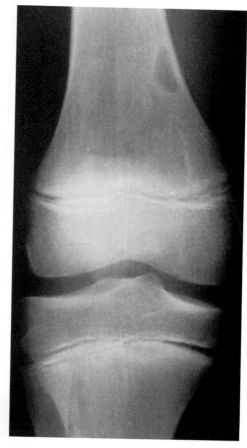

FIG. 3-1 A well-circumscribed, sclerotic, marginated fibrous cortical defect is noted in the posteromedial aspect of the distal femoral metaphysis. Note the immature skeleton.

A

B

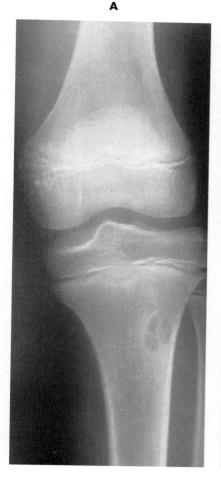
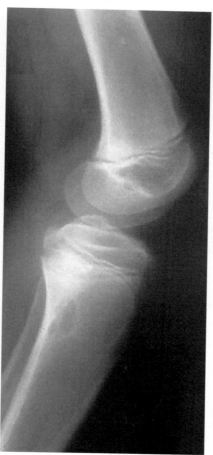

FIG. 3-2 A and **B,** A fibrous cortical defect is observed in the posterolateral portion of the proximal tibial metaphysis in this young patient.

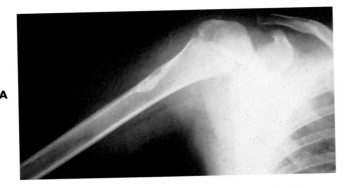

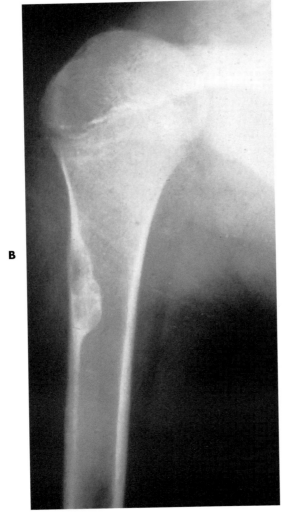

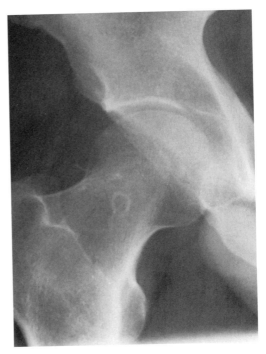

FIG. 3-4 The femoral neck represents another common site for the development of a fibrous cortical defect.

◆ The defect is metaphyseal (Fig. 3-5, *A* and *B*).
◆ It typically appears as a round, ovoid, or flame-shaped radiolucency.
◆ Its margins are well-defined with a thin zone of sclerosis (Fig. 3-6).

FIG. 3-3 **A** and **B,** A fibrous cortical defect is identified in the proximal lateral metadiaphyseal region of the humerus. Note the sharp zone of transition between the defect and the adjacent normal bone.

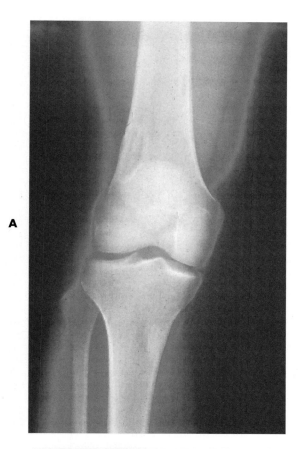

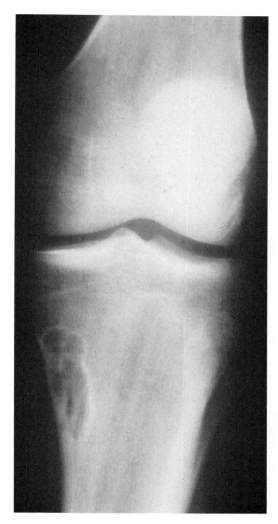

FIG. 3-6 The margin of a fibrous cortical defect is well-defined and bounded by a narrow zone of sclerosis.

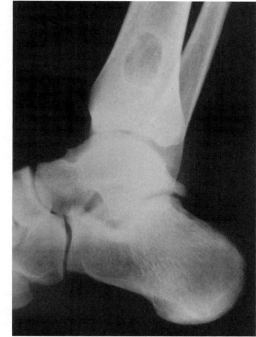

FIG. 3-5 A, The metaphysis is a favored location for occurrence of a fibrous cortical defect, as seen in this lateral distal metaphysis of the femur. **B,** A fibrous cortical defect is observed in the distal tibial metaphysis.

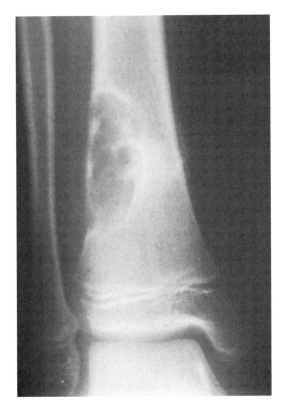

FIG. 3-7 A fibrous cortical defect averages 1 to 2 cm in length and generally parallels the long axis of the involved bone.

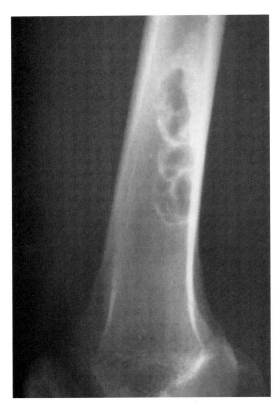

FIG. 3-8 A nonossifying fibroma may range from 2 to 7 cm in length.

- Its size averages from 1 to 2 cm, and the length of the lesion parallels the long axis of the bone (Fig. 3-7).

Nonossifying Fibroma (NOF)
- Not necessarily a true tumor, but may represent a fault in ossification

Clinical Presentation
- Usually discovered incidentally
- Asymptomatic
- Seen in children and young adults between the ages of 8 and 20 years
- Probably the most common bone lesion encountered
- Reportedly occurs in up to 20% of children

Radiographic Features
- It typically appears as a clearly defined area of radiolucency.

- It varies in size from 2 to 7 cm (Fig. 3-8).
- The lesion is ovoid and usually eccentrically located several centimeters shaftward from the metaphysis (Fig. 3-9).
- The defect may appear multilocular, with scalloped endosteal margins (Fig. 3-10).
- The endosteal margin of the tumor is characterized by a narrow, dense, sclerotic appearance (Fig. 3-11).
- It is found in or directly beneath a thin or expanded cortex.
- Long bones of the lower extremities are the most common sites of involvement, and the lesion exhibits a special affinity for the distal metaphysis of the femur (Fig. 3-12).
- The lesion may heal spontaneously with bone sclerosis, but some of the larger lesions may persist into adulthood.

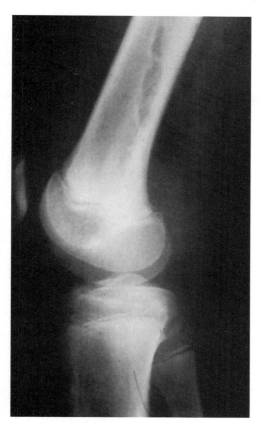

FIG. 3-9 The lesion is somewhat ovoid and usually eccentrically located several centimeters shaftward from the metaphysis.

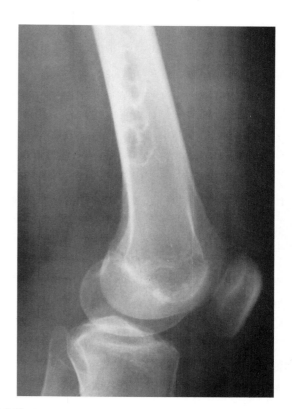

FIG. 3-10 A nonossifying fibroma may appear multilocular with scalloped endosteal margins.

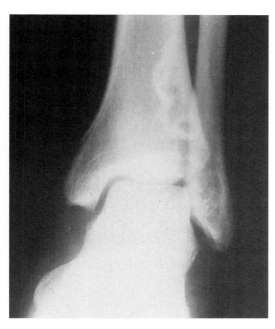

FIG. 3-11 The endosteal border is characterized by a narrow, dense, sclerotic appearance.

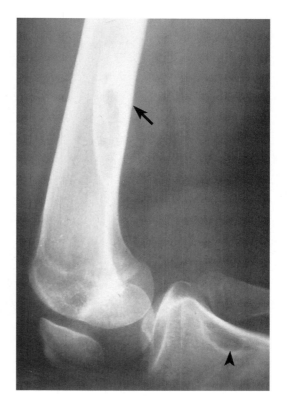

FIG. 3-12 In long bones of the lower extremities, nonossifying fibromas exhibit a special affinity for the distal femur (*arrow*). Note an additional nonossifying fibroma in the proximal tibia (*arrowhead*).

Osteoma

◆ Develops only in intramembranous bone

Clinical Presentation

◆ Most common sites of origin are the inner and outer tables of the skull, paranasal sinuses, and mandible.
◆ Patients are usually asymptomatic.
◆ Development occurs from the inner table of the skull and may produce symptoms of increased intracranial pressure.
◆ It often develops in the sinuses, most commonly frontal (Fig. 3-13) or ethmoid areas.
◆ Sinus involvement may interfere with nasal drainage.
◆ The lesion is seen in adults.
◆ It does not usually progress to a malignant course.

Radiographic Features

◆ Round, smooth, and homogenously radiopaque
◆ Lesions generally 2 cm in diameter or less

Osteoid Osteoma

◆ An osteoid osteoma is an osteoblastic lesion that contains a central nidus consisting of a mass of osteoid tissue.

◆ The nidus is usually less than 1 cm in diameter and surrounded by a zone of reactive sclerosis.
◆ The nidus may be intracortical (80%), intramedullary, or subperiosteal and is a source of pain.

Clinical Presentation

◆ The patient usually has a history of discretely localized, intermittent osseous pain that lasts several weeks or months and is worse at night, ameliorated by activity, and often relieved by the use of aspirin.
◆ In the case of spinal involvement, osteoid osteoma produces a painful, rigid scoliosis, with the lesion appearing on the concave aspect of the curve.
◆ The lesions are most frequently observed in the second and third decades of life, and males are affected twice as often as females.

Radiographic Features

◆ Although any bone may be involved, the tibia (Fig. 3-14) and femur (Fig. 3-15) are most commonly affected.
◆ Other common sites of involvement are the fibula, humerus, and vertebral arch (Fig. 3-16).

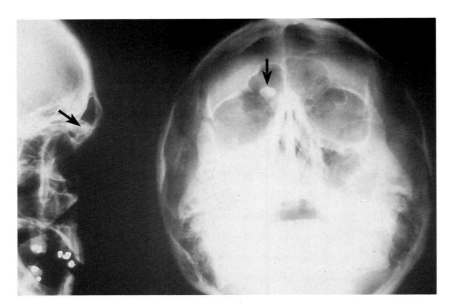

FIG. 3-13 An osteoma (*arrows*) most commonly develops in the frontal sinus.

TUMOR

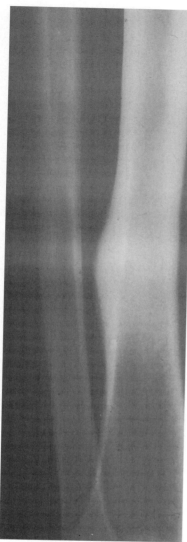

FIG. 3-14 The tibia is a common site for the development of an osteoid osteoma.

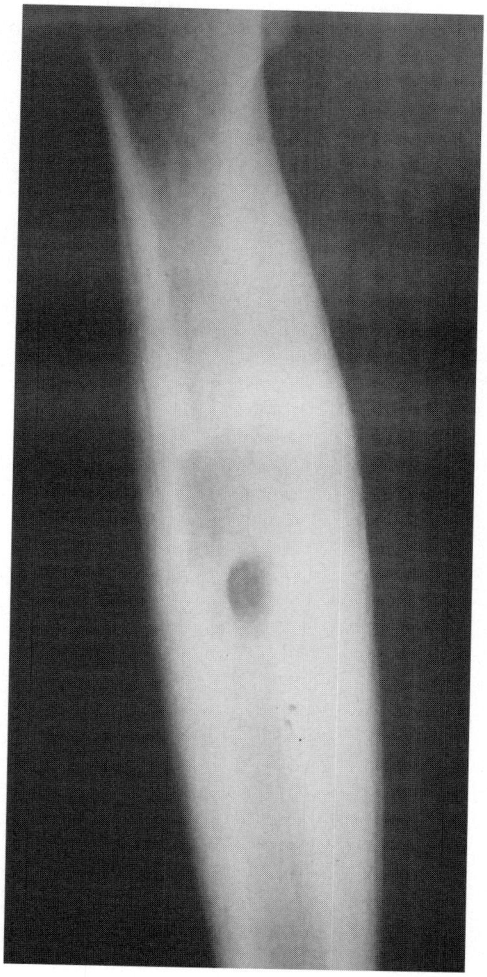

FIG. 3-15 The femur represents another frequent site for the development of an osteoid osteoma.

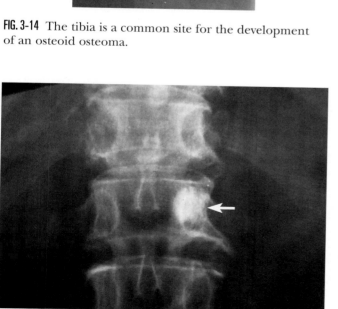

FIG. 3-16 An osteoid osteoma may develop in the neural arch, as seen in this lumbar pedicle (*arrow*).

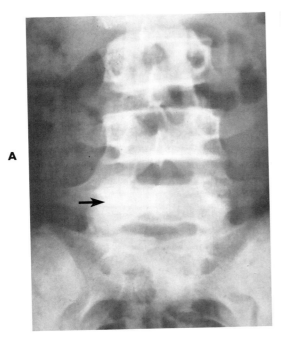

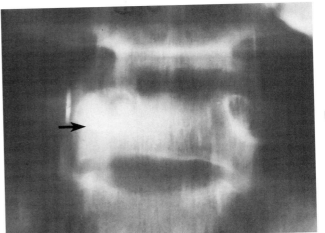

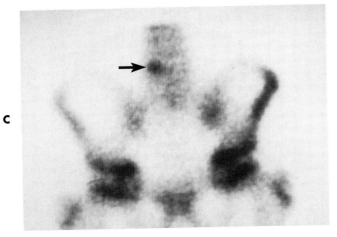

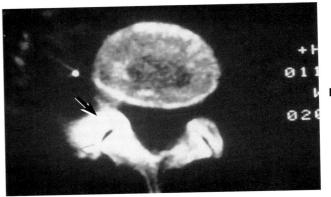

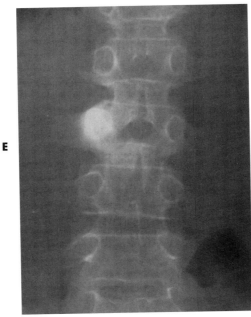

FIG. 3-17 **A,** The pedicle is a predilectory site for the development of an osteoid osteoma in the spine (*arrow*). **B,** A tomogram manifests the homogenous sclerosis associated with an osteoid osteoma, suggesting a "bright" pedicle (*arrow*). **C,** Increased radioisotopic uptake is noted in the presence of a pedicular osteoid osteoma (*arrow*). **D,** A computed axial tomographic scan exhibits the presence of an osteoid osteoma in the vertebral pedicle (*arrow*). **E,** Note the dense, homogenous sclerosis, representing the "bright" pedicle associated with osteoid osteoma of the neural arch.

- When arising in the spine, the pedicle is a predilectory site (Fig. 3-17, *A-D*) and frequently manifests as homogenously sclerotic ("bright") pedicle (Fig. 3-17, *E*).
- Other posterior elements that can be affected include the laminae (Fig. 3-18) and transverse processes.
- Its classical appearance is that of an intracortical, round, or oval area of radiolucency (Fig. 3-19).

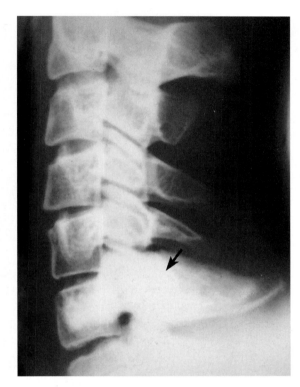

FIG. 3-18 The lamina of C7 manifests the presence of an osteoid osteoma (*arrow*).

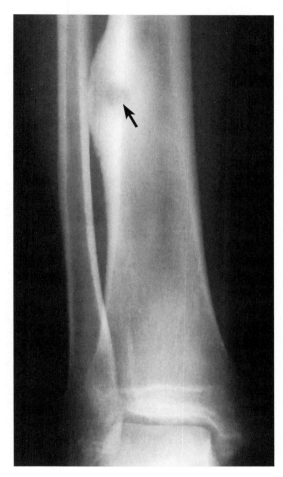

FIG. 3-19 A small intracortical round or oval area of radiolucency, the nidus, may be observed (*arrow*).

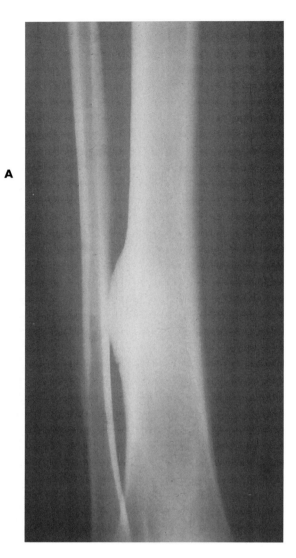

A

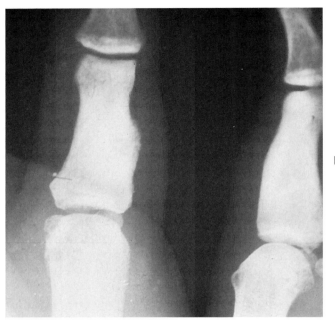

B

FIG. 3-20 A, The nidus may be radiolucent or entirely obscured by the surrounding sclerosis, as in this tibia. **B,** The nidus may be difficult to identify amidst the adjacent reactive sclerotic bone.

♦ The nidus may be entirely lucent or totally obscured by the surrounding sclerosis (Fig. 3-20, *A* and *B*).
♦ This condition must be differentiated from chronic osteomyelitis (Fig. 3-21).

Osteoblastoma

♦ A rare benign neoplasm consisting of osteoblasts and giant cells in a vascular connective tissue stroma

Clinical Presentation

♦ A palpable mass and moderate local tenderness may develop.
♦ With spinal involvement, neurologic deficits and even paraplegia may result.

♦ More males are affected than females.
♦ Peak age incidence is between 20 and 30 years.

Radiographic Features

♦ The spine, particularly the neural arch, is the most common site of involvement and accounts for approximately 50% of the cases (Fig. 3-22).
♦ Long bones and tubular bones of the hands are frequent sites of involvement.
♦ The vertebral body may also, on occasion, be affected.
♦ The tumor may appear as (1) an expansile, amorphous lesion; (2) a densely calcified mass; or (3) a combination of these presentations (Fig. 3-23).

Differential Diagnosis

♦ Lesions to be considered are osteoid osteoma and aneurysmal bone cysts.

Osteochondroma

♦ An osseous projection with a cartilaginous cap arising from the host bone cortex
♦ The most common benign tumor involving the skeleton
♦ Develops slowly during childhood and adolescence

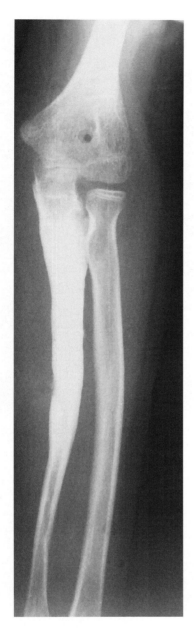

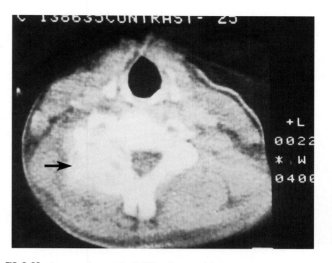

FIG. 3-22 Approximately 50% of osteoblastomas are observed in the neural arch (*arrow*).

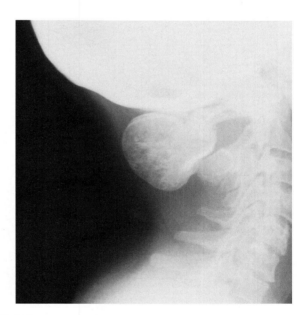

FIG. 3-21 Osteoid osteoma may be difficult to differentiate from this example of chronic osteomyelitis.

FIG. 3-23 An osteoblastoma may present as an expansile mass, containing amorphous or dense calcification, or a combination of both, as observed in this patient's posterior arch of atlas.

- Cortex continuous with the cortex of the host bone, and medullary portion continuous with the central spongiosa
- Cessation of tumor development with skeletal maturity

Clinical Presentation
- Osteochondromas may be solitary or multiple.

- They affect both genders equally.
- The most frequent complaint is a painless mass.
- The pressure exerted by the tumor on contiguous vascular or neurologic elements may produce symptoms, or the lesion may be entirely asymptomatic.
- Symptoms may follow mild trauma or fracture of the lesion.

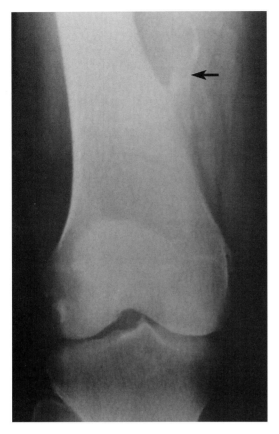

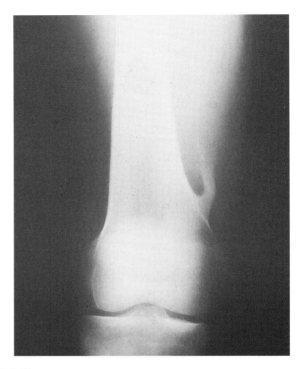

FIG. 3-24 A pedunculated osteochondroma (*arrow*) is seen arising from the medial metaphyseal surface of the femur.

FIG. 3-25 The most frequent site of involvement is the knee.

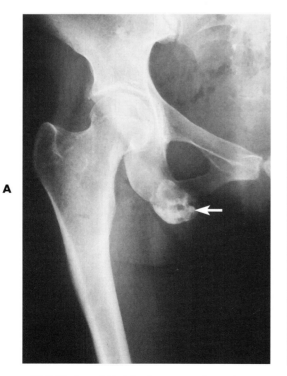

A

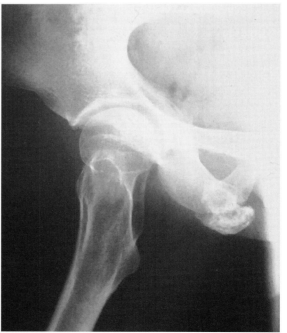

B

FIG. 3-26 A and **B,** Flat bones such as the pelvis may be affected by an osteochondroma. Note the ischial exostosis (*arrow*).

Radiographic Features

♦ Osteochondromas are most often found in tubular bones near the metaphysis (Fig. 3-24).

♦ The most common site of involvement is the knee (Fig. 3-25).

♦ Flat bones such as the pelvis (Fig. 3-26, *A* and *B*) and scapula (Fig. 3-27) may also be affected, especially after radiotherapy.

♦ Two varieties are distinguished: pedunculated and sessile.

PEDUNCULATED

♦ This variety is characterized by a long, narrow stalk (peduncle) with a cartilaginous cap (Fig. 3-28).

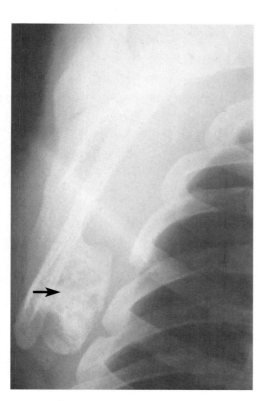

FIG. 3-27 The scapula may be another flat bone affected by an osteochondroma (*arrow*).

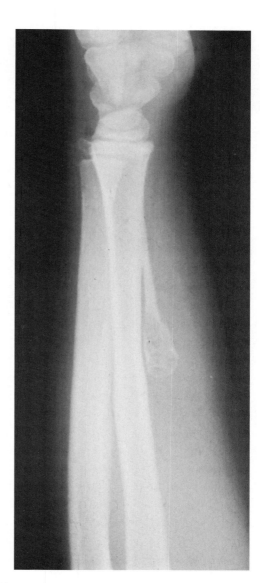

FIG. 3-28 Note the narrow osseous stalk and typical cartilaginous cap.

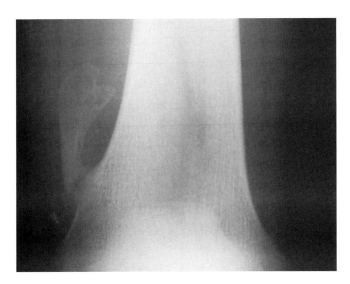

FIG. 3-29 The characteristic "coat-hanger" exostosis is exhibited in this osteochondroma of the distal femur.

- The direction of the peduncle is characteristically away from the adjacent joint because of muscle pull—hence, the term *coat-hanger exostosis* (Fig. 3-29).
- Pedunculated osteochondromas vary in size, extending to 8 cm in length.
- The cartilaginous cap may appear flocculent and is always well-defined, thus giving rise to the term *cauliflower exostosis* (Figs. 3-30 and 3-31).
- Irregular or streaky calcification with an ill-defined margin may suggest malignant degeneration into chondrosarcoma.

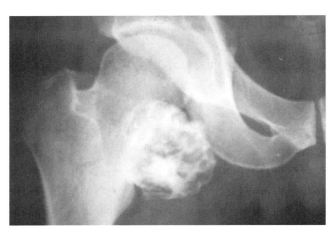

FIG. 3-31 Osteochondroma demonstrating a "cauliflower" exostosis.

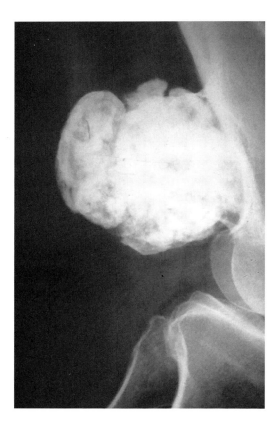

FIG. 3-30 A typical "cauliflower" exostosis is visualized in this osteochondroma.

SESSILE

- This variety is characterized by a broad-based lesion that forms a local widening or "bump" on the cortex (Fig. 3-32).
- Although more commonly seen in the pelvis, it is occasionally noted in long bones or the costal elements (Fig. 3-33, *A* and *B*).
- It may be extremely large and of an extremely irregular shape.
- The clinical importance of the tumor depends on the cartilage cap, which may present a small risk of malignant transformation to chondrosarcoma; the risk is probably less than 1% in solitary lesions but is significantly higher (20%) in multiple osteochondromatosis (hereditary multiple exostosis, diaphyseal aclasis).
- The patient with hereditary multiple exostosis may exhibit pedunculated and sessile varieties simultaneously (Fig. 3-34, *A-H*).

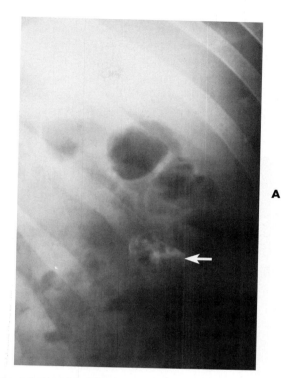

A

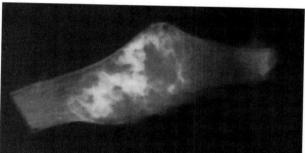

B

FIG. 3-33 A, Osteochondroma involving a rib (*arrow*). **B,** Resected osteochondroma.

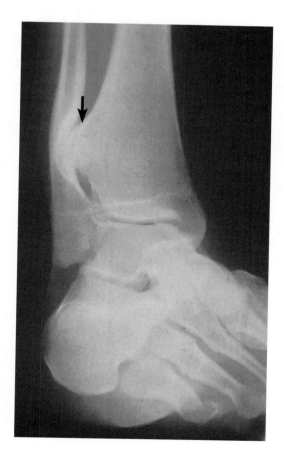

FIG. 3-32 A widening, or bump, on the cortex may be typical of the sessile variety of osteochondroma (*arrow*). Note the pressure erosion of the adjacent distal fibula by the expanding lesion.

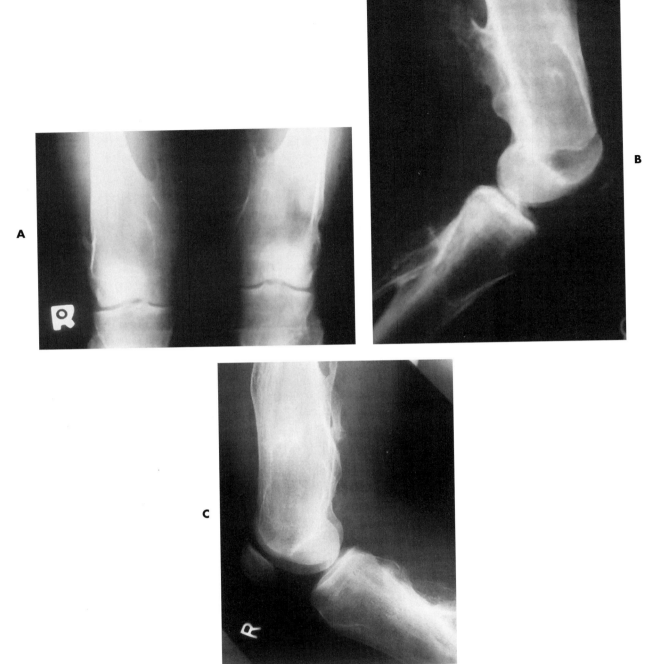

FIG. 3-34 A, An example of pedunculated and sessile varieties of osteochondromata, associated with hereditary multiple exostosis, seen in this anteroposterior radiograph of the knees. **B** and **C,** Lateral views of knees manifesting hereditary multiple exostosis. **D** and **E,** Anteroposterior and lateral views of a humerus demonstrating the sessile osteochondromata of this patient with hereditary multiple exostosis. **F,** Hereditary multiple exostosis as manifested in the proximal humerus and coracoid process of the scapula. **G,** An increase in radionuclide uptake (*arrow*) is seen in the proximal humerus of a patient with hereditary multiple exostosis. **H,** A posteroanterior bone scan reveals increased uptake caused by an osteochondroma in the proximal humerus (*arrow*).

D

E

F

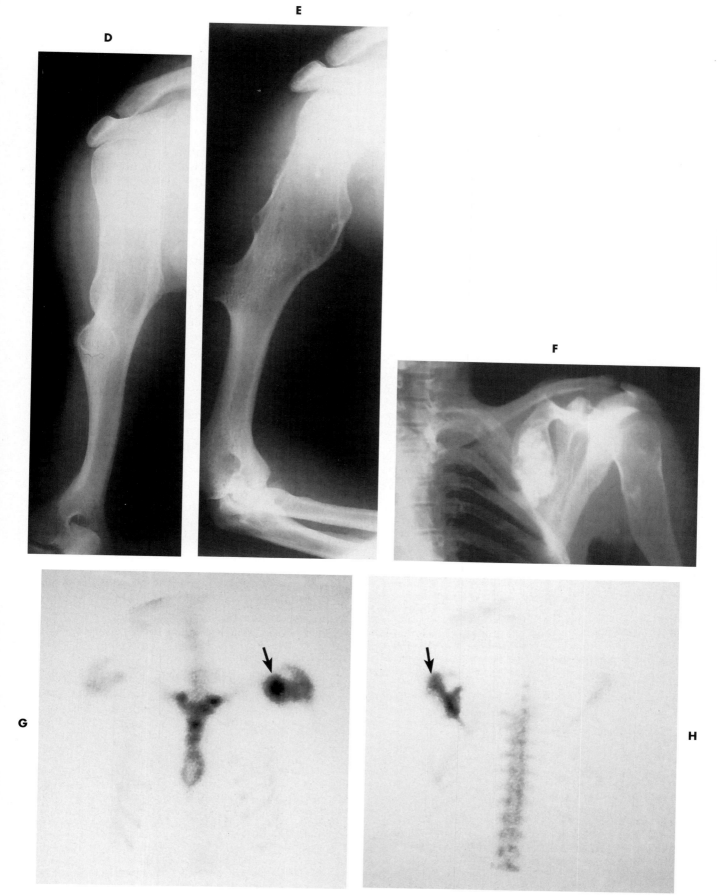

G

H

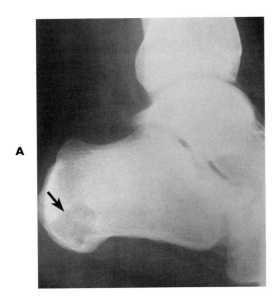

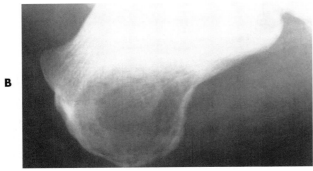

FIG. 3-35 A, Chondroblastoma of the posterior calcaneus (*arrow*). **B,** Another patient with a calcaneal chondroblastoma.

Chondroblastoma

- Arises only in the epiphyses

Clinical Presentation

- Features low-grade pain that is referred to a joint
- Characterized by tenderness and limitation of motion
- Possible weakness, numbness, and local atrophy
- Peak age incidence between 10 and 25 years
- A male-female preponderance of 2:1

Radiographic Features

- Originates in the physeal plate and extends into the epiphysis
- Usually a well-demarcated, spheroid, or ovoid radiolucent area
- May be eccentrically located in an epiphysis
- Ranges in size from 3 to 19 cm
- Possible sites of involvement: upper humerus, upper and lower femur, and tibia
- Short bones sometimes involved (Fig. 3-35, *A* and *B*)

Hemangioma

- This lesion is considered as a benign neoplasm or congenital malformation.
- It may be cavernous, capillary, or venous.

Clinical Presentation

- Patients are asymptomatic.
- Women are affected twice as frequently as men.
- It arises in the fourth or fifth decades.
- Lesions are usually single.
- The two most common sites of involvement are the vertebral bodies and the skull, particularly the facial bones.
- In the spine the thoracic and lumbar vertebral bodies are most commonly affected.
- Long bone occurrence has been reported.

Radiographic Features

- The typical vertebral body presentation is that of a coarsened, accentuated, vertically striped trabecular orientation, which results in a "corduroy cloth" appearance (Fig. 3-36, *A-D*).

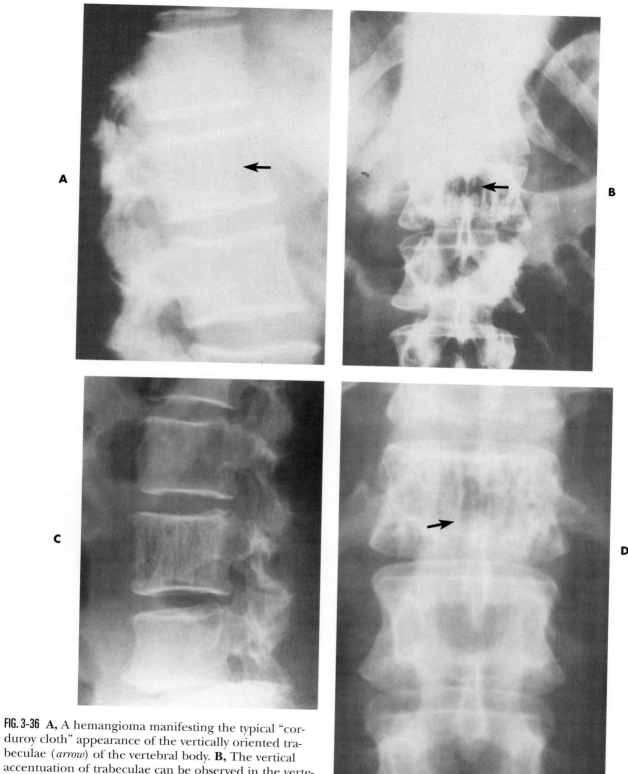

FIG. 3-36 A, A hemangioma manifesting the typical "corduroy cloth" appearance of the vertically oriented trabeculae (*arrow*) of the vertebral body. **B,** The vertical accentuation of trabeculae can be observed in the vertebral body (*arrow*). **C,** Hemangioma usually involves a solitary vertebral body (in this case, L4). **D,** A vertically striped vertebral body is identified. Note the prominent osseous trabecula (*arrow*).

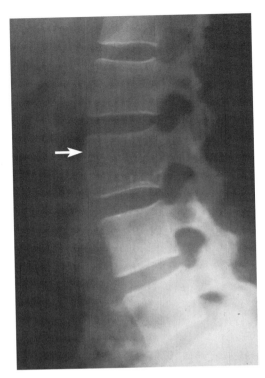

FIG. 3-37 A mild degree of vertebral body expansion (*arrow*) may be associated with hemangioma.

- Mild vertebral body expansion may be associated (Fig. 3-37).
- Cortical margins remain intact, although compression fractures may occur (Fig. 3-38, *A-C*).
- Occasionally, these fractures are complicated by spinal cord compression, with resultant neurologic symptoms and signs.
- In the mandible and skull the lesion is radiolucent, slightly expansile, and well-defined, with a radiating trabecular pattern of 1 to 7 cm in diameter that resembles a "wagon wheel."
- Long bone involvement, which is infrequent, may create a coarse "honeycomb" pattern (Fig. 3-39).

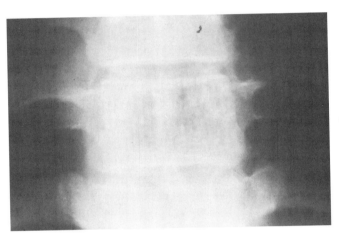

A

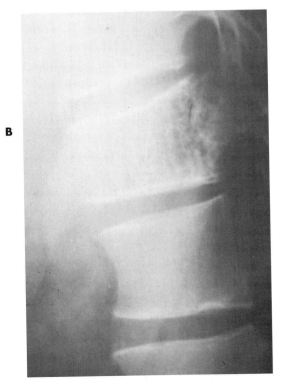

B

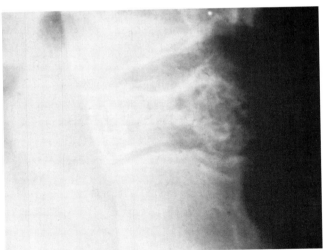

C

FIG. 3-38 **A,** The vertebral body cortex usually remains intact. **B,** A compression fracture may occur in a vertebral body affected by a hemangioma. **C,** A severe compression fracture of the vertebra may induce spinal cord compression.

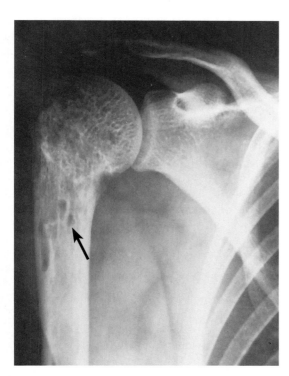

FIG. 3-39　Hemangioma involving a long bone may resemble a coarse "honeycomb" trabecular appearance (*arrow*), as observed here in the humeral metadiaphysis.

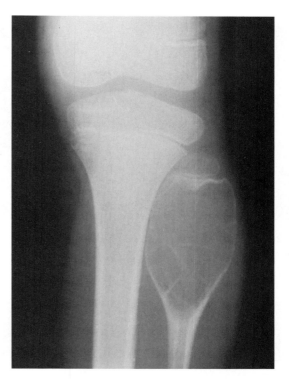

FIG. 3-40　Expansive bone destruction is observed in the aneurysmal bone cyst of the proximal fibular metaphysis.

Aneurysmal Bone Cyst (ABC)

- Unknown etiology
- Characterized by a ballooned cortical appearance; may arise secondary to hemorrhage into cancellous bone

Clinical Presentation

- The age distribution ranges from children to adults under the age of 30.
- Two females are affected for every male.
- Mild pain in the affected site may last for several months.
- A localized, tender, swollen area may also be present.
- The most common sites of involvement are the long bones, most often the femur and tibia.
- Aneurysmal bone cysts may be found at any spinal level and in any portion of a vertebra, including the body, posterior arch, and various processes.

Radiographic Features

- An area of expansive bone destruction is typical (Fig. 3-40).
- The overlying cortex remains sharply delineated by a thin, expanded shell (Fig. 3-41).

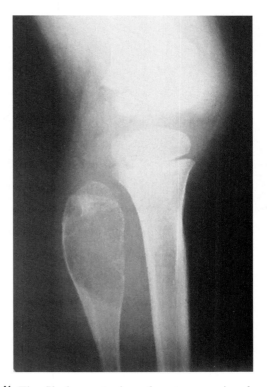

FIG. 3-41　The fibular metaphyseal cortex remains sharply delineated as a thin, expanded, intact shell.

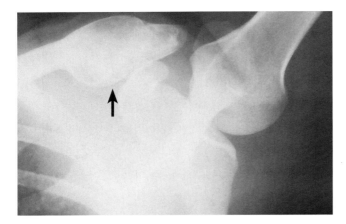

FIG. 3-42 An aneurysmal bone cyst is observed involving the distal end of the clavicle (*arrow*).

- In tubular long bones the lesion is eccentric and usually metaphyseal, but it may extend into the epiphysis after fusion of the secondary ossification centers (Fig. 3-42).
- Light trabeculation may be seen in the lesion (Fig. 3-43).
- With vertebral involvement the ABC has an expansile, trabeculated appearance and may attain a large size (Fig. 3-44).

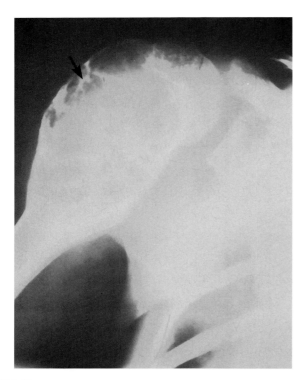

FIG. 3-43 Light trabeculations (*arrow*) may be observed traversing the lesion.

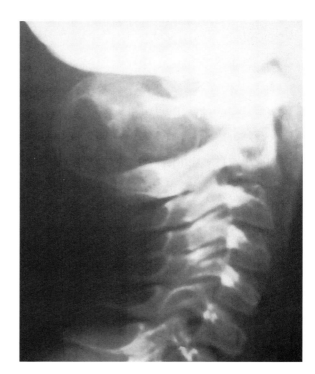

FIG. 3-44 Neural arch lesions may appear expansile and trabeculated, possibly attaining a large size, as noted in the posterior tubercle of this atlas.

Unicameral Bone Cyst (UBC): Solitary Bone Cyst, Simple Bone Cyst

- A true fluid cyst lined by fibrous and vascular tissues
- Etiology unknown
- Migration farther into the diaphysis as skeletal growth continues

Clinical Presentation

- More common in males than females
- In 80% of cases, age incidence between 3 and 14 years
- Often asymptomatic and discovered incidentally
- More than half the cases present following a pathologic fracture

Radiographic Features

- These cysts occur most often in the proximal metaphysis (Figs. 3-45 and 3-46).

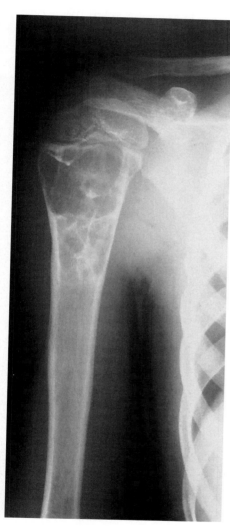

FIG. 3-45 Unicameral bone cysts frequently involve a proximal metaphyseal region.

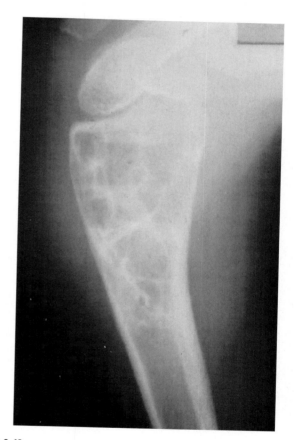

FIG. 3-46 The proximal humeral metaphysis of this skeletally immature patient exhibits a unicameral bone cyst.

TUMOR

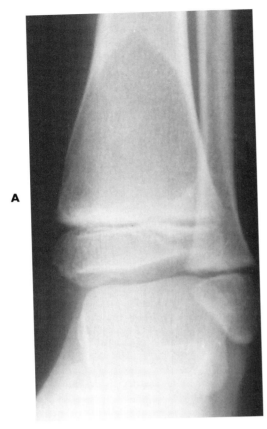

A

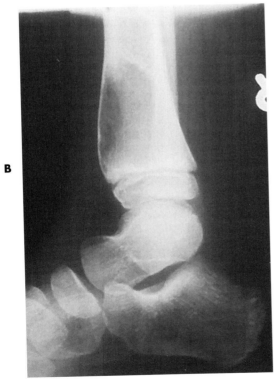

B

◆ Its typical appearance is that of a central radiolucent lesion that is broader at the metaphyseal end and narrower at the diaphyseal end (Figs. 3-47, *A* and *B*).
◆ The long axis of the lesion exceeds its diameter (Fig. 3-48).
◆ The lesion never crosses the physeal plate (Figs. 3-49, *A* and *B*; 3-50, *A* and *B*).
◆ The UBC is well-demarcated from normal bone.

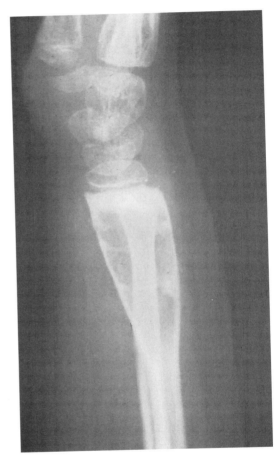

FIG. 3-48 The long axis of the lesion exceeds its diameter.

FIG. 3-47 **A** and **B,** Note the central radiolucent lesion, which is broader at the metaphyseal end and narrower at the diaphyseal end.

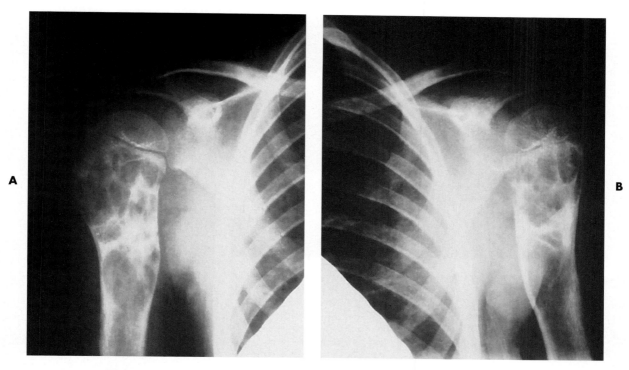

FIG. 3-49 **A** and **B,** A unicameral bone cyst never crosses the epiphyseal plate.

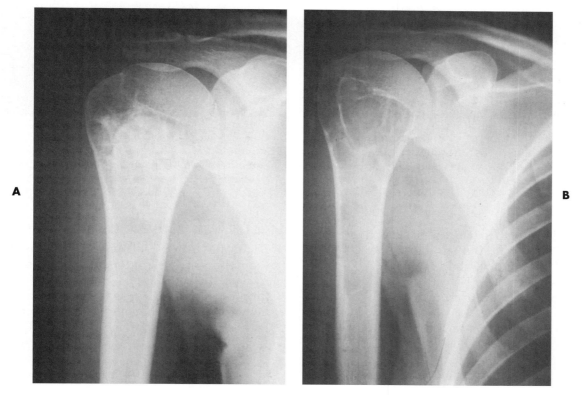

FIG. 3-50 **A** and **B,** The lesion is limited to the metaphyseal portion of the bone and does not traverse the epiphyseal plate.

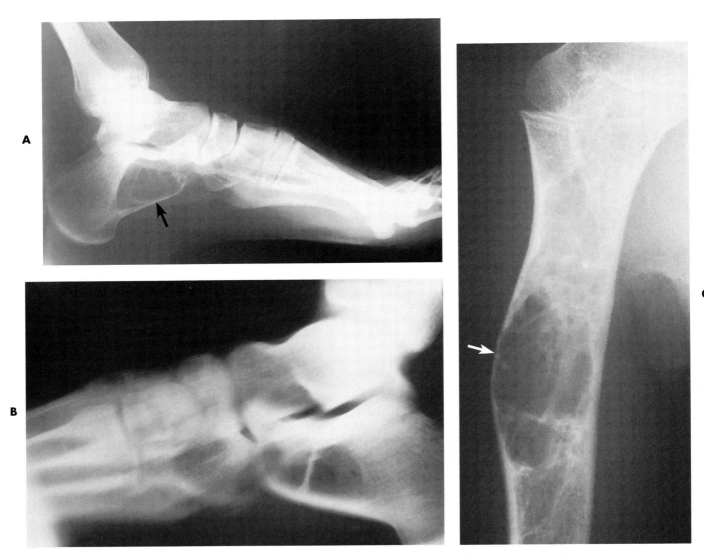

FIG. 3-51 A, The overlying cortex exhibits marked thinning (*arrow*). **B,** A tomogram of a unicameral bone cyst of the anterior calcaneus revealing a thin but intact overlying cortex. **C,** The overlying cortex may be slightly expanded (*arrow*), as seen in this young patient's humerus.

- The overlying cortex, which is greatly thinned (Fig. 3-51, *A* and *B*), is often slightly expanded (Fig. 3-51, *C*) but never broken.
- No periosteal reaction is evident unless a pathologic fracture has occurred (Figs. 3-52, 3-53, and 3-54).
- Fractures may demonstrate the "fallen-fragment sign," which is produced by the osseous fragment descending to the most dependent portion of the fluid-filled cyst, with the patient being radiographed in the upright posture.
- This lesion rarely demonstrates internal calcification.

Giant Cell Tumor (GCT): Osteoclastoma

- Highly vascular lesion consisting of spindle-shaped stromal cells interspersed among multinucleated giant cells
- Proportion of stroma cells to giant cells an indication of the malignant nature of the tumor, which represents 5% of all primary bone neoplasms
- Incidence of malignant degeneration estimated to be at 20%

Clinical Presentation

- Occurs mainly in adults who are 20 to 40 years of age

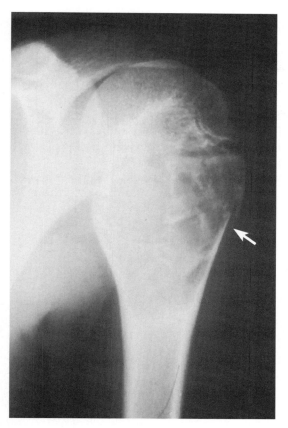

FIG. 3-52 Note the cortical disruption (*arrow*) caused by pathologic fracture in this unicameral bone cyst of the proximal humerus.

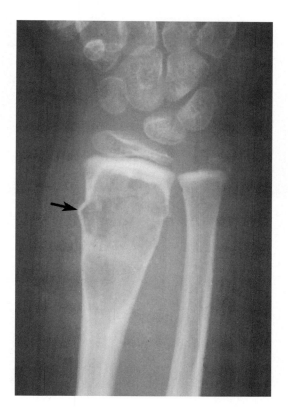

FIG. 3-53 A pathologic fracture (*arrow*) traverses this unicameral bone cyst of the distal radius and demonstrates cortical buckling.

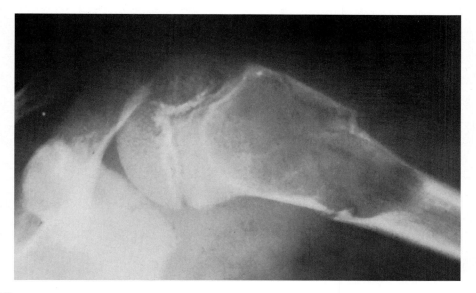

FIG. 3-54 Note the pathologic fracture through this unicameral bone cyst of the proximal humeral metadiaphysis in this young patient. Lateral cortical buckling is also observed.

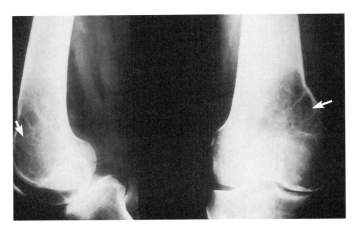

FIG. 3-55 A giant cell tumor is classically located in the distal femur (*arrows*).

- Affects both genders equally
- Characterized by a chronic, intermittent, dull pain, particularly at night
- Pain worsens with activity
- Possibly accompanied by a tender, palpable mass

Radiographic Features

- Tends to involve the long bones, with the classic locations being the distal femur (Figs. 3-55 and 3-56) and proximal tibia (Fig. 3-57)
- May also be seen in the distal end of the radius (Figs. 3-58; 3-59; 3-60, *A* and *B*) and the proximal humerus and radius (Fig. 3-61)

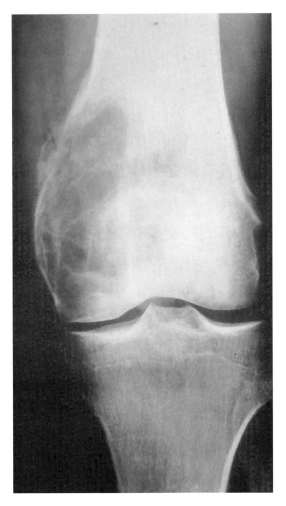

FIG. 3-56 Note the large giant cell tumor in the medial femoral condyle.

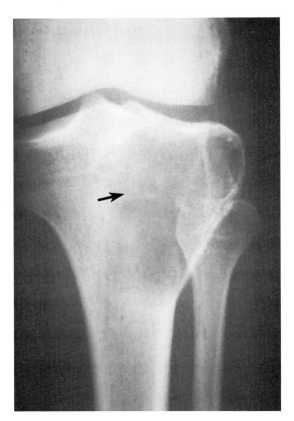

FIG. 3-57 A giant cell tumor is seen in the proximal tibia (*arrow*).

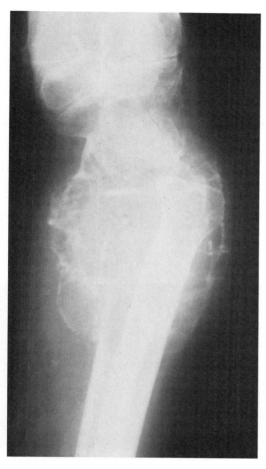

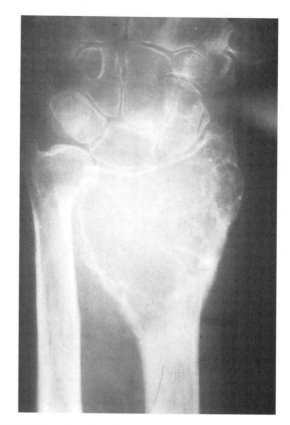

FIG. 3-58 A giant cell tumor is noted in the distal radius. Observe the marked cortical thinning and expansion.

FIG. 3-59 The distal radius demonstrates a giant cell tumor.

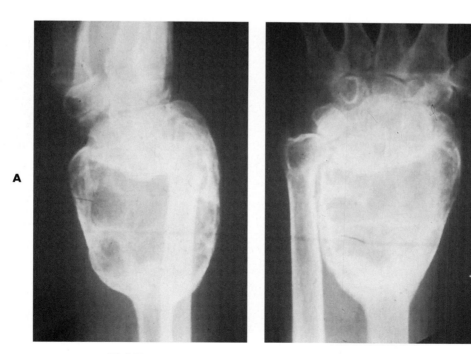

A

B

FIG. 3-60 **A** and **B,** Giant cell tumor of the distal radius.

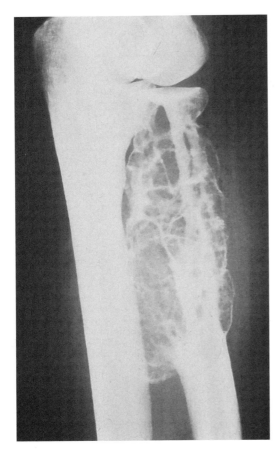

FIG. 3-61 A giant cell tumor of the proximal radius demonstrating the characteristic "soap bubble" appearance.

- GCT is extremely rare in the spine, except for the sacrum (Fig. 3-62)
- Sacral tumors often present with neurologic disturbances
- May be complicated by pathologic fracture (Fig. 3-63)
- Appears as an expansile, radiolucent lesion that is virtually always subarticular (Fig. 3-64)
- Closed physeal plate
- Lesion usually round, frequently eccentric, and possibly involving the entire diameter of the terminal end of the bone (Fig. 3-65)
- Thin and expanded cortex that remains well-defined

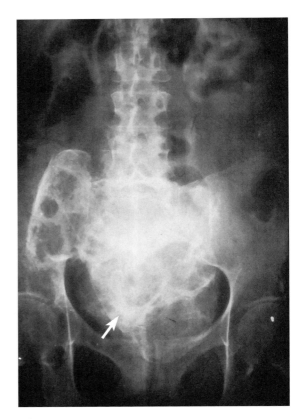

FIG. 3-62 Rare sacral giant cell tumor (*arrow*).

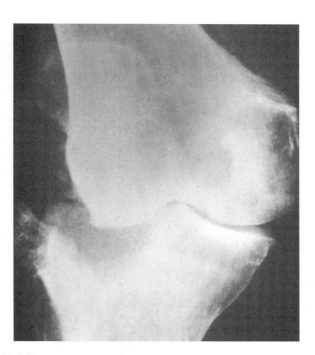

FIG. 3-63 Pathologic fractures may be a complication of the giant cell tumor.

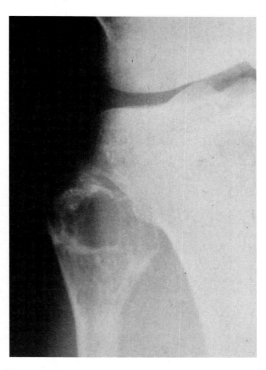

FIG. 3-64 Giant cell tumors appear expansile and radiolucent and are always subarticular in location.

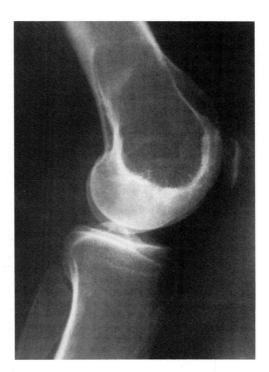

FIG. 3-65 Lesions may appear round and eccentric, involving the entire diameter of the terminal end of the bone.

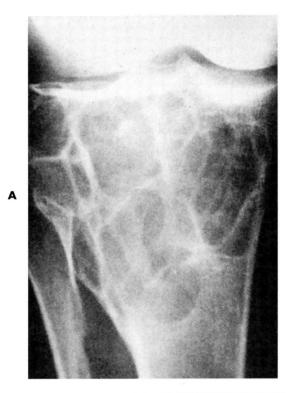

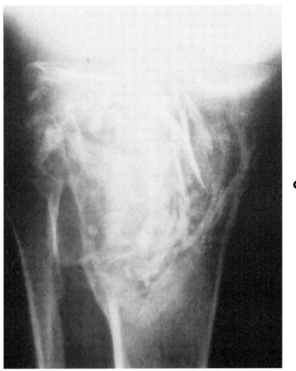

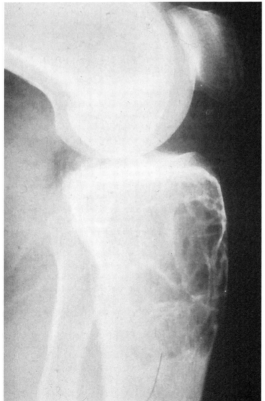

FIG. 3-66 A-C, Septations in the lesion may render a "soap-bubble" appearance.

- Trabecular septations in a lesion common, rendering a "soap-bubble" appearance (Fig. 3-66, *A-C*)

MALIGNANT VARIETY

- Determining whether a GCT is benign or malignant is not possible based on radiographic evidence alone.
- Lesions with intact outer margins and sharp inner surfaces suggest a more favorable prognosis.
- Those with indistinct inner margins or outer cortical interruptions denote more aggressive tendencies (Figs. 3-67, 3-68, 3-69, and 3-70).
- Distal radial lesions are more likely to become malignant (Fig. 3-71).

Enchondroma (Central Chondroma)

- Benign, cartilaginous tumor of bone, characteristically located in the medullary canal
- Varying degrees of calcification possible in the lesion

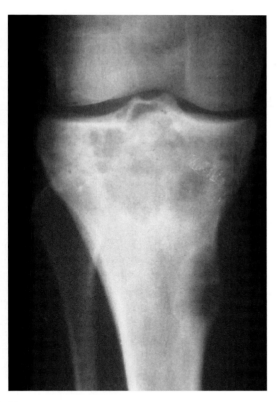

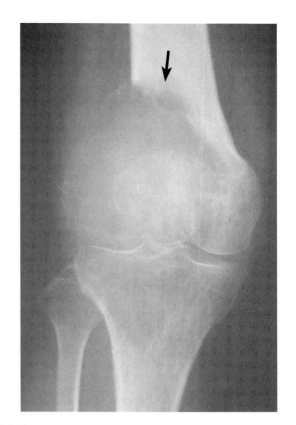

FIG. 3-67 Giant cell tumors manifesting indistinct inner margins or outer cortical interruptions suggest more aggressive behavior.

FIG. 3-68 Note the wide zone of transition between the lesion and adjacent normal bone (*arrow*).

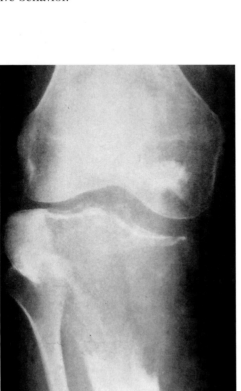

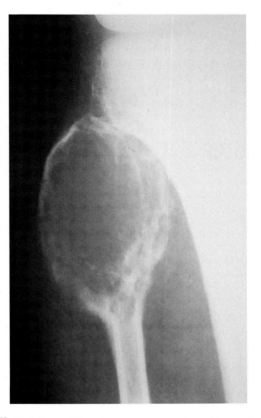

FIG. 3-69 Involvement of the epiphyseal end of the bone and indistinct margination of the lesion suggest an aggressive nature. Note the complete destruction of the cortex of the proximal medial tibia.

FIG. 3-70 Epiphyseal involvement suggests a diagnosis of giant cell tumor in this fibular head.

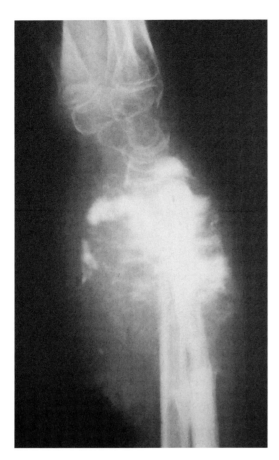

FIG. 3-71 Distal radial involvement has a higher tendency to result in malignant degeneration, as depicted in this radiograph. Observe the massive soft tissue extension of the tumor.

Clinical Presentation

- Occurs between the second and fifth decades of life
- No apparent gender predilection
- Fusiform, painless swelling of one or more digits when lesions occur in the hands (especially when lesions are multiple)
- Represents the most common benign tumor of the hands, comprising 35% to 50% of cases
- Lesion asymptomatic unless a pathologic fracture occurs

Radiographic Features

- May be solitary (Fig. 3-72) or multiple (Ollier's disease) (Fig. 3-73); central in location
- Appears to favor the small tubular bones of the hands (Fig. 3-74, *A* and *B*) and, less commonly, the feet (Fig. 3-75, *A* and *B*)

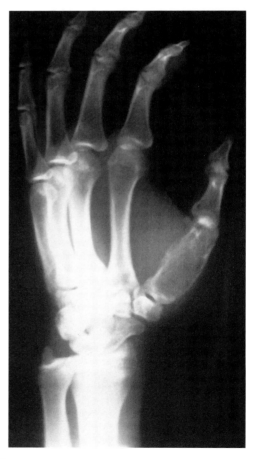

FIG. 3-72 A solitary enchondroma involving the first metacarpal is noted.

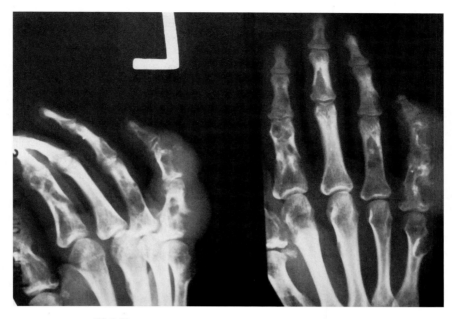

FIG. 3-73 Ollier's disease: multiple enchondromas.

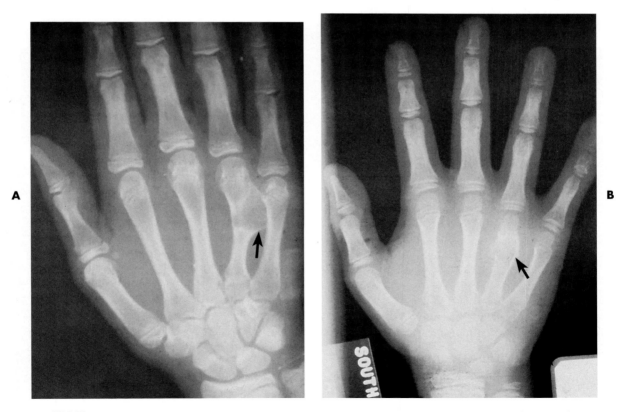

FIG. 3-74 A and **B,** Enchondromas favor the small tubular bones, particularly of the hands (*arrows*).

- Proximal phalanges, metacarpals, and middle and distal phalanges affected with decreasing frequency
- Pathologic fracture possible (Fig. 3-76)
- Rarely affects thumb
- May affect any bone preformed by cartilage
- Lesions found in the vertebrae, skull, and patellae uncommonly
- Malignant transformation into chondrosarcoma more frequently associated with those lesions discovered in the shoulder and pelvic girdles
- Is metaphyseal and centralized in the medullary canal
- Typically oval or round and lucent, producing varying degrees of cortical expansion
- Remains well-demarcated, with no soft tissue or periosteal involvement
- Invariable development of internal necrosis, which produces varying degrees of "spotty" or "speckled" calcification in the matrix of the lesion; classically characterizes the identity of the enchondroma, with the exception of the phalanges
- In long bones, "spotty" internal calcification often observed
- Ollier's disease not hereditary; does not demonstrate an increased rate of malignant degeneration (Fig. 3-77)

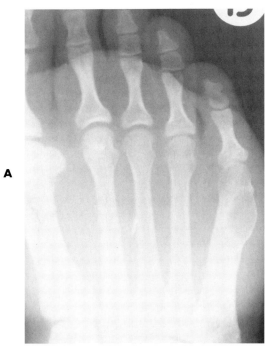

A

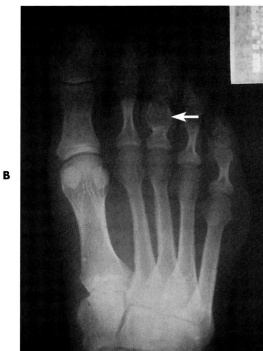

B

FIG. 3-75 A and **B,** Less commonly, enchondromas may be present in the small tubular bones of the feet (*arrow*).

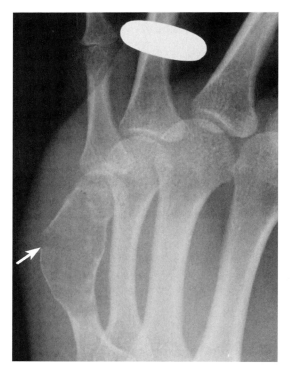

FIG. 3-76 Enchondromas may manifest pathologic fractures, as observed in this fifth metacarpal (*arrow*).

- Presence of multiple enchondromata associated with soft tissue hemangiomas known as *Maffucci's syndrome* (Fig. 3-78)

Bone Island (Enostoma)

- Characterized by a discrete sclerotic focus of compact lamellar bone located in normal spongiosa
- Incidental finding
- Common in the ischium, ilium, sacrum, and proximal femur
- May be found in the humerus, vertebra, talus, scaphoid, and ribs
- Skull only location in which bone islands do not occur

Clinical Presentation

- Found at any age but far more common in adults
- Asymptomatic
- May remain unchanged in size over many years
- Not clinically significant

Radiographic Features

- They are intramedullary, ovoid, round, or oblong radiopaque densities that are aligned with the long axis of stress vectors in the trabecular architecture (Fig. 3-79).

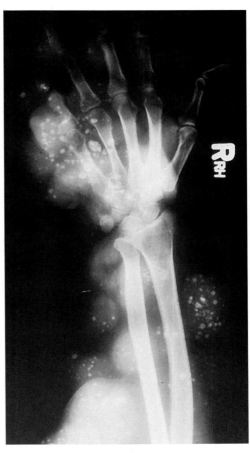

FIG. 3-78 The presence of multiple enchondromas associated with soft tissue hemangiomas is known as *Maffucci's syndrome.*

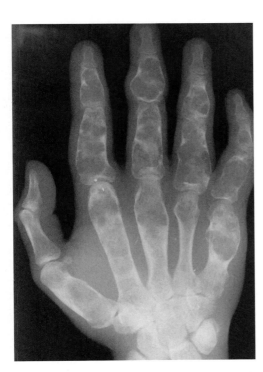

FIG. 3-77 Ollier's disease is not hereditary. Although dramatic in appearance, it does not possess an increased rate of malignant degeneration.

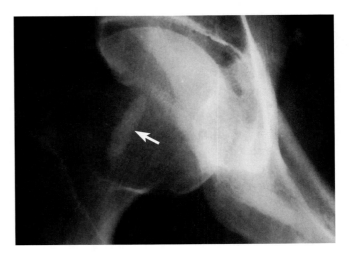

FIG. 3-79 Bone islands usually align with the stress vectors in trabecular bone (*arrow*).

- Margins are sharply demarcated and may have thornlike radiating spicules.
- The majority are seen in the femoral neck and intertrochanteric ridge.

MALIGNANT TUMORS OF BONE

In contrast to benign neoplasms, malignant lesions are frequently characterized by pain that is moderate to severe. Soft tissue involvement is common. A periosteal reaction may be characterized by the presence of laminations, a "sunburst appearance," or a Codman's triangle pattern. Metastasis to organs and soft tissue structures is not uncommon.

Fortunately, primary malignant neoplastic bone disease is seen somewhat less prevalently in general practice. However, the gravity and disclosure of these conditions is nonetheless important because management of these pathologies frequently requires a radical approach. All practitioners should therefore be sensitive to the potential presence of these diseases. Examples of primary malignant neoplastic bone disease can be found in the following pages.

Differentiation of Malignant Versus Benign Bone Tumors

- The following three features of the lesion are examined:
  - Cortical destruction
  - Periostitis
  - Zone of transition
- Only the zone of transition is accurate to a rate of 90% or greater.

CORTICAL DESTRUCTION

- The appearance can be misleading.
- Benign processes such as infection can produce extensive cortical destruction and mimic a malignancy.
- ABCs also cause extreme thinning of the cortex, sometimes rendering the cortex radiographically undetectable.

PERIOSTITIS

- Periosteal response occurs in a nonspecific manner when the periosteum (the osteoblastic inner cambium layer) is irritated.
- Irritation can be the result of a malignant tumor, infection, or trauma. (Callus formation in a fracture is the most benign form of periosteal reaction.)
- Primary malignant bone tumors produce a periosteal reaction that is high-grade and acute; hence the periosteum does not have time to consolidate, resulting in a laminated "onion-skin," amorphous, or "sunburst" appearance.

ZONE OF TRANSITION

- The zone of transition is the most reliable indicator in determining benign versus malignant lesions.
- The *zone of transition* is defined as the interface between the lesion and adjacent normal bone.
- The zone of transition is usually easier to characterize than the periostitis. In addition, it is always present to evaluate, whereas many lesions (benign or malignant) produce no periostitis.

Narrow Zone of Transition
- It is so well-defined that it can be traced with a fine-point pen.
- If a lesion possesses a thin sclerotic border, it is an example of a narrow zone of transition and is benign.

Wide Zone of Transition
- A wide zone of transition is an imperceptible merging of normal and abnormal bone.
- If a lesion has a wide (long) zone of transition, it is considered aggressive but not necessarily malignant (i.e., infection).
- Lesions with a wide zone of transition tend to display a moth-eaten or permeative pattern of destruction.
- These lesions typically include round cell tumors such as multiple myeloma, Ewing's sarcoma, reticulum cell sarcoma, and metastasis.
- Infection can produce a similar appearance.

Differentiating Types of Tumors

- Differentiation is facilitated by the fact that most malignant diseases adhere to somewhat strict age groups and bone location (Table 3-1).

Primary Malignant Neoplasia

OSTEOSARCOMA (OSTEOGENIC SARCOMA)

- It is the second most common primary malignant tumor of bone (twice as common as chondrosarcoma and three times as common as Ewing's sarcoma).
- It represents 20% of all primary bone malignancies.
- It is characterized by neoplastic, osteoblastic cellular production of osteoid and bone.
- It has a male-predominance ratio of 2:1.
- Approximately 75% of cases occur between the ages of 10 and 25 years.
- Approximately 25% of these tumors arise after the age of 70.
- Most osteogenic sarcomas that arise after age 40 occur secondary to other disease states such as Paget's disease (Fig. 3-80) or postirradiation

TABLE 3-1
Age of Peak Incidence and Location of Skeletal Neoplasia

	Tumor	Age (years)	Location
BENIGN	Fibrous cortical defect	4-8	Metaphysis
	Nonossifying fibroma	8-20	Diametaphysis
	Osteoma	20-40	Intramembranous
	Osteoid osteoma	5-30	Metaphysis
	Osteoblastoma	3-78	Vertebral column
	Osteochondroma	5-20	Metaphysis
	Chondroblastoma	10-25	Epiphysis
	Hemangioma	40-60	Axial skeleton
	Aneurysmal bone cyst	10-30	Vertebral column
			Metaphysis
	Unicameral bone cyst	3-14	Metadiaphysis
	Giant cell tumor	20-40	Metaphysis
			Epiphysis
	Enchondroma	20-60	Metaphysis
			Diaphysis
	Bone island	25-70	Epiphysis
			Metaphysis
MALIGNANT	Osteosarcoma	10-25, 60-75	Metaphysis
	Chondrosarcoma	30-60	Metaphysis
	Fibrosarcoma	30-45	Metadiaphysis
	Ewing's sarcoma	5-20	Diaphysis
	Multiple myeloma	40-80	Metadiaphysis
			Any skeletal structure

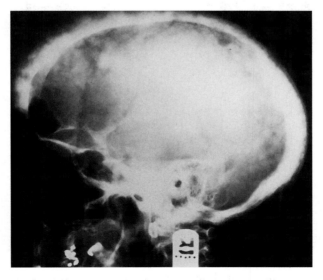

FIG. 3-80 Osteosarcomatous degeneration of a pagetoid skull is demonstrated.

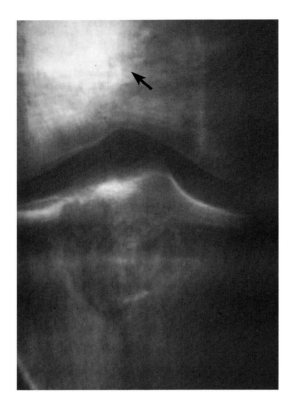

FIG. 3-81 Osteosarcoma has a predilection for the distal femoral metaphysis (*arrow*).

therapy, which represent the two most common antecedent lesions.

◆ It commonly presents as painful swelling of the involved limb.
◆ Pain may be of insidious onset, aching in nature, and may become excruciating.

Common Sites

◆ Metaphysis of distal femur (Fig. 3-81)
◆ Proximal tibial metaphysis (Fig. 3-82)
◆ Proximal humeral metaphysis
◆ Less than 7% arise in the spine

Laboratory Assessment

◆ Consistent elevation of serum alkaline phosphatase
◆ Aggressive tumor, with evidence of bone destruction, subperiosteal elevation, and ensuing soft tissue invasion

Radiographic Features

◆ Three patterns of pathogenesis:
  • Sclerotic (50%)
  • Lytic (25%)
  • Mixed (25%)
◆ A dense ivory medullary lesion with some degree of permeative destruction is noted.
◆ Approximately 90% of long bone osteosarcomas are metaphyseal.
◆ It demonstrates cortical disruption, with an associated large soft tissue mass.

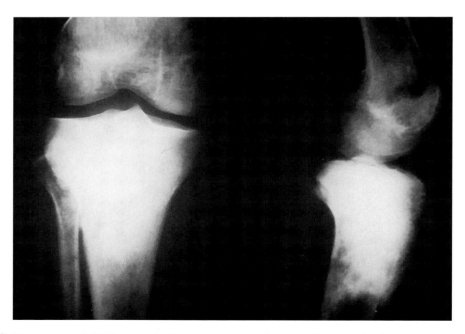

FIG. 3-82 The proximal tibial metaphysis represents another predilectory site for osteosarcomatous onset.

♦ The mass is eccentric and lobulated, with rough, irregular margins and is described as a *cumulus cloud appearance.*

♦ The periosteum is often stimulated by the rapidly growing tumor to form reactive new bone in the form of Codman's triangles (Fig. 3-83, *A* and *B*), "hair-on-end" (Fig. 3-84), or a "sunburst" pattern (Fig. 3-85).

♦ The "sunburst" or "sunray" periosteal response is characteristic.

♦ Hematogenous metastasis to the lungs is common.

♦ Multiple large pulmonary parenchymal lesions are termed *cannonball metastasis.*

♦ Spontaneous pneumothorax is a common clinical sequela.

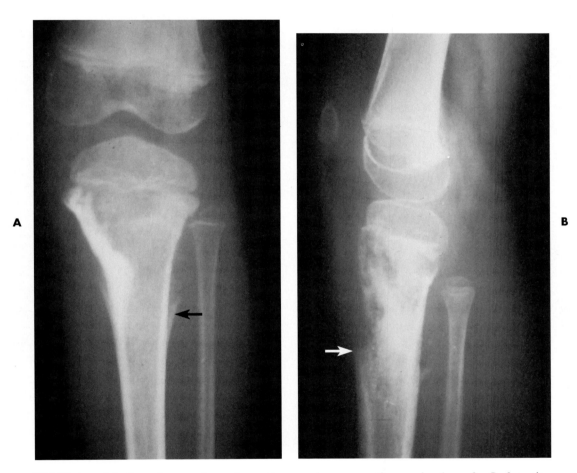

FIG. 3-83 **A** and **B,** Reactive new bone formation can be seen as the production of a Codman's triangle (*arrows*).

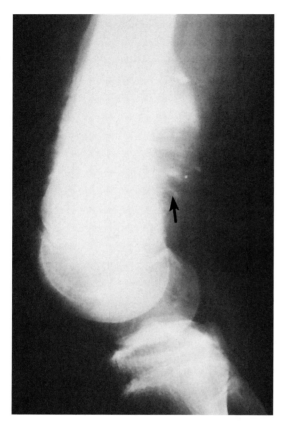

FIG. 3-84 Associated periosteal reaction in osteosarcoma is observed as a "hair-on-end" appearance (*arrow*).

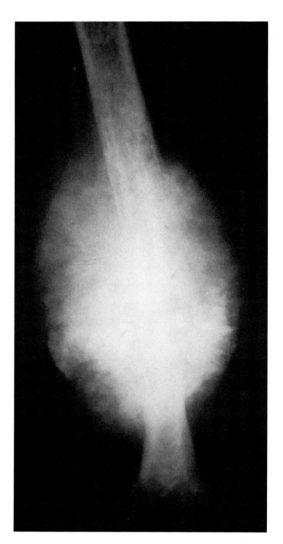

FIG. 3-85 A "sunburst" or "sunray" pattern may also be a radiographic feature associated with a primary osteosarcoma.

Prognosis

◆ The traditional 5-year survival rate is 20%, with amputation of the lesion if surgically accessible (Fig. 3-86, *A* and *B*).

CHONDROSARCOMA

◆ It is a malignant cartilaginous tumor, which is the third most common primary malignancy of bone.
◆ It is of chondrogenic origin, arising from a pre-existent enchondroma, osteochondroma, or de novo in any bone embryologically preformed in cartilage.
◆ It is slow growing, is less aggressive, and posesses a more favorable prognosis than osteosarcoma.

Common Sites

◆ Innominate (27%)
◆ Proximal femur (22%)

◆ Ribs (14%)
◆ Less-frequent sites
  • Shoulder girdle
  • Facial bones
◆ In long bones, the tumor begins in the metaphysis and usually extends into substantial portions of the diaphysis.
◆ In general, the closer the lesion is to the axial skeleton, the greater is its malignant potential.

Clinical Presentation

◆ It commences at a more advanced age, with a peak incidence between 30 and 60 years.
◆ The ratio of males to females is 3:1.
◆ Local dull pain and swelling are the usual presenting symptoms.

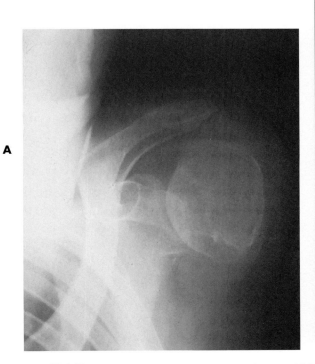
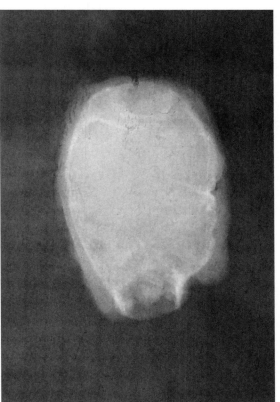

FIG. 3-86 A, A traditional 5-year survival rate of 20% is noted following surgical amputation, as is the case with this affected humerus. **B,** Radiograph of the resected humeral head.

Radiographic Features

♦ It is recognized by osseous destruction, with an irregular, amorphous, and flocculent calcific matrix (Figs. 3-87 and 3-88).

♦ Chondrosarcomas, in general, may demonstrate a number of appearances that at times make them difficult to diagnose with any assurance.

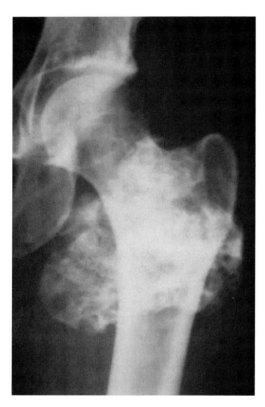

FIG. 3-87 A chondrosarcoma exhibiting irregular, amorphous, and flocculent calcification in its matrix.

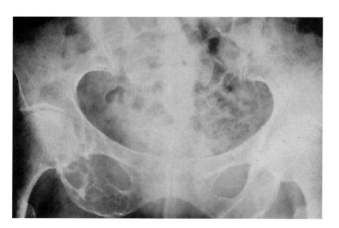

FIG. 3-88 Chondrosarcoma of the pelvis. Note the destruction of the ischium on the reading left, with some internal calcification noted in the primarily radiolucent matrix.

♦ The diagnosis of chondrosarcoma is reserved for patients over 40 years of age, unless a patient manifests an enchondroma or osteochondroma that becomes painful or develops a destructive appearance.

Prognosis

♦ The 5-year survival rate, if the condition is treated, is approximately 50%.

FIBROSARCOMA

♦ This is a rare malignant tumor of fibroblastic tissue.

♦ Approximately 75% arise de novo.

♦ Approximately 25% can develop at a site of a preexisting benign condition, including Paget's disease, GCTs, osteomyelitis, and benign lesions such as bone cysts.

♦ Mostly affects long bones
  · Femur (33%)
  · Tibia (17%)
  · Humerus (12%)

♦ Classic locations include the femoral condyles or the humeral epicondyles.

Clinical Presentation

♦ The mean age is 38 years, but patients may range in age from 4 to 83 years.

♦ A misconception exists that the condition only occurs in older people.

♦ Gender distribution is equal.

♦ Severely progressive pain and swelling are the chief complaints.

Radiographic Features

♦ It is typically eccentric in long bone metaphysis.

♦ It usually does not elicit reactive new bone formation and is therefore almost always lytic in appearance.

♦ It possesses no distinct pathognomonic features.

♦ The lytic appearance may take any form, from permeative or moth-eaten to a fairly well-defined area of lysis.

♦ It tends to be aggressive and demonstrates ill-defined "fuzzy" margins.

♦ Breaking through the expanded cortical shell leads to the formation of a contiguous soft tissue mass that lacks calcifications or ossifications, differentially diagnosing it from osteosarcoma and chondrosarcoma.

♦ Margins of the tumor are poorly defined, and usually there is no overlying periosteal reaction until the entire cortex is destroyed.

♦ The periosteal reaction is decidedly less with fibrosarcoma than osteosarcoma.

- Although the periosteal reaction is rare, an extremely large soft tissue mass is common.
- In its latter stages, fibrosarcoma, like osteosarcoma, hematologically metastasizes, producing secondary foci in other skeletal regions, as well as in the pulmonary parenchyma.

Prognosis

- The 5-year survival rate is 27%.
- The 10-year survival rate is 20%.

EWING'S SARCOMA

- A rare malignant tumor of bone
- A distinct, small round cell sarcoma comprised of undifferentiated mesenchymal cells in the medullary cavity
- Other round cell tumors such as myeloma and reticulum cell sarcoma

Clinical Presentation

- It is most frequent in the appendicular skeleton and pelvic girdle.
- Pain and swelling are presenting complaints; encountering an asymptomatic Ewing's sarcoma is unusual.
- It often features a palpable, tender mass that is rapidly growing.
- The most common age at the time of occurrence is between 10 and 30 years.
- A male preponderance exists.
- Blacks appear resistant to this tumor.

Radiographic Features

- Central diaphyseal area of tubular bones of the lower limb
- Mottled, patchy, streaky, or "moth-eaten" lytic lesion that may involve the entire diaphysis
- Ruptures through the cortex because it is aggressive and destructive
- Gives rise to periosteal reactive new bone formation; classically manifests as the multilayered "onion-skin" appearance
- "Onion skin" periosteal reaction characterized by laminated, alternating thin bands of lucency and radiodensity (Fig. 3-89, *A-C*)
- Possibility of also demonstrating a spiculated, "trimmed-whisker" periosteal response
- "Trimmed-whisker" periosteal reaction characterized by perpendicular spicules thinner than those of osteosarcoma (Fig. 3-90)
- Hematogenous dissemination occurring early

MULTIPLE MYELOMA

- Most frequent primary malignant skeletal tumor

- Characterized by the proliferation of plasma cells in the marrow cavity and the overproduction of monoclonal immunoglobulins or Bence Jones protein
- Represents approximately half of all primary malignant bone tumors
- A multicentric disease, involving several sites
- Primarily characterized by widespread osteolytic bone destruction
- Remains confined to the skeleton

Clinical Presentation

- The peak age incidence is between 50 and 59 years.
- The male to female ratio is 2:1.
- The most prominent single symptom is deep, vague low-back pain.
- Pain is the initial symptom; it increases, becoming more prevalent during the day and easing in the evening.
- Physical activity enhances the pain.
- Weight loss, fever, and anemia may also be associated.
- Increased susceptibility to infections of all types complicates the condition.

Radiographic Features

- Presenting skeletal lesions are found primarily in bones containing red marrow.
  - Vertebrae (60%)
  - Ribs (59%)
  - Skull (40%)
  - Pelvis (40%)
- The initial sign is universal diffuse osteopenia resembling osteoporosis.
- Multiple myeloma is classically characterized by numerous foci of osteolytic "punched-out" bone destruction in the absence of surrounding sclerosis (Fig. 3-91).
- Diffuse osteoporosis is common, and pathologic fractures, especially of the vertebrae, are often seen (Figs. 3-92 and 3-93).
- Lesions are frequently regular in size and shape and vary up to 5 cm in diameter.
- It is one of the only lesions that is not characteristically "hot" on a radionuclide bone scan; therefore radiographic bone surveys are performed instead of radionuclide bone scans when evidence of myeloma is clinically suspected.
- There is preservation of the vertebral pedicles until quite late.
- *Raindrop skull* is defined as multiple osteolytic "punched-out" lesions of multiple myeloma, as seen in the tables of the skull (Fig. 3-94, *A* and *B*).

A   **B**   **C**

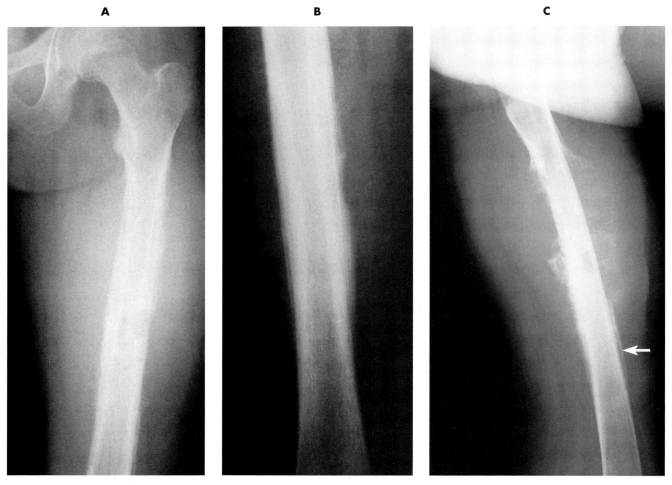

FIG. 3-89 A-C, Examples of "onion skin" periosteal reaction in Ewing's sarcoma. Note the alternating narrow bands of radiolucency and radiodensity (*arrow*).

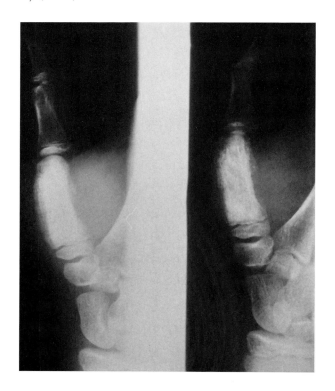

FIG. 3-90 The "trimmed whisker" periosteal reaction is characterized by perpendicular periosteal spicules.

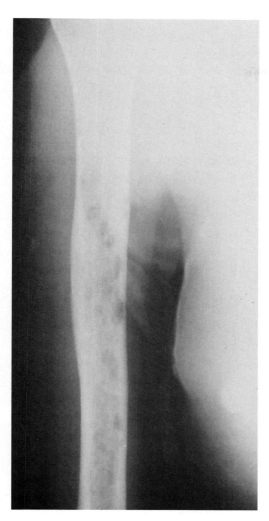

FIG. 3-91 Numerous foci of osteolytic "punched out" bone lesions typical of multiple myeloma. Note the absence of surrounding sclerosis around the radiolucent defects.

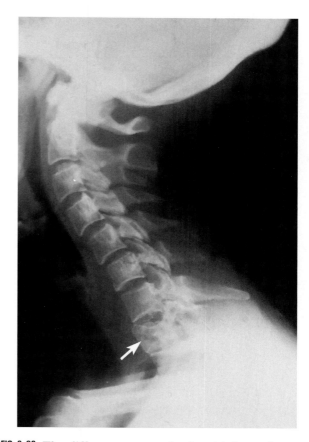

FIG. 3-92 The diffuse osteoporosis of multiple myeloma commonly results in a pathologic vertebral body fracture (*arrow*).

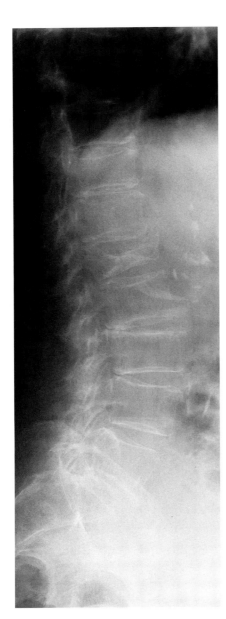

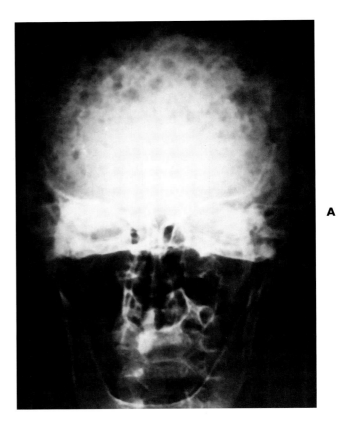

A

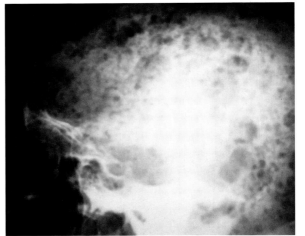

B

FIG. 3-93 Marked universal osteopenia accompanies a vertebral body compression fracture at L1 in this patient with advanced multiple myeloma. The decrease in anterior and posterior body height suggests an etiology other than postmenopausal osteoporosis.

FIG. 3-94 A and B, Multiple myeloma of the skull may render a "raindrop" skull appearance as a result of the multiple "punched out" lesions, as observed in these anteroposterior and lateral views.

TABLE 3-2 *Differential Diagnosis of Multiple Myeloma Versus Osteolytic Metastasis*		
Feature	**Multiple Myeloma**	**Osteolytic Metastasis**
Osteopenia	Uniformally diffuse	Focal
Pedicles	Affected late	Affected early
Lesions	Uniform size and shape	Any size or shape
Bone scan	Negative	Positive (usually)

Laboratory Analysis

- Globulins appear in the serum.
- Abnormal Bence Jones protein may be found in the urine.
- Bone marrow aspiration is the most important diagnostic procedure.

Differential Diagnosis

See Table 3-2 for the differential diagnosis.

PLASMACYTOMA

- Rare
- A solitary focus of myeloma
- Usual presentation: expansile metaphyseal lesion
- May be complicated by pathologic fracture
- Can occur in a rib or acetabular roof
- Virtually all patients with plasmacytomas proceed to develop multiple myeloma.

Prognosis

- Poor; survival is seldom more than 2 years.
- The 5-year survival rate is 7.5%.

Secondary Malignant Neoplasia: Metastatic Bone Disease

Malignant metastatic neoplastic disease arguably represents the most common sinister condition that presents to practice. Metastatic neoplastic bone disease is characterized radiographically by lesions with ill-defined margins, variations in size, distribution, a wide zone of transition, and early loss of cortical integrity. The prognosis is frequently poor but continues to improve. Early identification and diagnosis of malignant metastatic disease is crucial to the ultimate success or failure in case management.

- It is discovered mainly in older people.
- It occurs when primary malignant tumors spread to adjacent and distant sites of the body.
- Most metastatic tumors in bone arise from carcinomas, and any carcinoma may metastasize to bone.

- Metastasis to bone may produce an osteolytic, osteoblastic, or mixed osteolytic and sclerotic (osteoblastic) type of lesion.
- Metastatic deposits are most frequently found in the red marrow bones (i.e., the spine, ribs, pelvis, skull, and upper ends of the humerus and femur).
- Although any bone may be affected, tumors uncommonly disseminate distal to the knees and elbows.
- Bone metastasis arises after longstanding primary disease, resulting in a poorer prognosis.
- Metastasis may be the first recognizable indication of a primary malignant disease.
- This disease may metastasize to bone hematogenously, lymphatically, or by direct extension from adjacent diseased tissues (e.g., when carcinoma of the cervix extends to the pelvic wall or by lymph nodes that have been known to become enlarged sufficiently enough to erode nearby periosteum and invade the adjacent bone).
- Involvement of the spinal column usually occurs via hematogenous spread, either through the systemic circulation or by way of the vertebral venous complex.
- Metastasis usually involves multiple levels of the spine, although solitary lesions occur in approximately 10% of patients.
- When contiguous vertebrae are involved, the intervertebral disc is usually spared because cartilage is resistant to invasion.
- This relative preservation of the disc allows metastatic disease to be differentiated from inflammatory processes, in which case the disc is invariably compromised.
- Diarthrodial joint spaces are normally spared, suggesting that hyaline cartilage is resistant.
- Tumors originating from the prostate, breast, lung, kidney, and colon produce approximately 80% of all skeletal metastasis.

◆ In females, lung and breast carcinoma may be responsible for 70% of all cases, with the remainder originating in the thyroid, kidney, and uterus.

◆ In males the prostate produces 60% of metastases, and the lung contributes an additional 25%.

◆ The sigmoid colon, pancreas, cervix, and stomach infrequently exhibit skeletal metastasis.

THREE PRINCIPAL PATHWAYS OF DISSEMINATION

Hematogenous

◆ This is the most common pathway for tumor embolic spread, especially via venous networks.

◆ This pathway accounts for the almost exclusive involvement of the axial skeleton because it has the greatest percentage of hematopoietic tissue.

◆ Most tumor cells exit the primary site via capillary veins.

◆ Less than 0.1% of circulating tumor emboli survive.

◆ A colony of metastatic cells in a host organ cannot generate a significant metastatic focus until separate vascularization is acquired.

Lymphatic

◆ Adjacent osseous structures may be eroded by hypertrophied lymph nodes.

Direct

◆ The primary tumor is situated adjacent to osseous surfaces, which it can invade.

◆ This pathway can be seeded locally following surgical section.

THE RADIOGRAPHIC APPEARANCES

Osteolytic

◆ If the process of destruction predominates, the lesion appears osteolytic.

◆ Lytic defects are produced by the mechanical effect of tumor growth resulting in selective reabsorption of medullary bone.

Osteoblastic

◆ If bone formation predominates, the lesion assumes an osteoblastic appearance.

◆ Neoplastic cells produce enzymes that may stimulate osteoid production from osteoblasts, causing an osteoblastic lesion.

Mixed osteolytic-osteoblastic

◆ When destruction and formation are equivalent, a mixed osteolytic-osteoblastic lesion is the result.

Clinical Presentation

◆ Metastatic bone disease usually occurs in people over 40 years old, although it may develop at any age.

◆ There is no particular gender distribution because metastatic bone disease depends on the type and location of the primary tumor.

◆ The prostate and lung are the most common primary tumor sites in males.

◆ The lung and breast are the most common primary sites of malignancy in females.

◆ Back pain is often the presenting complaint of a patient with an undetected primary malignant tumor that has metastasized to the spine.

◆ Pain is usually described as constant, dull, usually unrelieved by rest, and often worse at night.

◆ Pain is not always apparent at night but may be related to physical exertion (i.e., the result of pathologic fracture).

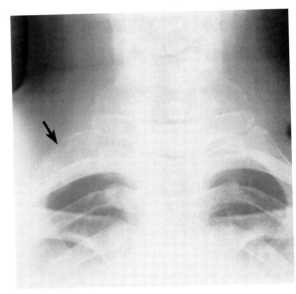

FIG. 3-95 Osteolytic metastasis in the proximal end of the first rib (*arrow*).

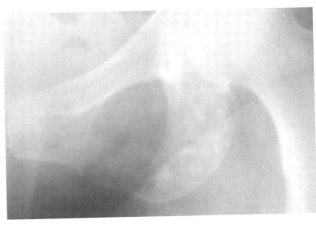

FIG. 3-96 Osteolytic metastasis manifesting in the ischium.

- Pain occurring suddenly or after minor trauma may be the result of a pathologic fracture in 15% to 20% of patients.
- Patients may be relatively asymptomatic until secondary lesions have already disseminated.
- Unexplained weight loss, anemia, intermittent pain, fever, and cachexia occur later.
- The lung, breast, prostate, and kidney are the most common sites of primary tumors that metastasize to the spine and produce spinal cord compression.
- In patients over the age of 40 who have dull, unremitting spinal pain and signs of neurologic deficit, metastatic bone disease must rank high on the index of suspicion.

Sites of Involvement

- The most common sites of metastatic spread are as follows:
  - Lungs
  - Liver
  - Skeleton
- Metastatic disease is the most frequent form of malignant neoplasm appearing in the skeleton.
- The most frequent sites of metastatic spread are as follows:
  - Vertebral column
  - Ribs (Fig. 3-95)
  - Pelvis (Fig. 3-96)
  - Proximal humerus (Fig. 3-97, *A-C*)
  - Femora

A

B

C

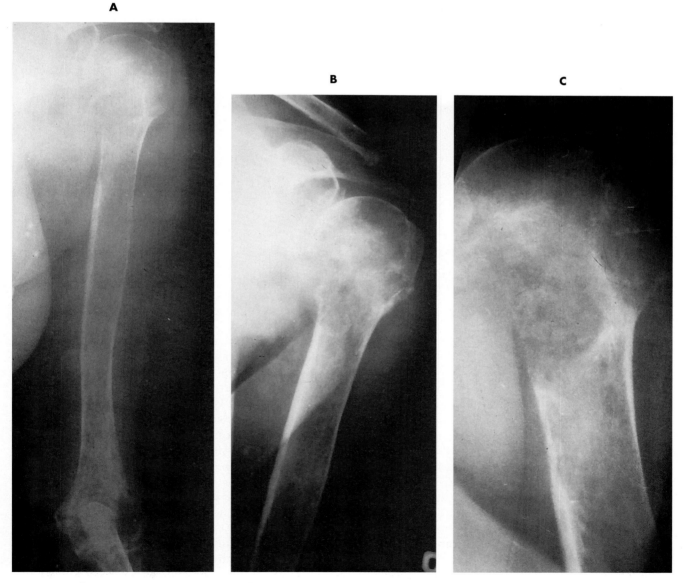

FIG. 3-97 A-C, The progressive effect of osteolytic neoplastic bone disease in the proximal humeral metaphysis.

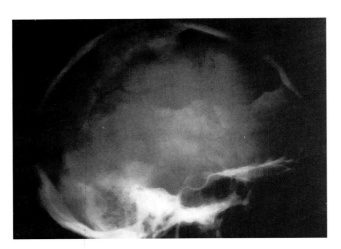

FIG. 3-98 Osteolytic metastasis in the calvarium.

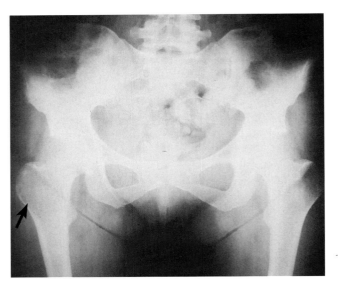

FIG. 3-100 Large, solitary, "blow out" osteolytic metastasis from a renal primary, as observed in the region of the greater trochanter and intertrochanteric ridge (*arrow*).

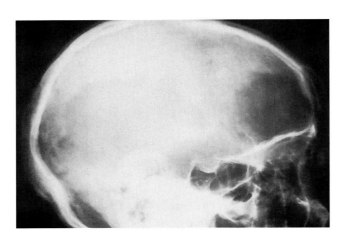

FIG. 3-99 Calvarial osteolytic metastasis.

• Sternum
• Calvarium (Figs. 3-98 and 3-99)

Radiographic Features

◆ The response of bone to the metastatic spread of carcinoma can be described as osteolytic, osteoblastic, or mixed osteolytic-osteoblastic.

OSTEOLYTIC METASTASIS

◆ Lytic metastasis is the most common malignancy of bone.
◆ Approximately 75% of all skeletal metastases are osteolytic in appearance.

◆ Approximately 80% of lytic metastases occur in the axial skeleton.
◆ Osteolytic metastasis is characterized by decreased bone density or bone destruction.
◆ Osteolytic metastasis commences in the medullary space and quickly spreads to involve cortical bone.
◆ Eventually, the entire bone becomes weakened and is predisposed to pathologic fracture.
◆ Lesions may be single or multiple.
◆ Usually, no periosteal reaction is associated with these tumors. When a reaction is apparent, it is likely a response to a pathologic fracture rather than the tumor.
◆ Renal or thyroid malignancies tend to produce a large, single metastatic "blow out" lesion (Fig. 3-100).
◆ Lesions may coalesce to form a "moth-eaten" or permeative lytic pattern (Figs. 3-101, *A* and *B*; 3-102).
◆ Focal rib expansion (Fig. 3-103) or destruction may produce an extrapleural sign in chest studies.
◆ In the spine, any portion of a vertebra may be involved.

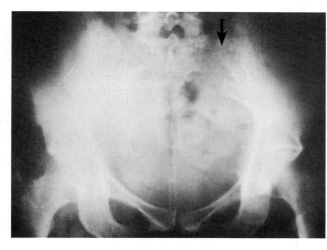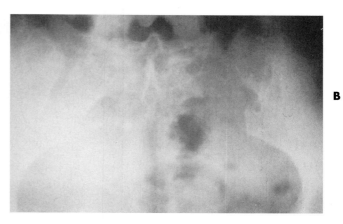

FIG. 3-101 A and **B,** A "moth-eaten" permeative lytic pattern in the sacral ala (*arrow*). Note that the disease respects the integrity of the adjacent sacroiliac joint.

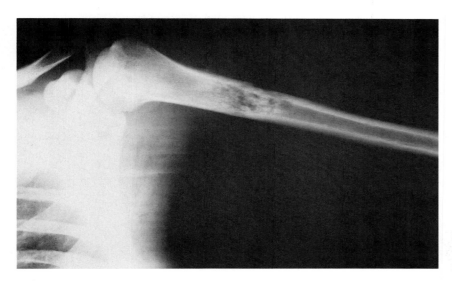

FIG. 3-102 An osteolytic permeative "moth-eaten" pattern in the proximal metadiaphyseal region of the humerus.

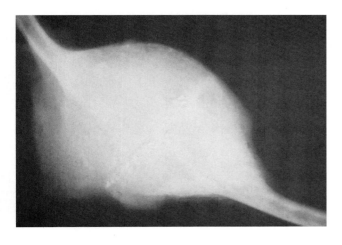

FIG. 3-103 The focal osteolytic rib expansion may produce an extrapleural sign in chest radiographic studies.

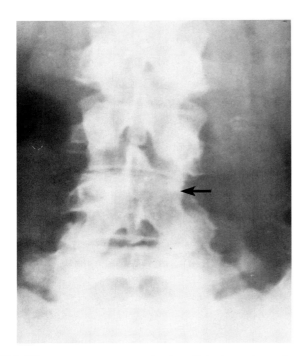

FIG. 3-104 Osteolysis of a vertebral pedicle (*arrow*) produces the "one-eyed" vertebra sign.

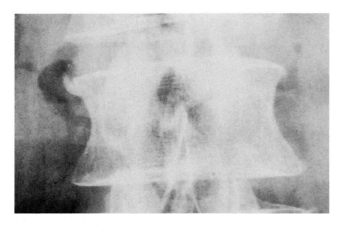

FIG. 3-105 Osteolysis of a solitary vertebral pedicle may also be termed the *winking vertebra sign.*

- Lytic involvement of one pedicle results in the "winking" or "one-eyed" vertebra sign (Figs. 3-104 and 3-105), and lytic destruction of both pedicles in a segment has been termed the *blind vertebra sign* (Fig. 3-106).

- A pathologic compression fracture with decreased anterior and posterior body height is frequently seen in the presence of osteolytic metastasis and multiple myeloma (Figs. 3-107, *A* and *B*; 3-108; 3-109, *A* and *B*; 3-110; 3-111, 3-112, *A-C*; and 3-113).

- A compression fracture may result in back pain, acute gibbus deformity, and possible neurologic deficit.

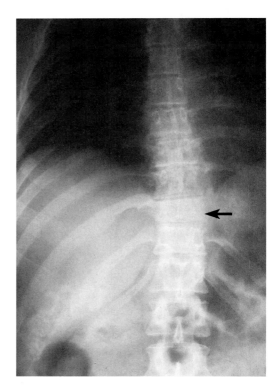

FIG. 3-106 Osteolysis of both vertebral pedicles in a segment has been termed the *blind vertebra sign* (*arrow*).

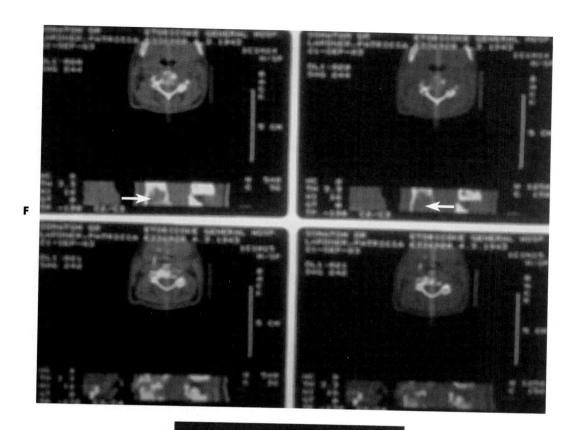

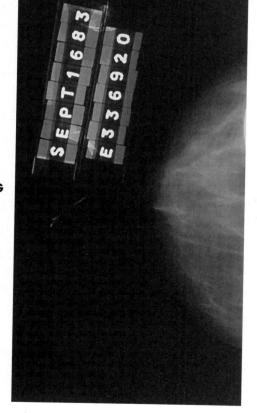

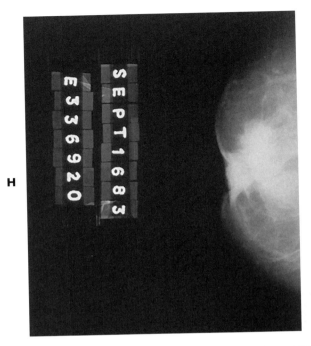

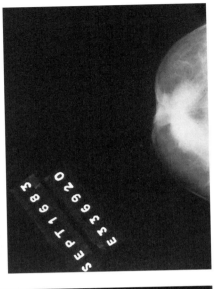

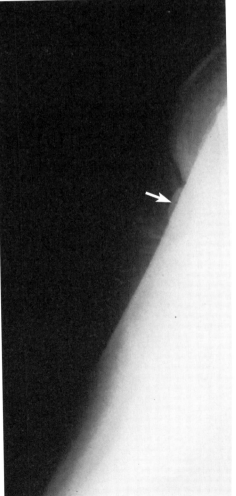

FIG. 3-117, cont'd. H and **I,** Mammograms of the contralateral breast exhibiting a horse-shoe shaped, 5-cm carcinoma and nipple retraction. **J,** A tangential mammogram of the affected breast demonstrating obvious nipple inversion (*arrow*). (Courtesy Henry Mayers, DC, Mississauga, Ontario.)

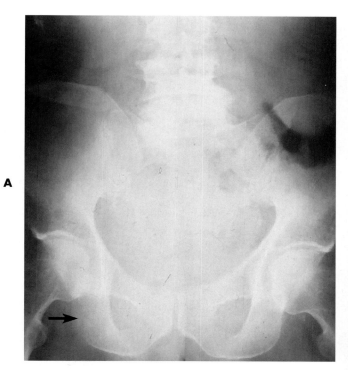

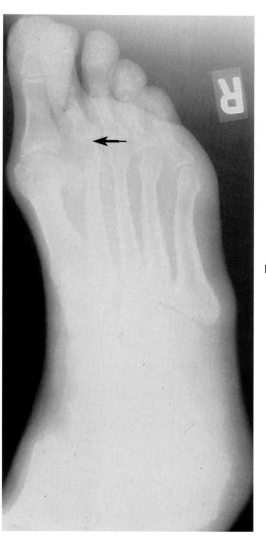

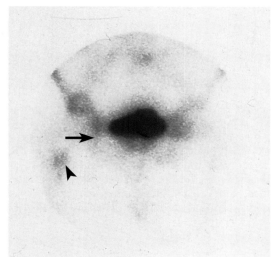

FIG. 3-118 A, A large metastatic, osteolytic focus in the superior ramus of the ischium is observed (*arrow*). The overlying cortex is also severely compromised. **B,** A smaller osteolytic focus is contained in the second metatarsal head (*arrow*). **C,** A radionuclide bone scan reveals increases in isotopic uptake in the superior ramus of the ischium (*arrow*), as well as the lesser trochanter (*arrowhead*). *Continued.*

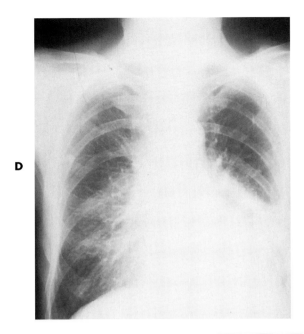

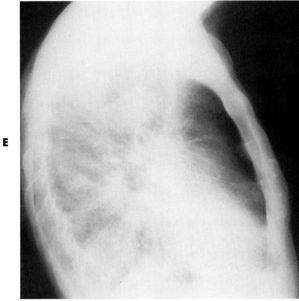

OSTEOBLASTIC METASTASIS

- Osteoblastic metastasis is generally characterized by focal or diffuse increases in osseous density (Fig. 3-119, *A-D*).
- This appearance accounts for approximately 15% of all skeletal metastasis.

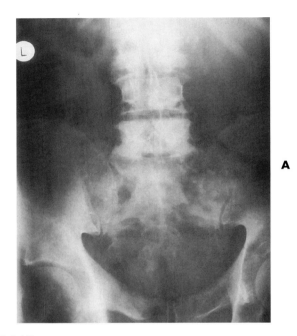

FIG. 3-119 A, Anteroposterior view of the lumbopelvic region manifesting increased osseous density in multiple vertebral body levels in a 64-year-old man. The metastasis originated from a primary site in the prostate. **B,** Lateral projection of the same patient, exhibiting osteoblastic metastasis at multiple lumbar levels. **C** and **D,** Posteroanterior and lateral views of the chest demonstrating multiple, randomly disseminated foci through-

FIG. 3-118, cont'd. D and **E,** Posteroanterior and lateral views of the chest exhibit a large cavitating primary bronchogenic carcinoma in the left lower lobe. It is responsible for the previously observed skeletal defects.

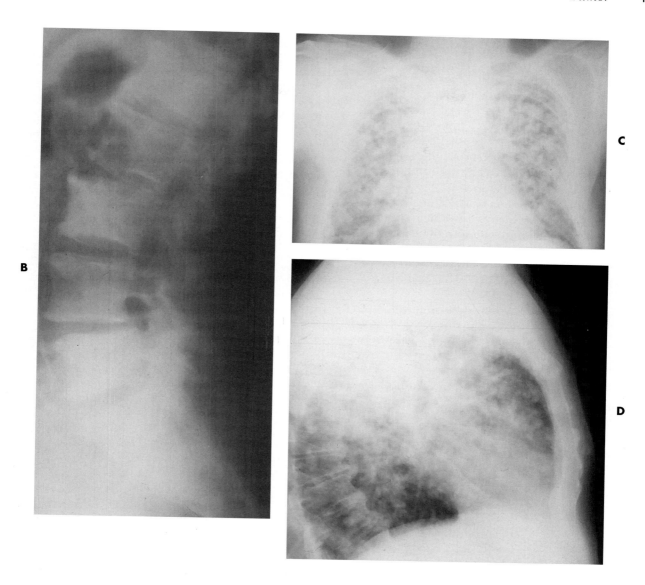

B

C

D

- Osteoblastic metastasis usually produces a pattern of multiple discrete lesions (Fig. 3-120, *A-D*).
- Osteoblastic metastasis can occur as isolated rounded foci of sclerotic density or as diffuse sclerosis involving a large area of bone.
- Tumor cells do not produce bone themselves but enzymatically stimulate osteoblasts to do so.
- Tumors originating in the prostate in males and in the breast in females after radiotherapy frequently produce this pattern.
- Other tumors related to blastic change include those arising in the bladder, stomach, lung, gastrointestinal tract, and osteosarcoma.
- This appearance may develop after lytic metastatic tumor irradiation.
- Normal trabecular architecture is lost when osteoblastic lesions coalesce.
- In the spine, "ivory" vertebral formation (Figs. 3-121, 3-122, and 3-123) must be differentiated from Paget's disease and Hodgkin's lymphoma.

Differential Diagnosis

- With osteoblastic metastasis, the vertebral body maintains its size and shape.
- With Paget's disease, squaring and enlargement of the vertebral body is observed.
- Hodgkin's lymphoma demonstrates anterior body scalloping as a result of pressure erosion by adjacent lymph nodal hypertrophy.
- A sclerotic pedicle may be the result of metastatic disease or may arise as a result of biomechanical stresses secondary to a neural arch defect or congenital dysplasia.

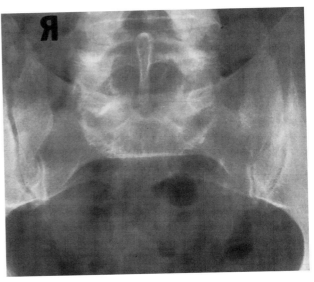

A

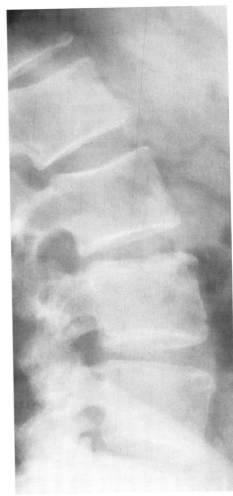

B

FIG. 3-120 **A** and **B,** A spot anteroposterior lumbosacral and lateral lumbar spine of a 64-year-old man exhibiting no evidence of bone disease. **C** and **D,** A similar study of the same patient 5 years later, demonstrating several discrete osteoblastic lesions in the medial portion of the left innominate bone, which proved to be metastasis from the prostate. Other foci are observed in the lumbar vertebral bodies at all levels. (Courtesy Dr. Andrew Pulinec, Toronto, Ontario.)

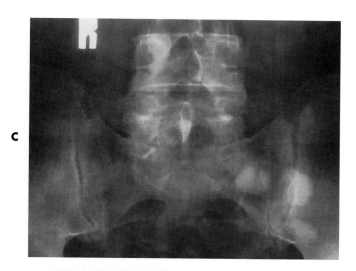

C

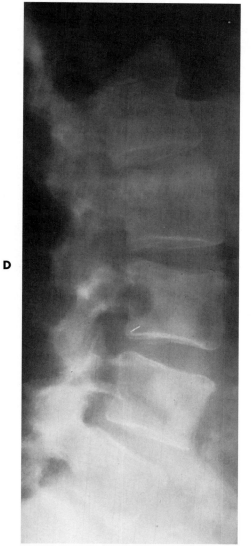

D

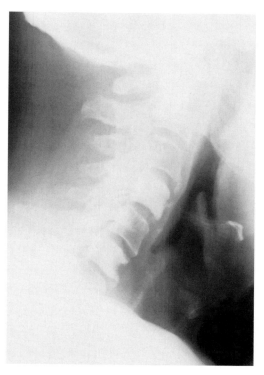

FIG. 3-121 Evidence of "ivory" vertebral formation in the cervical spine.

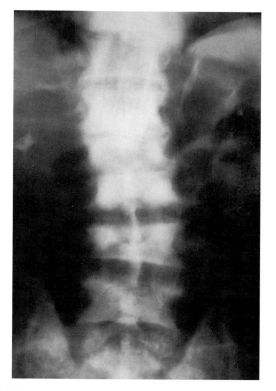

FIG. 3-122 Multiple "ivory" vertebrae in the lumbar spine.

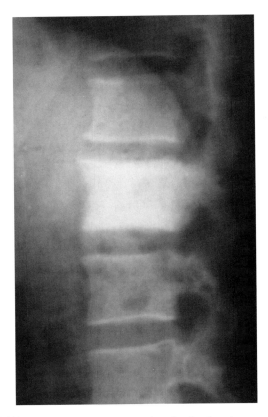

FIG. 3-123 A solitary "ivory" vertebra in the lumbar region secondary to primary prostatic malignant disease.

MIXED OSTEOLYTIC-OSTEOBLASTIC METASTASIS

- Approximately 10% of skeletal metastases are mixed.
- Tumors from the breast, lung, kidney, and liver and those developing after lytic lesion irradiation may produce this pattern.
- A combination of bone destruction and sclerosis is found (Fig. 3-124), with destruction usually predominating (Fig. 3-125, *A* and *B*).
- The tumor usually possesses a mottled appearance as a result of the mixed destructive and sclerotic areas (Fig. 3-126).

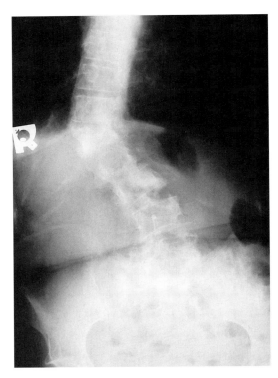

FIG. 3-124 A combination of osteolytic and osteoblastic metastatic, neoplastic bone alterations are exhibited in this lumbopelvic study.

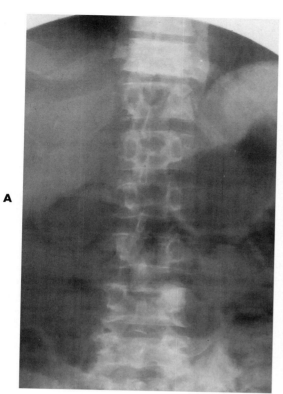

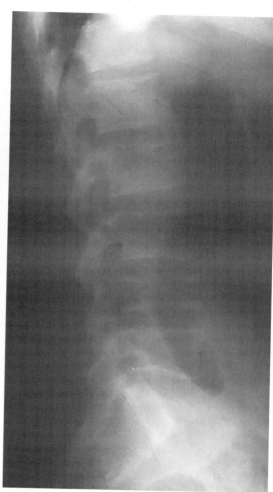

FIG. 3-125 **A** and **B,** Anteroposterior and lateral views of the lumbar spine demonstrate the presence of mixed osteolytic and osteoblastic bone change. Osteolysis usually predominates.

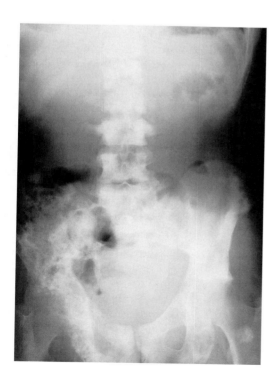

FIG. 3-126 Mixed metastasis may produce a mottled appearance as a result of the combination of bone lysis and sclerosis.

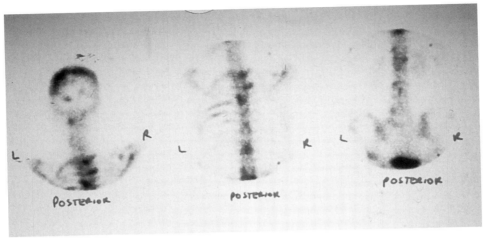

FIG. 3-127 A bone scan demonstrating the random uptake of radioisotope. Note the absence of uptake symmetry and variation of sizes of the foci throughout the skeleton.

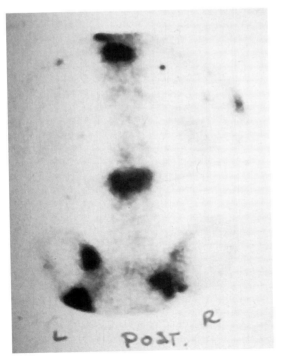

FIG. 3-128 Bone scan exhibiting the lack of symmetric distribution and size of the malignant lesions. This pattern has been alluded to as the *lit Christmas tree effect*.

Imaging

- The degree of bone destruction needed to be seen on x-ray film varies with the patient's age, the amount of osteoporosis, and the location of the lesion (i.e., an older patient with osteoporosis requires a relatively greater bone change than a younger patient to visualize a pathology).
- A lesion requires 30% to 50% bone destruction to be visualized on plain film.
- Tomography requires a 15% to 20% change in bone density to be appreciated.
- A radionuclide bone scan (bone scintigraphy) requires only a 3% alteration in bone metabolic activity to be demonstrated.
- Currently, radiographic skeletal studies remain the most commonly used tool for the detection of skeletal metastasis. However, the development of a phosphate compound labelled with technetium 99m (Tc 99m) has made the radioisotope bone scan unquestionably more sensitive than radiographic skeletal studies in detecting early metastatic disease (Figs. 3-127 and 3-128).
- Because neoplastic processes may be detected long before radiographic features appear, bone scanning has changed the examination and management procedures of patients whose spinal pain is suspected to be caused by metastatic disease.
- Tc 99m studies possess only a 3% margin of error. Therefore Tc 99m sensitivity approaches 97%.
- Scintigraphy is featured by focal, or more commonly, diffuse areas of increased radionuclide accumulation in the skeleton.

- "Hot" areas signify accelerated areas of bone metabolic activity, regardless of the etiology. Therefore scans should be correlated with a skeletal survey, tomography, computerized tomography (CT), and clinical laboratory data for a greater degree of diagnostic specificity.
- Exceptions are tumors such as multiple myelomas that are associated with little osseous repair.
- The use of CT is especially diagnostic for pelvic, sacral, and spinal metastasis because skeletal lesions may be obscured by overlying soft tissue structures and contents.
- Magnetic resonance imaging (MRI) may permit the evaluation of the feasability of tumor resection and the extent of radiotherapy.
- Osseous biopsy remains the only definitive method of determining the presence and origin of metastatic disease. However, it is seldomly required to render a diagnosis.

Laboratory Analysis

- Elevated titer of serum alkaline phosphatase
- In presence of malignant prostatic carcinoma, serum alkaline phosphatase and serum acid phosphatase usually elevated, as well as prostate-specific antigen (PSA)
- Hypercalcemia usually present in osteolytic metastases

Additional Considerations

- Metastatic disease may assume virtually any appearance and can mimic a benign lesion or primary bone tumor.
- Metastasis must be included in any differential diagnosis of a bone lesion in patients over 40 years of age.

- Metastatic bone disease must frequently be differentiated from musculoskeletal derangement, metabolic disorders, infection, and primary malignant tumors.
- Osteolytic metastases in the spine must be differentiated from multiple myeloma.
- Cartilage is resistant to the invasion of tumor cells, and the preservation of the intervertebral disc with destruction of the surrounding vertebral bodies is highly suggestive of metastatic bone disease.
- Intervertebral disc is invariably involved with infectious spondylopathy.

Summary

- Making a definitive diagnosis of metastatic bone disease is sometimes difficult.
- The importance of considering all pertinent information obtained from the case history and physical, radiographic, and laboratory examinations cannot be overemphasized.
- Special studies, such as radionuclide and CT scanning, may also be required to provide enough information for an accurate diagnosis.
- It is never unreasonable to assume that a patient over 40 years of age can have back pain produced by metastatic disease.
- Patients who suffer from skeletal pain and have a history of primary malignant neoplasm should always be observed closely.
- Unexplained skeletal pain in patients with primary malignant tumors in which the usual diagnostic processes prove futile warrants more sophisticated testing.

TUMOR

Blood (Vascular)

This category of skeletal disorder has been believed to denote a group of closely related conditions mainly characterized by avascular necrosis. This classification of bone disease is now regarded to possess a rather heterogenous variety of etiologies. Generally, the osteochondroses are comprised of a number of conditions affecting the primary and secondary growth centers of the immature skeleton. In long bones the secondary growth centers are affected, whereas in small, flat bones a predilection for the primary growth centers is typical. Although various etiologies have been postulated for the development of such disorders, trauma appears to be an influencing factor. A selection of avascular necrotic conditions may be studied in the following pages.

SICKLE CELL ANEMIA

- Red blood cells assume a reversible sickle shape at reduced oxygen tension (35-45 mmHg).

Etiology
- Abnormal, genetically transmitted hemoglobin (hemoglobin S)

Clinical Presentation
- Cause of anemia: rapid destruction of abnormal red blood cells
- Jaundice
- Cholelithiasis
- Increased hematopoietic activity in response to anemia

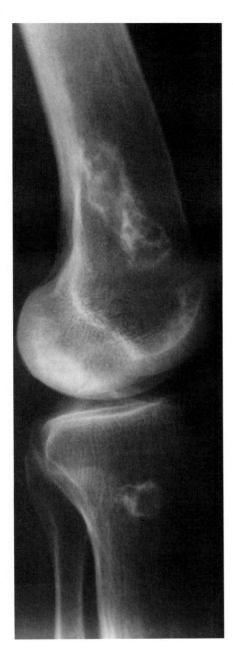

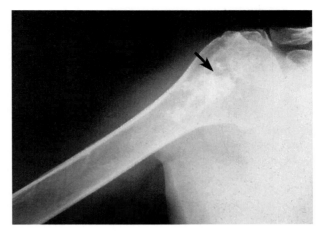

FIG. 4-7 Bone infarction of the proximal humerus. Note the serpigenous medullary metaphyseal sclerosis (*arrow*).

FIG. 4-6 Bone infarctions of the knee. The distal femur and proximal tibia each exhibit focal medullary avascular necrosis.

- Common sites: distal femur (Figs. 4-5, *A* and *B*), proximal tibia (Fig. 4-6), and proximal humerus (Fig. 4-7)
- Some common predisposing factors: trauma, hemoglobinopathy, Caisson disease, corticosteroids, collagen disease, radiation, alcoholism, Gaucher's disease, pancreatitis, and gout.
- Differential diagnosis must include enchondroma

OSTEOCHONDROSES

- It had long been felt that this classification of bone disorders denoted a group of related conditions characterized by avascular necrosis.
- The current prevailing opinion is that this classification of bone diseases is heterogeneous and has varied etiologies.
- Generally, the osteochondroses consist of a variety of conditions affecting primary and secondary growth centers of the immature skeleton.
- Various names are ascribed to epiphyseal avascular necroses, usually with the eponym being the first person to describe the disorder (see diagram).

Scheuermann's Disease (Vertebral Epiphysitis, Juvenile Kyphosis)

- Primarily affects the secondary ossification centers of the thoracic vertebrae (the ring epiphyses of the vertebral bodies)

Pathology

- It was originally linked to epiphyseal atrophy and disruption caused by excessive tensile forces acting from above and below by the annular fibers, resulting in epiphyseal vascular ischemic insult. It probably has a traumatic etiology.
- Today, it is considered a traumatic growth arrest with end-plate fracture and nuclear herniation (Schmorl's nodes) observed during the adolescent growth period.

◆ Genetic factors may play a role. This theory has led some authors to conclude that certain individuals may have an intrinsic weakness of the end plates, predisposing these individuals to posttraumatic interosseous discal herniation, which produces intravertebral cartilaginous nodal formation.

◆ Although opinion is mixed regarding the exact etiology, cartilaginous nodal formation produced by posttraumatic and/or genetic disruption of the growth plates seems most probable.

◆ The cumulative effect is multiple Schmorl's nodes, anterior body wedging (5 degrees or greater) resulting in a trapezoidal appearance, irregular end plates, and loss of disc height.

Clinical Presentation

◆ Occurrence primarily in males 13 to 17 years of age

◆ Gradually increasing kyphosis

◆ Mild to severe pain, usually evident on palpation or after physical exertion

◆ Possibly entirely asymptomatic, being noticed only incidentally later in life in x-ray studies

Radiographic Features

◆ Generalized kyphotic configuration of the spine, which is exclusively thoracic in 75% of patients

◆ Irregularities of vertebral end-plate contour (Fig. 4-8): sclerosis, roughening, and multiple Schmorl's nodes

◆ Involvement of only two to three vertebrae early in the process

◆ However, should observe at least three contiguous segments involved

◆ Wedging of anterior one third of vertebral bodies by compression fracture possible but not a universal finding (trapezoidal, which contributes to increased kyphosis) (Fig. 4-9)

◆ Spontaneous healing occurring between 18 and 20 years of age

Legg-Calvé-Perthes Disease

◆ A self-limiting disorder that affects the femoral capital epiphysis

◆ Avascular necrosis postulated to be of traumatic etiology, either micro- or gross trauma

Clinical Presentation

◆ It affects children between 4 and 8 years.

◆ The male to female ratio is 5:1.

◆ About 10% of patients exhibit bilateral involvement.

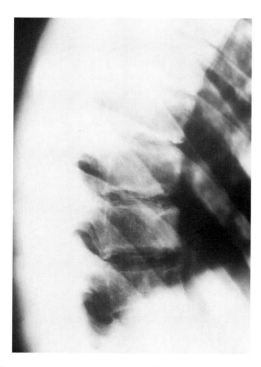

FIG. 4-8 Scheuermann's disease. Observe the irregular, roughened end plates at multiple levels.

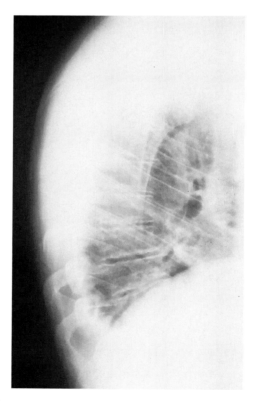

FIG. 4-9 Scheuermann's disease. An increase in the kyphosis is noted, resulting from mild anterior vertebral body wedging in the midthoracic region.

- The degree of symptomatology may be inconsistent with the radiographic appearance.

Radiographic Features

- Early changes may include soft tissue edema around the hip joint, possibly displacing normal fat planes.
- Intracapsular fluid distension may produce lateral displacement of the femoral head, thereby increasing the medial acetabular-femoral joint space.
- The affected epiphyseal center may appear smaller than its counterpart.
- However, asymmetric epiphyseal development may be regarded as a normal roentgen variant.
- A thin arclike zone of lucency may develop in the subchondral bone adjacent to the articular cortex in the superior aspect of the epiphysis. This zone is termed the *crescent sign* (Fig. 4-10).
- The crescent sign represents a stress-type fracture through necrotic, osteoporotic subcortical spongiosa.

- If the crescent sign becomes accentuated, it may resemble a vacuum phenomenon, and this appearance is best delineated in the lateral projection of the hip.
- Progressive fracture and compression of the epiphyseal center result in its flattening.
- The femoral neck widens secondarily.
- Increased sclerosis of the femoral head arises as a consequence of new bone production on preexisting dead trabeculae. This is termed the *snow-cap appearance* (Fig. 4-11).
- Fragmentation of the femoral head may ensue during the revascularization process.
- Reconstitution is slow, often requiring 2 to 3 years.
- Healing is usually complete, but residual permanent deformity, such as shortening and broadening of the femoral head, results in a "mushroom-cap" appearance.
- Premature degenerative joint disease is a common sequela to this deformity.

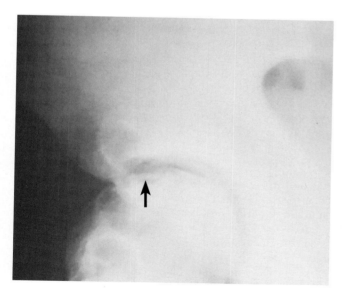

FIG. 4-10 Legg-Calvé-Perthes disease: crescent sign. Note the radiolucent subcortical cleft in the superior portion of the femoral capital epiphysis (*arrow*).

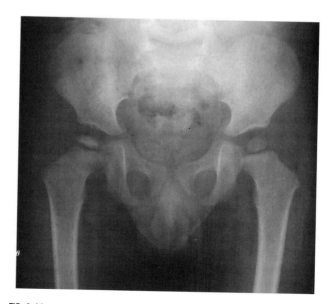

FIG. 4-11 Legg-Calvé-Perthes disease: pediatric. Note the underdevelopment of the affected femoral capital epiphysis (on the reading left), exhibiting dense, homogenous, increased sclerosis.

♦ Ischemic necrosis of the femoral (Fig. 4-12, *A* and *B*) and humeral head (Fig. 4-12, *C* and *D*) may arise as a sequela to corticosteroid therapy, and the radiographic features parallel avascular necrotic disease as a result of other etiologic factors.

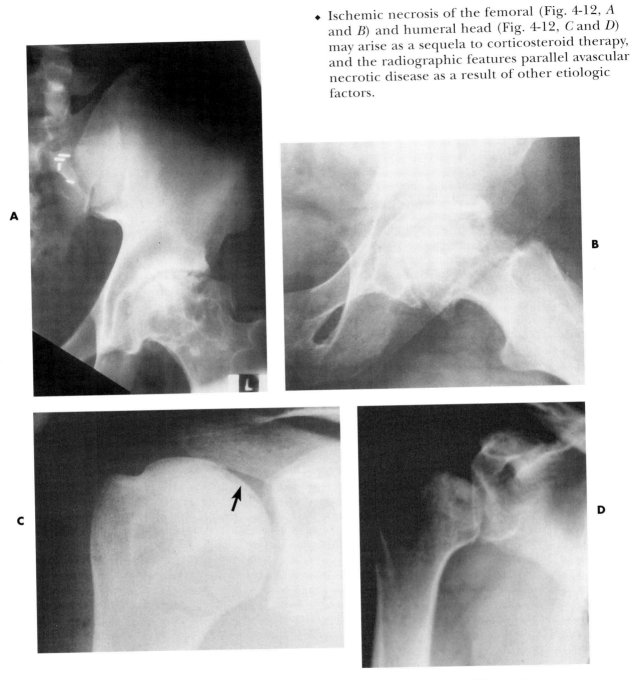

FIG. 4-12 Steroid therapy–induced ischemic necrosis. **A** and **B,** Femoral head. Observe the femoral head collapse, with cortical disruption seen at the lateral head and neck junction. Also note the degenerative arthritic changes (i.e., marked diminution of the joint space and subarticular sclerosis). **C,** Humeral head: crescent sign. Observe the subchondral radiolucent arc (*arrow*), paralleling the contour of the articular cortex. **D,** Humeral head: avascular necrosis. Observe the advancing collapse and fragmentation of the subarticular spongiosa.

Osgood-Schlatter's Disease

- Generally regarded as a traumatically induced force distributed to the tibial tuberosity through the patellar tendon

Clinical Presentation

- Commonly observed in males between the ages of 10 and 15 years
- Bilateral in 25% of patients
- Pain and focal swelling intensified by activity

Radiographic Features

- Soft tissue edema over the tuberosity may displace the infrapatellar fat pad.
- Localized irregularity in the osseous contour and increased density may be observed.
- Single or multiple osseous fragments of the anterior tibial tubercle may be seen (Fig. 4-13, *A-C*).
- Slight to moderate elevation of the inferior aspect of the tubercle may be noted.

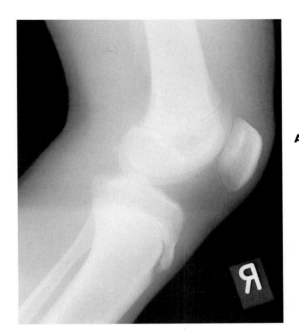

A

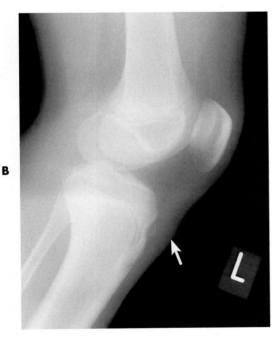

B

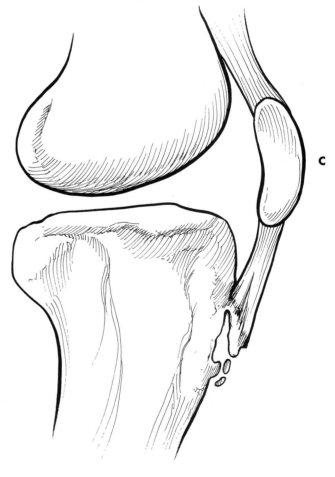

C

FIG. 4-13 Osgood-Schlatter's disease in a 12-year-old boy. **A,** Normal right knee. Observe the normal secondary ossification center of the tibial tuberosity. Although it has not yet completely fused, it has a smooth and regular contour. **B,** Affected left knee. Fragmentation of the secondary ossification center is evident. Soft tissue edema (*arrow*) is observed over the tuberosity. **C,** This diagram depicts the classic fragmentation and avulsion of the tibial tuberosity. (**B** courtesy Brian Kleinberg, DC, Concord, Ontario.)

◆ Marginal irregularity, difference in size, multiple ossicles, elevation, and increased density with lack of clinical findings may represent a normal variant of ossification.

Osteochondritis Dessicans

◆ Characterized by an isolated focus of osseous necrosis, most commonly involving the lateral aspect of the medial condyle of the distal femur
◆ Trauma is postulated as a cause.
◆ There is a gradual separation of a small, semilunar-shaped segment of articular cartilage and subarticular spongiosa, which becomes necrotic and may migrate into the articular cavity, leaving behind a residual subarticular pit.

Clinical Presentation

◆ It occurs most commonly in young males shortly after epiphyseal closure.
◆ About 20% of cases are bilateral.
◆ If a loose body is manifested, periodic attacks of pain and locking during knee extension may occur.
◆ If the fragment remains in situ, the disorder may remain asymptomatic.

Radiographic Features

◆ A narrow crescentic radiolucent cleft may outline an area of articular cartilage and subarticular spongiosa (Fig. 4-14, *A-G*).
◆ If separation of the fragment occurs, a loose body ("joint mouse") will subsequently result, migrating into the articular space and producing a lucent residual subarticular pit in the condyle.
◆ However, the fragment may remain in its cavity, in which case revascularization and reconstitution are promoted.

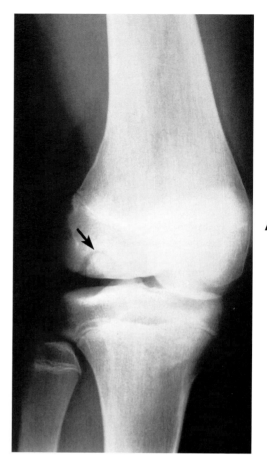

A

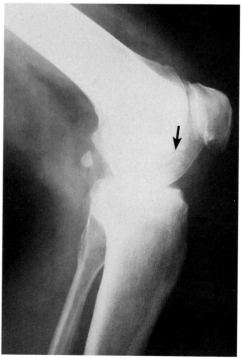

B

FIG. 4-14 Osteochondritis dessicans of the knee. **A** and **B,** Note the crescentic radiolucency (*arrows*) in an unusual location. Lateral femoral condylar involvement possesses an incidence of only 15%. The fragment of articular cartilage and subarticular spongiosa remains in situ.

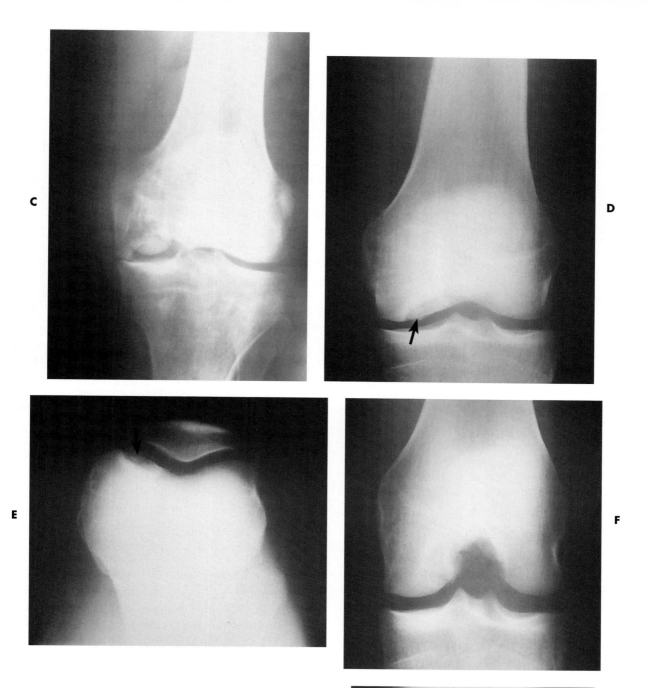

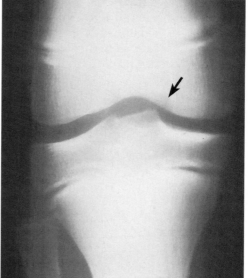

FIG. 4-14, cont'd. **C,** A defect of the lateral aspect of the medial femoral condyle is visualized. **D,** An in situ fragment (*arrow*) is surrounded by a lucent arc in a characteristic site at the lateral aspect of the medial condyle. **E,** Same case. The tangential "skyline" projection demonstrates the nonmigratory status of this fragment (*arrow*). **F,** Same case. Tunnel projections often provide optimal visualization of the necrotic femoral fragment. **G,** The necrotic undisplaced fragment is observed in its characteristic location (*arrow*).

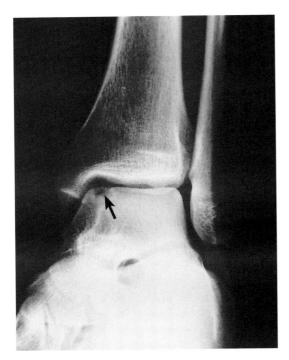

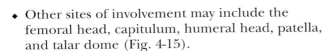

FIG. 4-15 Osteochondritis dessicans of the ankle. Note the in situ osseous fragment at the superomedial aspect of the talar dome (*arrow*). (Courtesy Michel Charbonneau, DC, Montréal, Québec.)

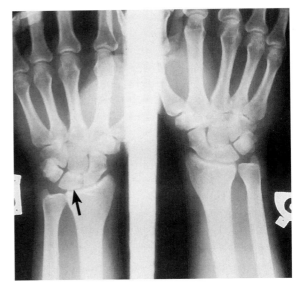

FIG. 4-16 Kienböck's disease. Intraosseous lucencies are observed in the carpal lunate (*arrow*).

- Other sites of involvement may include the femoral head, capitulum, humeral head, patella, and talar dome (Fig. 4-15).

Kienböck's Disease

- Repeated incidents of trauma disrupt the vulnerable vascular supply of the carpal lunate.
- A negative ulnar variance is observed in 75% of patients with this disorder.

Clinical Presentation

- It is most frequently encountered in males between 20 and 40 years of age.
- The right hand is most commonly affected, and a history of long-standing trauma from manual labor is typical.

Radiographic Features

- Small, linear stress fractures or compression fractures may be demonstrated.
- The lunate may exhibit irregular cortical margins, interosseous lucencies (Fig. 4-16), and increased density relative to the other carpal bones.
- Later changes may include fragmentation and lunate collapse (Fig. 4-17).

- Secondary degenerative joint disease of the radiocarpal articulations may ensue.

Freiberg's Disease

- Infarction of the second metatarsal head is attributed to repeated traumatic episodes.
- The third metatarsal head may be affected.

Clinical Presentation

- Prevalence in females between the ages of 13 and 18 years
- Commonly unilateral

Radiographic Features

- Periarticular soft tissue edema results in metatarsophalangeal joint-space widening.
- A focal increase in osseous density may be observed, and the cortical margins may become irregular.
- Subarticular pseudocysts may be displayed.
- Later, fragmentation of the metatarsal head occurs.
- Secondary degenerative joint disease may ensue.
- Healing is usually incomplete, and flattening and irregularity of the head may persist (Figs. 4-18, 4-19, and 4-20).

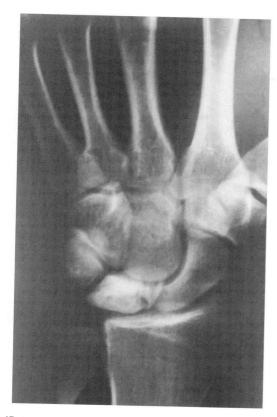

FIG. 4-17 Kienböck's disease. Fragmentation of the carpal lunate with collapse and associated sclerosis is observed in advanced disease.

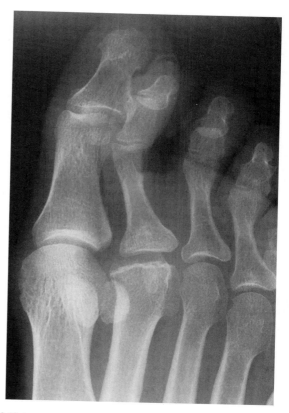

FIG. 4-18 Freiberg's disease. Note the flattened and irregular articular contour of the head of the second metatarsal.

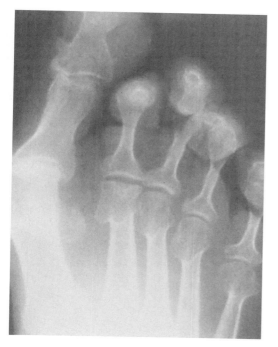

FIG. 4-19 Freiberg's disease. Dorsiplantar view of the head of the second metatarsal exhibits a flattened and irregular articular surface. Note the intact joint space and uninvolved articular surface of the opposing phalanx.

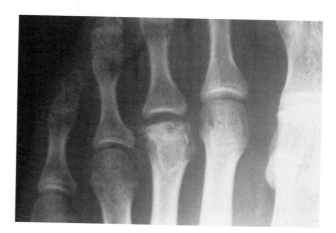

FIG. 4-20 Freiberg's disease. Flattening and pseudocystic formation are evident in the head of the third metatarsal.

Infection

Infection of bone is termed *osteomyelitis*. This disorder is most frequently associated with a bacterial origin, but other pathogens such as fungi, viruses, and parasites have been linked to the formation of osteomyelitis. Various components of the osseous system may be subject to infectious processes.

Infection infiltrating the cortex, or osteitis, may occur as an isolated finding but is more commonly associated with osteomyelitis of the cancellous bone. Osteitis may also be evident in disorders such as Reiter's syndrome, psoriatic arthropathy, and ankylosing spondylitis. Infectious processes occurring in the periosteal portion of bone may result in infective osteitis and proceed to osteomyelitis. With damage to the periosteum, interruption of the blood supply to the cortex can result in its necrosis. The periosteum may become disrupted, leading to adjacent soft tissue suppurative infiltration.

Periostitis may also be observed in neoplastic, inflammatory, metabolic, and traumatic disorders. Infection of parosseous soft tissues may be a direct result of osteomyelitis or a potential source of its formation. Soft tissue infection may arise in the subcutaneous, periarticular, muscular, or fascial structures. Articular infections denote septic states that may arise as isolated foci disseminated from adjacent osseous structures. It uncommonly develops as a complication extending from an adjacent area of osteomyelitis. Joint infection is discussed further in this chapter.

SUPPURATIVE OSTEOMYELITIS

Etiology

◆ Approximately 90% of all bone and joint infection is due to *Staphylococcus aureus*.

FOUR PATHWAYS OF DISSEMINATION

◆ Hematogenous spread—organism reaches distant sites through dissemination in the bloodstream
◆ Contiguous source—infection extends into bone from an adjacent infected site (i.e., cutaneous, sinus, and dental)
◆ Direct implantation—penetrating injuries (i.e., stepping on a nail)
◆ Postoperative—contamination of surgical sites

Clinical Presentation

◆ Most frequent ages from 2 to 12 years
◆ Males predominate
◆ Sites: large tubular bones of extremities (e.g., femur)
◆ High-risk populations
  · Intravenous drug abusers
  · Diabetic patients
  · Patients receiving steroid therapy
  · Hemodialysis patients

Pathogenesis

◆ Infants, children, and adults manifest different presentations as a result of their different vascular anatomy (Fig. 5-1).

INFANTS (UP TO 1 YEAR)

◆ Metaphyseal and diaphyseal vessels can penetrate the forming physis.
◆ Therefore the physis presents no barrier to the spread of infection into the epiphysis and adjacent joint.
◆ This explains the high incidence of septic arthritis in association with infantile osteomyelitis.

CHILDREN (BETWEEN 1 YEAR OF AGE AND TIME OF PHYSEAL FUSION)

◆ Blood flow through the metaphysis is slow and turbulent, establishing a favorable environment for microbial growth.
◆ Epiphysis possesses its own blood supply.
◆ No metaphyseal vessels can penetrate the completed physis, resulting in a predilection for metaphyseal involvement while the epiphysis and adjacent articulation are spared.

INFECTION

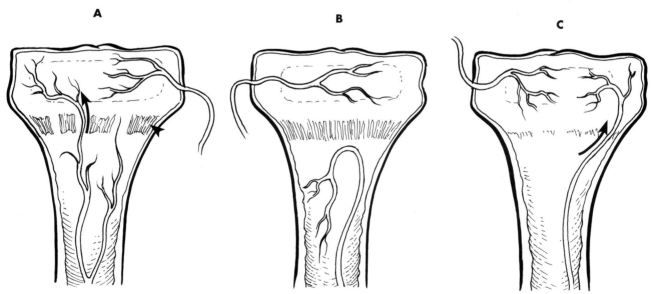

FIG. 5-1 Diagram illustrating the blood supply and the pathogenesis of osteomyelitis. **A,** In infants, metaphyseal and diaphyseal vessels can penetrate (*arrow*) the newly forming physeal plate (*arrowhead*), facilitating the spread of a metaphyseal or diaphyseal infection into the epiphysis and ultimately leading to septic arthritis. **B,** Children possess a fully formed physis, providing an effective barrier that prevents the vascular spread of metaphyseal osteomyelitis into the epiphysis. **C,** In the adult bone, after complete physeal fusion has occurred, metaphyseal vessels can again enter (*arrow*) the epiphysis, promoting subarticular infection and septic arthritis.

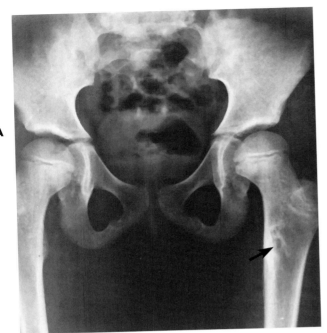
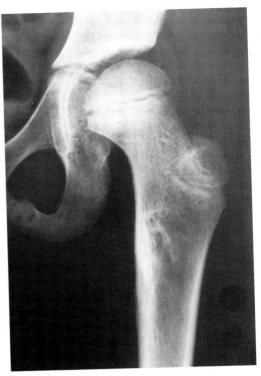

FIG. 5-2 A-D, Suppurative osteomyelitis of the proximal femur. This infection was the result of a biopsy of a nonossifying fibroma. The study follows a 6-month progression of the infection. **A** and **B,** Note the focal radiolucency surrounded by a narrow rim of sclerosis (*arrow*) in the metadiaphysis.

ADULTS

- Physis has fused.
- Metaphyseal vessels can extend as far as the subarticular bone.
- This facilitates the organisms' access to the subarticular bone and joint, resulting in increased incidence of septic arthritis secondary to osteomyelitis in adults.

Hematogenous Osteomyelitis

- The organism establishes a focus in medullary bone, inducing a localized vascular and cellular response (Fig. 5-2, *A-D*).
- Edema causes increased intramedullary pressure, resulting in capillary compression, leading to medullary infarction and necrosis.
- The necrotic bone is referred to as a *sequestrum.*
- The sequestrum can appear quite dense.
- This is actually an illusion; the sequestrum maintains a normal density, while the surrounding bone becomes demineralized (osteopenic) as a consequence of inflammatory hyperemia.
- In addition, the inflammatory hyperemia contains bone-destroying proteolytic enzymes.

- Eventually, the process extends to the endosteum, travelling through the haversian canal system to reach the subperiosteal space and stripping the periosteum from the bone. This then results in periostitis.
- Pus and edema elevate the periosteum, producing a shell of new bone termed the *involucrum* that resembles a thick bony collar. This is the body's attempt to "wall off" the infectious process.
- Chronic osteomyelitis (Fig. 5-3) may form draining sinus tracts referred to as a *cloaca* to allow decompression of internal fluid buildup.

Radiographic Features

- Characteristically, no early plain film findings are observed.
- A radiographic latent period can extend up to 3 weeks.
- With clinical suspicion of infection, a bone scan is warranted, even if plain film examination appears normal.
- A bone scan (bone scintigraphy) is ten times more sensitive than plain film.

- Favors metaphyses of the tibia (Fig. 5-10), femur, and fibula
- A focal abscess representing a lysis of bone surrounded by inflammatory granulation tissue
- Surrounding bone becomes sclerotic (Fig. 5-11)
- Manifests as an ovoid radiolucency with a thick rim of heavy, reactive sclerosis

- A central lucency usually in excess of 1 cm in diameter (osteoid osteoma with a central lucent nidus smaller than 1 cm; may possess a central "target" calcific fleck)
- Except for the size of this radiolucency, radiographically impossible to differentiate Brodie's abscess from osteoid osteoma

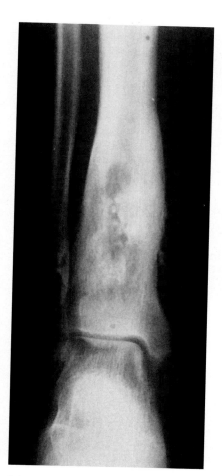

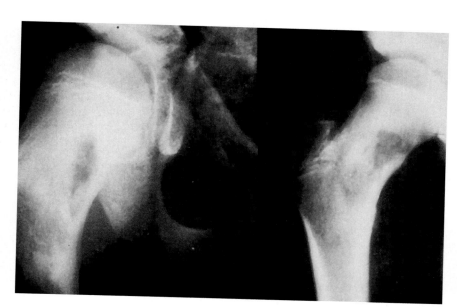

FIG. 5-11 Brodie's abscess of the proximal femur. Observe the dense, homogenous sclerosis surrounding a large, radiolucent nidus.

FIG. 5-10 Brodie's abscess in the distal tibia. Note the large lucent nidus (in excess of 1 cm), surrounded by dense sclerosis in the distal metaphyseal portion of the tibia. This is one of the favored sites of this lesion.

INFECTIOUS ARTHROPATHIES

Tuberculous (Nonsuppurative) Arthritis

- The infectious agent is called *Mycobacterium tuberculosis.*
- It produces a chronic, indolent infection having an insidious onset and a slow, progressive course.
- Prepubertal children are most often affected, but patients of all ages are susceptible.
- Occurrence is frequent in patients from substandard socioeconomic areas and recent immigrants from endemic third-world nations.
- Tuberculous osteomyelitis of long bones is uncommon.
- The spine is favored. However, other potential sites include the knee and hip (limp develops).
- It is usually monoarticular.

Pathophysiology

- Tuberculous arthritis may affect the joint by hematogenous spread or secondarily via invasion of a tuberculous abscess from neighboring bone.
- The organism can lodge in the synovium or adjacent metaphysis.
- This is followed by the proliferation of inflammatory granulation tissue, known as *pannus.*
- Synovitis is the first stage, appearing radiographically as joint distention or pseudowidening (Fig. 5-12, *A* and *B*).
- Pannus interferes with the nutrition of cartilage and results in marginal bone erosions.

- Adjacent bone undergoes marked deossification, with fibrous ankylosis being the ultimate result.

Clinical Presentation

- Skeletal tuberculosis exhibits accelerated progression in children and debilitated geriatric patients.
- Unlike suppurative (pyogenic or septic) osteomyelitis, which has a fairly rapid onset, tuberculous osteomyelitis arises as an insidious chronic infection.
- There is an insidious onset characterized by night sweats, prostration, and an absence of fever.
- Typically, symptoms are produced late in the disease. Pain and tenderness may be the first complaints.
- Tenderness, soft tissue swelling, joint effusion, and increased skin temperature are experienced over the affected joint.
- With progression, muscle contractures may lead to severe range-of-motion limitation, followed by muscle atrophy and deformity.
- A clinical feature that aids in the differential diagnosis is the notable lack of associated inflammatory signs.
- Characteristically, tuberculosis is much more destructive and difficult to control.

Laboratory Analysis

- A Mantoux test and sputum culture (along with chest radiographs) are usually diagnostic for active, primary tuberculosis.

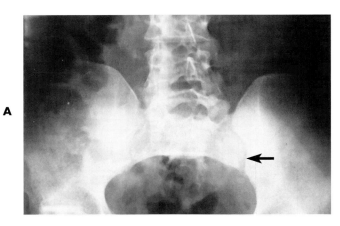
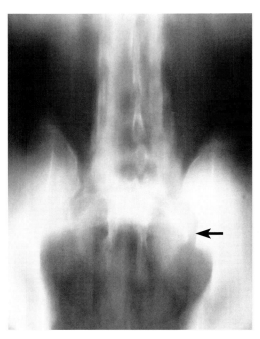

FIG. 5-12 Tuberculosis of the sacroiliac joint. **A,** Joint distention (*arrow*), known as *pseudowidening.* **B,** Tomogram (same patient) demonstrating further evidence of joint pseudowidening (*arrow*).

Radiographic Features

- An x-ray diagnosis may be difficult and often impossible.
- Joint aspiration is definitive.
- The first radiographic finding is one of joint effusion, which is secondary to the synovitis and characterized by initial joint-space widening.
- Granulation tissue (pannus) is produced.
- Articular cartilage becomes destroyed as a result of pannus, and nonuniform destruction of the articular surface produces joint-space narrowing.
- Increased vascularity of this low-grade inflammatory process leads to hyperemic periarticular osteoporosis.
- Osteoporosis is exacerbated by the effect of tuberculous toxins and disuse atrophy.
- The earliest sign of bone destruction is seen as marginal erosions at nonweight-bearing surfaces, resembling features seen in rheumatoid arthritis.
- Sequestra in opposing articular surfaces that are in contact with one another are called *kissing sequestra* and usually surrounded by a zone of reactive sclerosis.
- *Kissing sequestra* is defined as tuberculous involvement of opposing joint surfaces, resulting in extensive sequestered tubercular debris.
- Periosteal reaction is rare (much more common in pyogenic arthritis).
- Further progression of the disease may result in ankylosis, which is fibrous and therefore not visualized radiographically.
- Bony ankylosis is rare, but it is common in pyogenic arthritis.

- The result of long-standing tuberculous arthritis may be gross disorganization of the joint (Fig. 5-13).

PHEMISTER'S TRIAD

- Slow, progressive joint-space narrowing
- Juxta-articular osteoporosis secondary to tuberculous toxin production, hyperemia, and disuse atrophy
- Peripheral marginal erosive defects of articular surfaces (erosions may simulate those observed in rheumatoid arthritis)

Differential Diagnosis

- Osteoporotic compression fracture
  - There is no destruction of bone, only compression of it.
- Tumor
  - Neoplasms may produce paravertebral soft tissue masses. However, intervertebral discs are rarely affected.

Tuberculous Spondylitis (Pott's disease)

- This disease is characterized by the presence of back pain, decreased ranges of motion, and focal tenderness.
- The patient may demonstrate neurologic involvement, especially after vertebral body collapse.
- In children, 70% of the patients are between the ages of 1 and 5 years.
- The duration of symptoms before treatment is 1 to 2 years.
- There is a preference for the thoracic and lumbar spine.

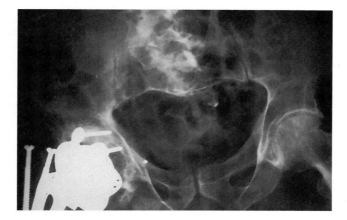

FIG. 5-13 Tuberculosis of the iliofemoral joint. A nonsuppurative arthropathy may result in a gross disorganization of an articulation. This may ultimately require surgical stabilization.

- This disease highly favors the thoracolumbar junction (i.e., L1 is the favored site of involvement).
- Infection extends to the spine from the pulmonary parenchyma via the venous plexus (Fig. 5-14).
- This disease is pathologically identical to suppurative spondylitis, but it is much slower in its progression.
- The earliest focus is the subchondral vertebral end plate because the adult disc is avascular.

- The area of involvement undergoes caseous necrosis, which becomes radiographically visible as a lytic lesion in 2 to 5 months.
- The weakened and collapsing vertebral end plate allows the infection to spread to the disc via direct extension (Fig. 5-15).
- This extension of the infection into the disc slowly destroys the cartilage, resulting in a visible loss of disc height.
- With progression, vertebral end plates and eventually the body are destroyed (Figs. 5-16, 5-17, and 5-18).

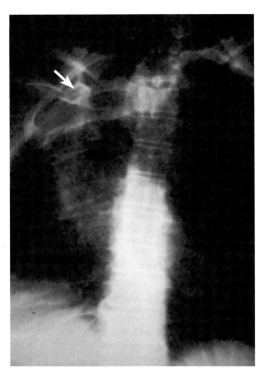

FIG. 5-14 Tuberculosis of the lung. A classic Ghon lesion is observed unilaterally in the apical parenchyma (*arrow*). Note the ipsilateral tracheal deviation secondary to fibroadhesive traction. Primary disease may spread to spinal structures as a result of hematogenous extension.

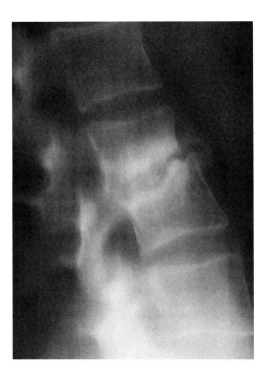

FIG. 5-15 Tuberculosis of the spine. The infection fails to respect intervertebral cartilage, permitting contiguous vertebral body destruction.

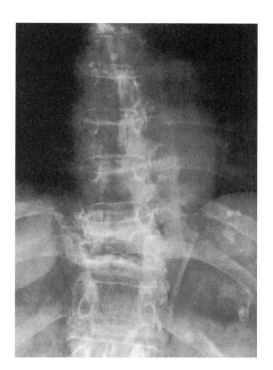

FIG. 5-16 An anteroposterior view of the thoracolumbar junction in a patient with a known paraspinal tuberculous abscess. Note the loss of height of the T10 and T11 vertebral bodies, as well as the marked bony sclerosis. These findings suggest a relatively chronic destructive process. (From Andersson BJ, Thomas W: *Lumbar spinal stenosis*, St Louis, 1992, Mosby.)

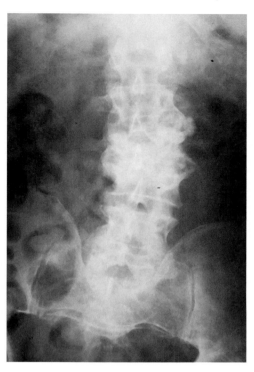

FIG. 5-17 Tuberculosis of the lumbar spine. Observe the midlumbar vertebral body collapse in progressive disease.

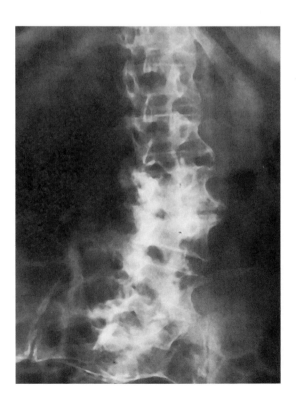

FIG. 5-18 Tuberculosis of the lumbar spine demonstrating nonpyogenic vertebral body collapse.

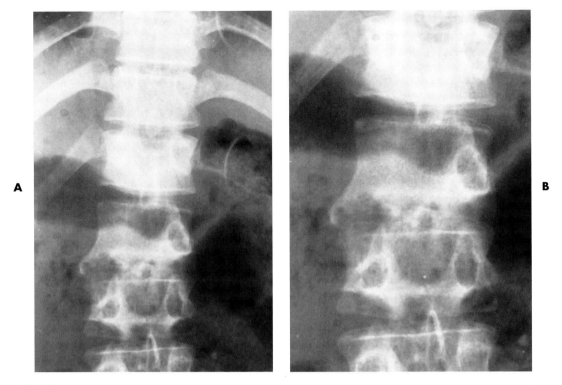

FIG. 5-19 Tuberculosis of the lumbar spine. **A,** Osteolysis of the L1 pedicle reveals extension of the disease into the neural arch. This occurs in only 2% to 4% of cases. **B,** Enhanced view of the same case.

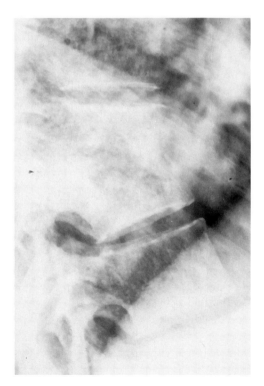

FIG. 5-20 Tuberculosis of the thoracic spine. Note the complete eradication of the disc space, leading to vertebral collapse.

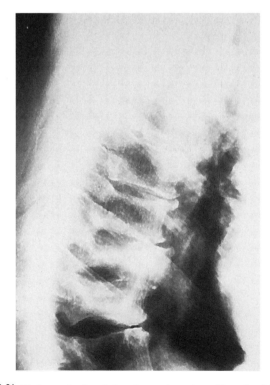

FIG. 5-21 Tuberculosis of the thoracic spine. Vertebral body collapse results in a mild gibbus formation.

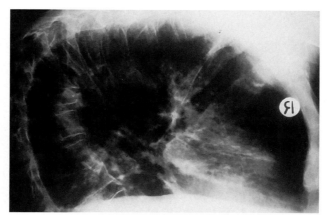

FIG. 5-22 Tuberculosis of the spine. Vertebral body collapse and subsequent severe gibbus deformity in this patient is the result of advanced infectious tuberculous spondylitis.

♦ Infection extends to the posterior vertebral elements in only 2% to 4% of patients (Fig. 5-19, *A* and *B*).

♦ Because the arches and articular processes are not generally affected, collapse of the body occurs anteriorly to a large extent (Fig. 5-20).

♦ Progressive vertebral collapse and disc disintegration result in severe spinal deformity (i.e., wedging with angular kyphosis, termed *gibbus deformity* (Figs. 5-21 and 5-22).

♦ A long-standing gibbus may result in a reversal of the height-width ratio of the uninvolved vertebral body immediately caudal to the gibbus as a result of tremendous biomechanical stress on that body. This is termed *long vertebra* (meaning the vertebra is taller than it is wide).

♦ A granulomatous abscess formation around the affected area may be visualized.

♦ This formation is normally unilateral and most frequently appears in the thoracic spine as a fusiform, paraspinal, soft tissue density.

PARASPINAL SOFT TISSUE INVOLVEMENT

Abscess formation

♦ Cervical spine
  • Increased retropharyngeal interspace (normal <7 mm)
  • Increased retrotracheal interspace (normal <21 mm)

♦ Thoracic spine
  • Unilateral, fusiform, soft tissue shadow represents a necrotizing, large anterolateral mass, the cold abscess, which indicates inactivity of the infectious process.
  • Displaces paraspinal line

♦ Lumbar spine
  • Anterolateral extension of a cold abscess to the psoas muscles (psoas abscess characterized by destructive, caseous granular necrotic debris that may be unilateral or bilateral; often a site for the precipitation of calcium salts manifesting in amorphous calcification)
  • Formation of draining sinuses from the abscess facilitated along fascial planes or muscle sheaths

Subligamentous dissection (rare)

♦ Massive and extensive paraspinal abscess formation with little osseous involvement

♦ Disc spaces spared as infection spreads contiguously beneath the anterior longitudinal ligament extending from one anterior vertebral body to another

♦ May result in anterior "gouge defects" as a consequence of pressure erosions simulating effects of an aortic aneurysm (i.e., Oppenheimer defect)

♦ Later stages characterized by disc-space narrowing and vertebral body collapse

Pott's paraplegia (rare)

♦ Observed in advanced spinal tuberculosis

♦ Represents a life-threatening complication

♦ Characterized by multiple vertebral body collapse with intervening disc disintegration

♦ Stimulates massive granulation tissue production

♦ This granulation tissue, along with vertebral body fragments, can sufficiently narrow the spinal canal to produce a pressure paraplegia.

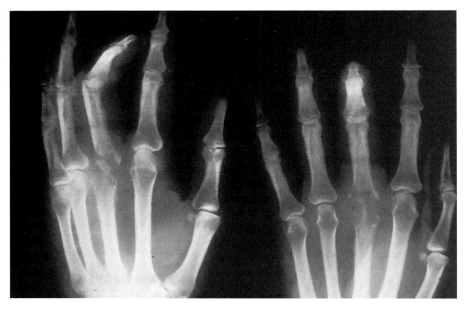

FIG. 5-23 Septic arthritis of the third metacarpophalangeal articulation. Destruction of the opposing articular surfaces and intervening joint space can be seen with associated adjacent soft tissue edema.

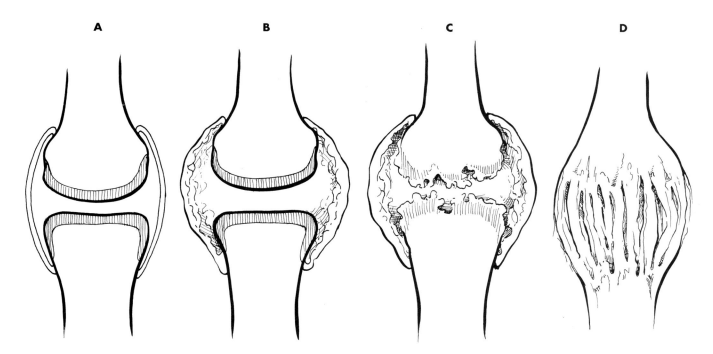

FIG. 5-24 Diagram illustrating the progression of septic arthritis. **A,** A normal joint, demonstrating synovial membrane and articular cartilage. **B,** Initial inflammation causes widening of the joint space and distension of the synovium and joint capsule. **C,** Articular cartilage and subchondral bone destruction occurs with the advancing inflammatory infectious process. **D,** Complete osseous ankylosis across the former joint space is a possible endstage result.

Pyogenic (Septic, Infectious) Arthritis

♦ Infection of a joint by pyogenic organisms may be produced by a blood-borne infection, compound injuries, surgical procedures performed on a joint, or direct extension into a joint from a focus of osteomyelitis adjacent to it.
♦ Pyogenic arthritis is usually monoarticular.
♦ It is most commonly observed in the knee, hip, and third metacarpophalangeal joint (Fig. 5-23).
♦ Most arthritic infections are due to *Staphylococcus aureus,* which is isolated by culture from the synovial aspirate.

Pathophysiology

♦ The organism lodges in the metaphysis because of its high vascularity.
♦ The organism spreads hematogenously to the vasculature of the synovial membrane.
♦ Entry into the joint results in soft tissue swelling and distention of the joint capsule by edema.
♦ Capsular distention ensues as a result of purulent exudate. The exudate interferes with cartilage nutrition, resulting in death of chondrocytes, producing a release of proteolytic enzymes, which result in progressive destruction of cartilage and bone (Figs. 5-24, 5-25, and 5-26).
♦ This may lead to joint dislocation.
♦ Eventually, if the articular cartilage is completely destroyed, bony ankylosis ensues (Fig. 5-27).

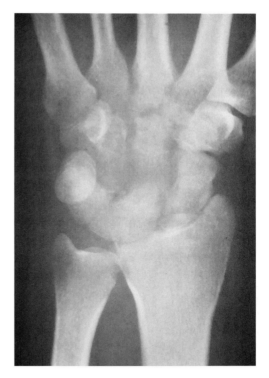

FIG. 5-26 Septic arthritis of the wrist. Advancing carpal involvement manifests as resorption, irregular osseous contours, and erosion of the metacarpal bases.

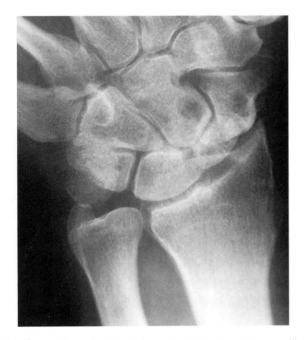

FIG. 5-25 Septic arthritis of the wrist. The "spotty carpal" sign, consisting of focal lucencies scattered throughout several carpals, denotes early wrist infection.

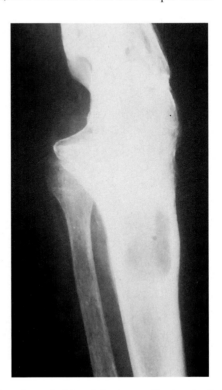

FIG. 5-27 Septic arthritis of the knee. End-stage infectious arthritis results in complete osseous ankylosis. Trabecular and cortical bone traverse and replace the joint space. Note the surgical excision of the patella.

Clinical Presentation

- Pyogenic arthritis presents with an acute onset, which results in pain, tenderness, swelling and redness, decreased ranges of motion, and constitutional symptoms such as fever and leukocytosis.

Laboratory Analysis

- The most common organisms involved are *Staphylococcus aureus* (90%), *Neisseria gonorrhoeae,* and *Streptococcus pneumoniae.*
- In children, *Streptococcus pyogenes* can be implicated.
- The organisms are usually isolated by a culture from pus following a joint fluid aspirate.

Radiographic Features

- The early stage is characterized by soft tissue swelling, joint capsular distention, displacement, and later, obliteration of juxta-articular fat planes. This is particularly apparent in the hip joint, where obliteration of the fat lines for obturator internus, iliopsoas, and gluteus medius is seen (Fig. 5-28).

- Abscess formation develops as a result of pus accumulation in adjacent soft tissues. This produces an increase in soft tissue density around the joint.
- Destruction of the articular cartilages invariably results in joint-space narrowing.

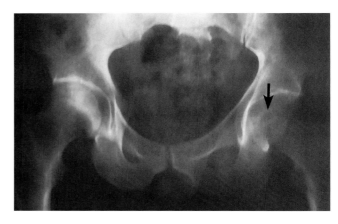

FIG. 5-29 Early septic arthritis of the hip exhibits a loss of the normal subchondral cortical white line (*arrow*).

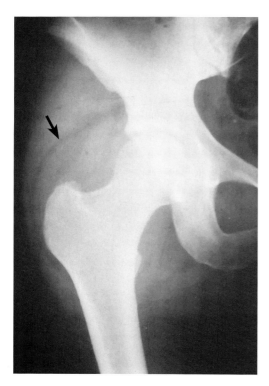

FIG. 5-28 Early infection demonstrates the displacement of the gluteus medius fat plane (*arrow*).

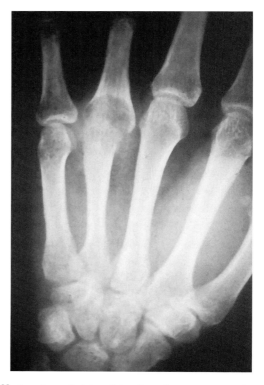

FIG. 5-30 Septic arthritis of the fourth metacarpophalangeal joint. Observe the complete destruction of the opposing articular surfaces and intervening joint space, with accompanying adjacent soft tissue edema.

♦ Early bone destruction is demonstrated at the capsular ligamentous-bone interface.

♦ There is an early loss of the normal subchondral cortical white line (Fig. 5-29). This is accompanied by an adjacent medullary metaphyseal "moth-eaten" pattern.

♦ A complete resorption of the articulating ends of long bones may ensue (Fig. 5-30).

♦ Juxta-articular osteoporosis arises as a consequence of regional hyperemia and disuse.

♦ As the infection subsides, articular surfaces may be remodelled, but there is usually some degree of residual articular deformity.

♦ The duration of these pathologic processes is brief compared with the extended time of progression attributed to nonsuppurative, granulomatous (tuberculous) arthritis.

♦ Healing may result in an irregular articular surface, or if the articular cartilages are completely destroyed, osseous ankylosis usually follows.

Differential Diagnosis

♦ Tuberculous arthritis (Table 5-1), gout, pigmented villonodular synovitis, hemophilia, and Reiter's syndrome should be considered.

TABLE 5-1
Differential Diagnosis of Pyogenic Versus Tuberculous Arthritis

	Pyogenic	Tuberculosis
Latent period	Short (7-10 days)	Extended (4-12 weeks)
Osteoporosis	Minimal, local	Advanced, generalized
Cartilage destruction	Weight-bearing areas	Nonweight-bearing areas (marginal erosions)
Ankylosis	Osseous	Fibrous
Most common sites	Knee, hip, third metacarpophalangeal joint	Spine, hip

INFECTION

Trauma

OUTLINE

Traumatic lesions of the skeleton are everyday occurrences for individuals of all ages. A fracture is created by force that has been directly applied to the bone at the site of the fracture (Fig. 6-1, *A*) or transmitted indirectly through some other portion of the body (Fig. 6-1, *B*), resulting in a fracture at a point remote from application of the force. If any doubt exists regarding the presence of a fracture, radiographs should be obtained. In addition to misdiag-

nosis of the patient, severe medicolegal implications may be encountered if fractures are overlooked.

Successful treatment of fractures starts with an accurate diagnosis, which requires a well-performed and accurately interpreted radiographic examination. Any examination of less than two radiographs at 90 degrees to each other is considered incomplete. Once a fracture is identified, the clinician should assess the remainder of the radiograph for

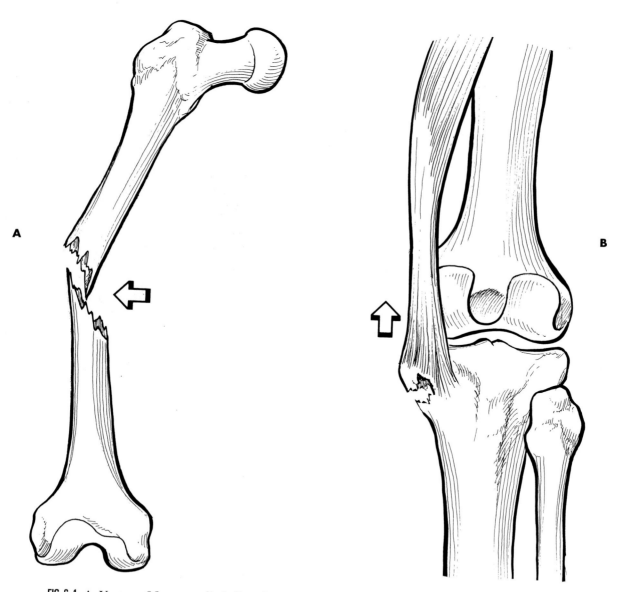

FIG. 6-1 A, Vector of force applied directly to an osseous structure, resulting in its fracture. **B,** Vector of force transmitted through tendons or ligaments, resulting in an indirect bone fracture.

additional signs of trauma. A minority of cases harbor a second finding that is often as clinically relevant as, or even more than, the initial finding.

Before a discussion of fractures specific to various region of the body, the following general information is presented: types of fractures, fracture orientation, spatial relationships of fractures, traumatic joint disruptions, fracture repair, complications, interpretation of radiographs in the evaluation of fracture healing, and guidelines for determining whether a fracture is old or new.

TYPES OF FRACTURES

Open

- Penetrates the skin over the fracture (Fig. 6-2)
- At one time was termed a *compound fracture*

Closed

- Does not break the skin (Fig. 6-3)
- At one time was termed a *simple fracture*

Comminuted

- Three or more bony fragments (Fig. 6-4, *A* and *B*)

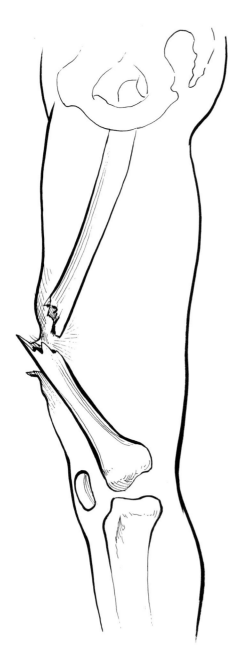

FIG. 6-2 An open, or compound, fracture. Note the bone fragment penetrating the skin surface.

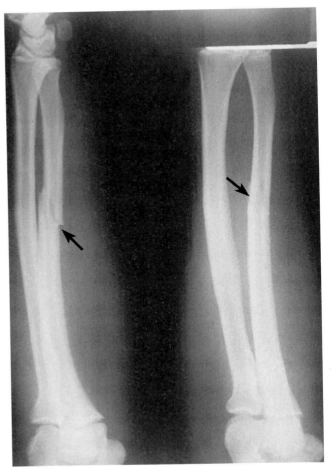

FIG. 6-3 A simple fracture of the ulna (*arrows*), whereby the overlying skin remains intact.

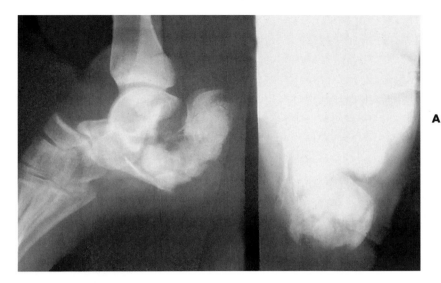

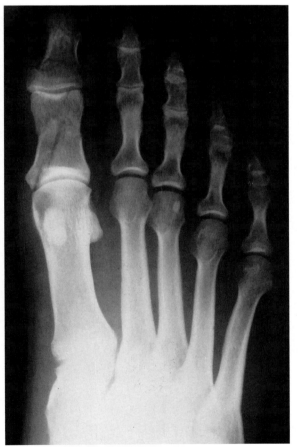

FIG. 6-4 **A,** A comminuted fracture exhibits more than two osseous fragments, as observed in these lateral and tangential views of the calcaneus. Note the talocalcaneal dislocation as well. **B,** Comminuted fracture of the first proximal phalanx.

Noncomminuted

- Penetrates completely through the bone, separating it into two fragments

Avulsion

- Tearing away of a portion of the bone by a forceful muscular or ligamentous traction (Fig. 6-5)
- Frequent sites: tuberosities of tubular bones and lower cervical spinous processes

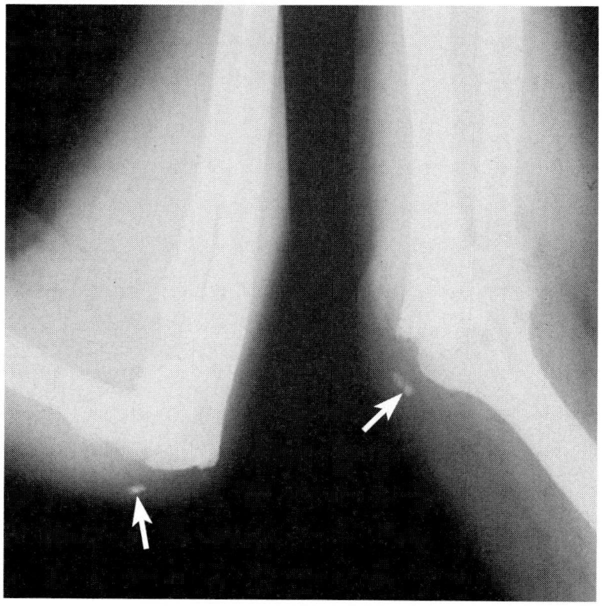

Impaction

- A portion of bone is "driven" into its adjacent segment (Fig. 6-6).
- Because of the compressive forces, the radiolucent fracture line is seldom visualized; instead, a subtle radiopaque white line may be seen in the region of impaction.
- A common example of an impaction fracture is the traumatic telescoping of the humeral diaphysis into the humeral head after severe axial compression loading.

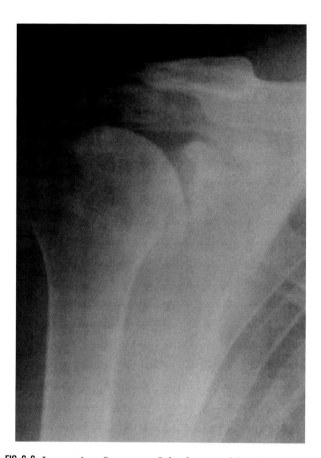

FIG. 6-5 Note the avulsive fragmentation of the triceps tendinous insertion. This occurs as a consequence of a forceful muscular or ligamentous action tearing away a portion of bone, as seen in the anteroposterior and lateral views of the elbow (*arrows*).

FIG. 6-6 Impaction fracture of the humeral head.

Compression

- This fracture occurs primarily in the spine after a forceful hyperflexion injury.
- The vertebral end plates are driven toward each other, creating compression of the intervening spongy bone (Fig. 6-7).
- This fracture may result in a gibbus deformity.

Incomplete

- Osseous disruption of only one side of the bone, resulting in buckling or bending of the bone
- Angular deformity common; however, no displacement expected

Examples of Incomplete Fractures

GREENSTICK FRACTURE

- This type of fracture occurs primarily in infants and children under the age of 10 as a result of the relatively greater component of pliable woven bone (Fig. 6-8, *A* and *B*).
- The bone is permitted to bend rather than snap, thus demonstrating a disruption of the cortex on only one side.
- The affected bone bends like a green twig.
- Greenstick fractures heal without any complication in most instances.

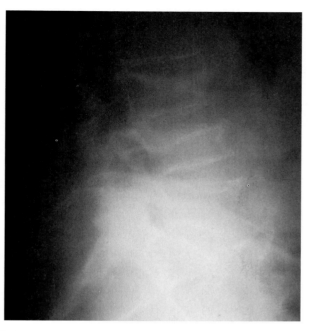

FIG. 6-7 Vertebral end plates are driven toward each other, producing a compression fracture of the intervening spongy bone. This usually follows a forceful hyperflexion injury of the spine. L3 and L4 are affected in this patient.

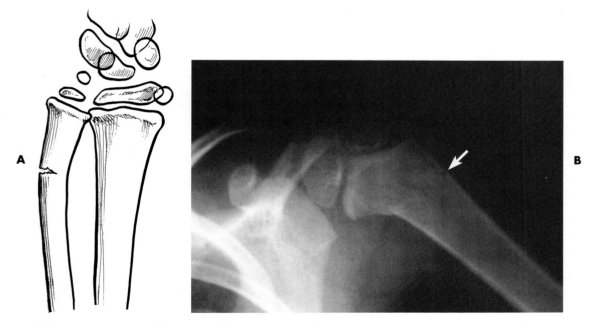

FIG. 6-8 A, A greenstick fracture of the ulna. Note the incomplete fracture causing a gapping on the convex aspect of the distal ulnar diaphysis. **B,** This 3-year-old girl sustained a greenstick fracture after falling off a swing at the playground. Note the lucent line (*arrow*), which partially traverses the proximal humeral metadiaphysis. The cortex at the site of the fracture demonstrates a mild convexity.

TRAUMA

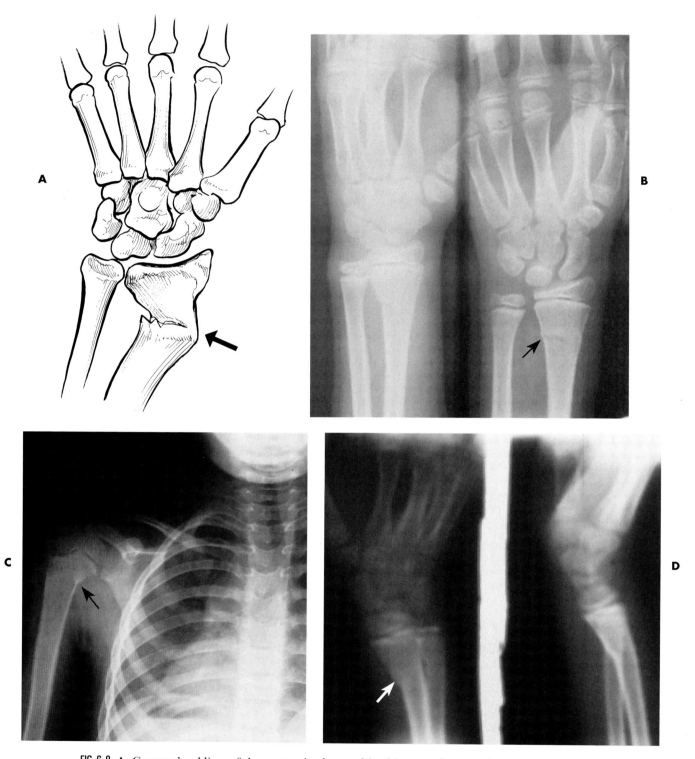

FIG. 6-9 **A,** Convex buckling of the cortex is observed in this torus fracture (*arrow*). **B,** Buckling of the cortex results in a torus-type fracture, as seen in the distal metaphysis of the radius (*arrow*). **C,** This torus fracture of the proximal humerus demonstrates cortical buckling (*arrow*). **D,** Disruption of the bony cortex is seen on the palmar aspect of the radius (*arrow*) and results in a torus fracture of the distal metaphysis.

TORUS FRACTURE

- The term *torus* is derived from the Latin root meaning "to bulge."
- The appearance has been likened to the lip or bulge at the base of a Greek column or pillar.
- This is a buckling of the cortex through forces applied to the long axis of the bone (Fig. 6-9, *A-C*).
- Most of these fractures occur in the metaphysis and are extremely painful.

Infraction

- One example is a central end-plate compression fracture (Fig. 6-10).

Chip

- Variety of avulsion fracture
- Consists of the separation of a small chip of bone from the corner of a phalanx, other tubular bone, or vertebral body (Fig. 6-11)

Pathologic

- Represents a fracture through a bone weakened by a localized or systemic disease process
- Pathologic fractures usually transverse and often demonstrate smooth, opposing fracture surfaces

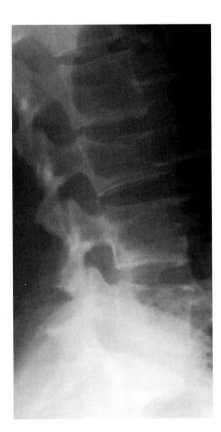

FIG. 6-10 Central infraction of the midsuperior vertebral end plate of L3 is observed in a 20-year-old woman.

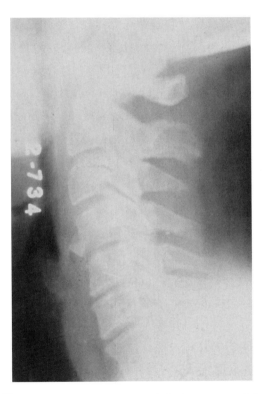

FIG. 6-11 An avulsion of the anteroinferior aspect of the C4 vertebral body resulting in a chip, or "teardrop," fracture.

TRAUMA

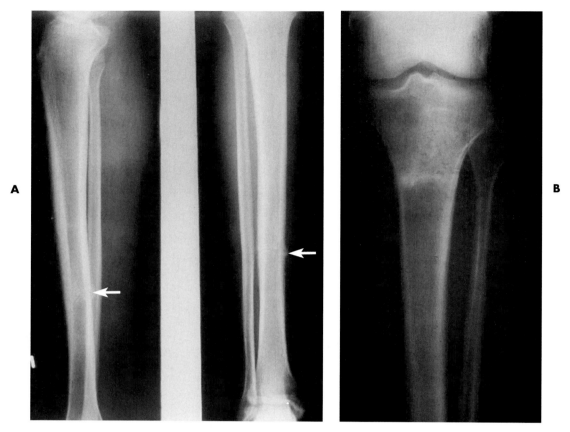

FIG. 6-12 A, Repetitive stress on a bone may result in its microfracture (*arrows*). This has been termed a *fatigue,* or *insufficiency, fracture.* **B,** Stress fractures of the posterior proximal metaphyseal region of the tibia are not uncommon. The horizontal sclerotic line observed in this tibia is highly suggestive of this phenomenon.

Stress

- This fracture is produced by repetitive stress, causing the gradual formation of microfractures and eventually an interruption in the bone structure at a greater rate than can be offset by the reparative process (Fig. 6-12, *A* and *B*).
- It represents an actual fatigue failure of the bone.
- A contemporary synonym for a stress fracture is an insufficiency fracture.

Occult

- This fracture contributes clinical signs of its presence in the absence of any radiologic evidence.
- A serial radiologic examination, usually within 7 to 10 days, often reveals resorption of bone at the fracture site.
- Bone radioisotope studies are frequently necessary to demonstrate the presence of these fractures.

- Bleeding within the bone secondary to trauma (bone edema) may be appreciated by a magnetic resonance imaging (MRI) evaluation, documenting the relative age of the trauma.

Pseudofracture

- This is not a true fracture.
- Histologically, pseudofractures are discrete regions of uncalcified osteoid caused by a variety of etiologies.
- Radiographically, they appear as linear lucencies on the convex surface of the bone, oriented at 90 degrees to the long axis of the diaphysis.
- Pseudofractures are discovered in association with bone-softening diseases such as Paget's disease, rickets, osteomalacia, and fibrous dysplasia.
- Various synonyms have been applied to pseudofractures, including Looser's lines, Milkman's syndrome, and umbau zonen.

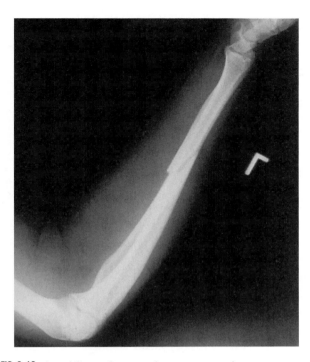

FIG. 6-13 An oblique fracture is seen traversing a course of approximately 45 degrees to the long axis of an otherwise healthy long bone.

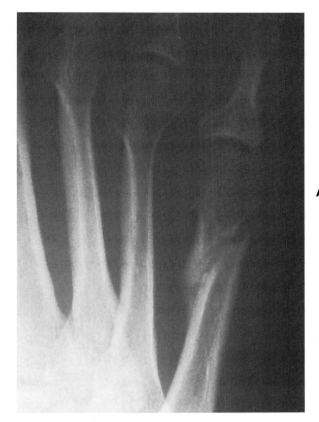

A

B

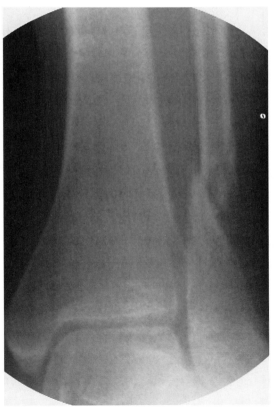

ORIENTATION

Oblique Fracture

- This fracture traverses the bone at approximately 45 degrees to the long axis of the diaphysis (Fig. 6-13).
- It is a common fracture.

Spiral Fracture

- Torsional forces create a spiral fracture (Fig. 6-14, *A* and *B*).
- The ends of a spiral fracture are pointed like a pen because of its circumferential involvement of the bone diaphysis, resembling a spiral staircase.

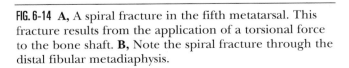

FIG. 6-14 **A,** A spiral fracture in the fifth metatarsal. This fracture results from the application of a torsional force to the bone shaft. **B,** Note the spiral fracture through the distal fibular metadiaphysis.

Transverse Fracture

- This fracture is oriented at a right angle to the long axis of a bone (Fig. 6-15, *A* and *B*).
- It is uncommon through healthy bone (except pediatric) but is observed in diseased bone (pathologic fracture).
- An example of this type of fracture is the "banana" transverse pathologic facture associated with Paget's disease.

SPATIAL RELATIONSHIPS OF FRACTURES

- Position of the fragments
  - The relationship of fracture fragments must be accurately described in the x-ray report.

Alignment

- The alignment of a fracture is described as the position of the distal fragment in relation to the proximal fragment.
- Fractures are in optimal alignment when there is no perceptible angulation in anteroposterior and lateral projections (Fig. 6-16, *A* and *B*).

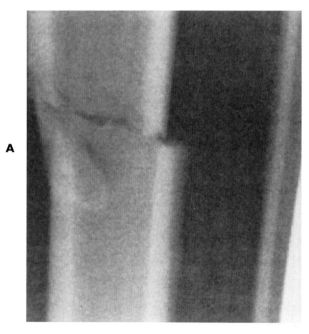

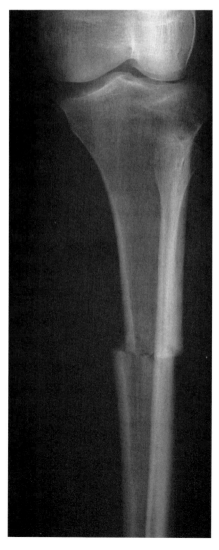

FIG. 6-15 A, A transverse fracture is oriented at a right angle to the long axis of a bone. **B,** A transverse fracture exhibits the characteristic perpendicular orientation to the long axis of the diaphysis.

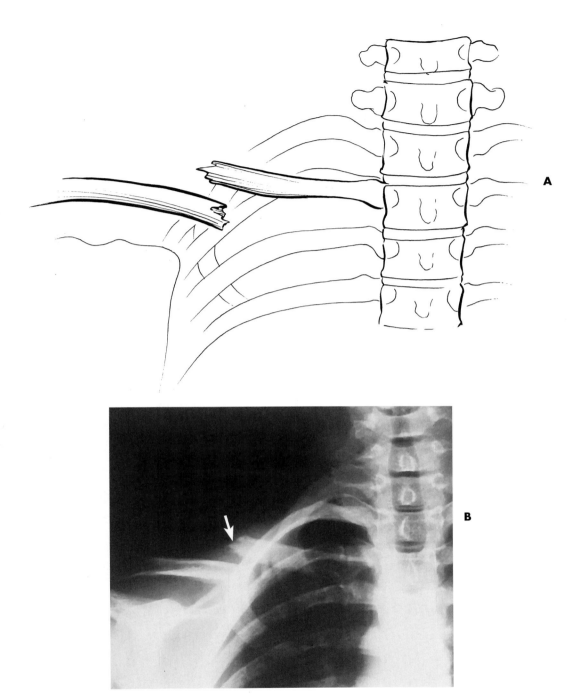

FIG. 6-16 A, Poorly aligned fracture fragments. **B,** A poorly aligned clavicular fracture (*arrow*).

Apposition

- The appositional state of the fracture site concerns the proximity of fracture fragments (Fig. 6-17).
- Acceptable apposition is denoted by near-complete surface contact of the fractured fragments.
- *Partial apposition* refers to partial osseous fragment contact.

Rotation

- Twisting forces on a fractured bone located circumferentially around its longitudinal axis produce rotational deformity (Fig. 6-18).
- Inclusion of the proximal and distal joints on the examination is necessary in determining rotation malposition.

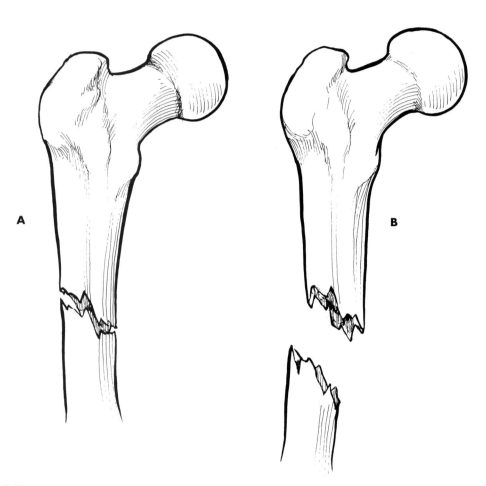

FIG. 6-17 A, Adequate fracture apposition. **B,** Poor apposition of the fracture.

TRAUMATIC JOINT DISRUPTIONS

Subluxation

- Subluxation arises when partial loss of contact occurs between the usual articular surface components of a joint.
- The joint surfaces are incongruous, but a portion remains apposed (Fig. 6-19).

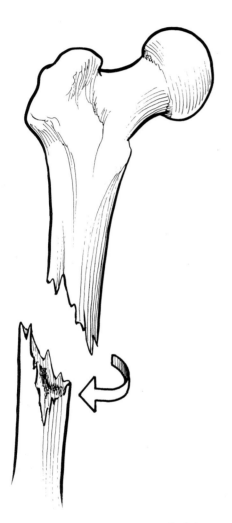

FIG. 6-18 Torsional forces that cause a spiral fracture.

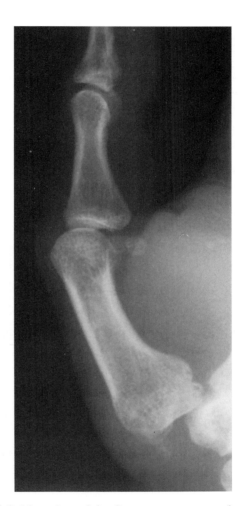

FIG. 6-19 Subluxation of the first carpometacarpal articulation.

Dislocation

- *Dislocation* refers to a complete loss of contact between the surfaces of a joint (Fig. 6-20).
- When associated with a fracture, this type of displacement is referred to as a *fracture-dislocation.*
- In the extremities a dislocated bone is always described in relation to the proximal bone.

Diastasis

- Diastasis represents displacement or frank separation of a slightly movable joint (syndesmosis).
- Examples include separations of the symphysis pubis (Fig. 6-21, *A* and *B*) and sutures of the skull.
- A separated skull suture may be referred to as a *diastatic fracture.*

FRACTURE REPAIR

Phases of Healing

CIRCULATORY (INFLAMMATORY) PHASE

- This phase is characterized by varying amounts of serous and/or sanguinous edema (hematoma) as a consequence of a rupture of vasculature and subsequent hemostasis.
- Tissue may be destroyed directly by the force of the injury or indirectly by devascularization secondary to the disruption of blood supply.
- Periosteal cells adjacent to the fracture site become activated and secrete a matrix around themselves that "elevates" the periosteum.
- The products of tissue necrosis incite an inflammatory reaction, hence the term *inflammatory phase.*
- This phase persists for 7 to 10 days after trauma.
- The earliest radiographic manifestation of repair is widening of the fracture line and blurring of

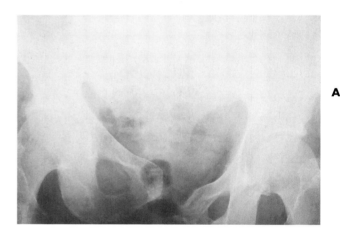

A

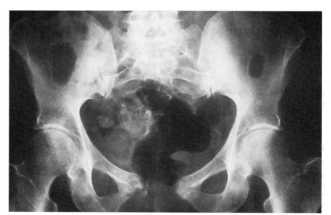

B

FIG. 6-20 Complete anteroinferior glenohumeral joint dislocation.

FIG. 6-21 A and **B,** Separation, or diastasis, of the symphysis pubis. The width of this joint space should never exceed 6 mm in women or 7 mm in men.

the apposing margins of the fracture fragments as a result of resorption of dead bone.

VASCULAR PHASE

- The next 10 days are characterized by a proliferation of capillary formation adjacent to the fracture site.
- Trauma in the muscle and stripping of the periosteum may also add to the initial fracture hematoma.
- This phase usually occurs within 10 to 14 days.

PRIMARY CALLUS (FIBROUS, FLUFFY, IMMATURE CALLUS) PHASE

- Callus is the plastic exudate and tissue that develops around the ends of the fracture fragments, ultimately uniting them.
- Cellular elements arise from injured bone, connective tissue, marrow, and muscle to form undifferentiated mesenchymal cells, representing the onset of a fibrous callus formation.

- Granulation tissue evolves from the replacement of the hematoma by undifferentiated mesenchymal cells, which serve as the precursor to the formation of the primary callus.

SECONDARY CALLUS (OSSEOUS, DENSE, MATURE CALLUS) PHASE

- High-speed deposition of osteoid occurs in the form of coarsely woven bone, deposited in a haphazard fashion in the area of the fracture.
- This osteoid subsequently organizes and mineralizes.
- The earliest radiographic visualization occurs after 14 days.
- Radiographically, callus fills the medullary cavity and arises from the marrow to "seal" it from the fracture site.
- Callus unites the gap between the two fracture ends and joins the cortical portions of the fractured bone (Fig. 6-22, *A* and *B*).

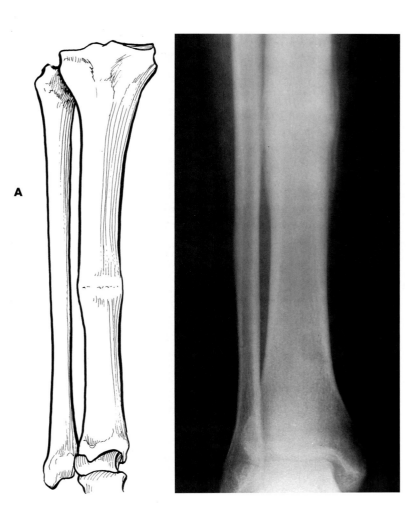

A

B

FIG. 6-22 A, Complete union of a fracture of the tibial diaphysis. Note the negligible deformity of the contour, denoting an optimal fracture-site union. **B,** Fracture of the tibial shaft demonstrating near-complete healing. A mild convexity of the cortex is visualized at the site of union and is a result of callus.

TRAUMA

- A clinical union is achieved when the callus is sufficiently developed to allow weight-bearing or normal stresses.
- The extent of the callus is roughly proportional to the amount of separation, or gap, between the fragments; the greater the gap, the more exuberant the eventual callus.
- Impacted fractures develop minimal peripheral callus.

REMODELLING PHASE

- This is the final phase in fracture repair involving the realignment and remodeling of bone and callus along lines of stress.
- Extra bone is deposited in stress lines and removed in areas in which stress is not applied (Wolff's law).
- The final stage of fracture healing is the restoration of the medullary cavity and bone marrow.
- The woven bone of the callus is eventually replaced by bone oriented along lines of stress.
- Distinct cortical bone and medullary cancellous bone develop at the site of the fracture and gradually remodel to form an outline similar to that of the bone before the fracture.
- In time, the bone may remodel to such a degree that no evidence exists of the previous fracture. This occurs frequently in children and adolescents but less commonly in adults.
- Mild residual deformity may be present.

Fracture Union

- The clinical union of fracture fragments occurs via the sufficient growth of bone across the fracture line. This occurs even before radiographic evidence of the fracture line is obliterated.
- The union is therefore best determined via clinical means.
- The clinical indications of fracture healing are stability, as determined by physical examination, lack of pain at the fracture site, and the ability to use the part without external support (i.e., in a fracture of the lower extremity, the ability to walk without a cast, crutch, or cane).
- The radiographic evidence of a union consists of a continuous external bridge of callus across the line of fracture uniting the fracture fragments.
- The callus is uniformly ossified and approaches the density of normal bone.
- These findings must be present on at least two projections taken at 90 degrees to each other.
- The time required for the clinical union of an uncomplicated fracture varies chiefly with the age of the individual and the bone involved.

- In an adult, 3 to 4 weeks may be required for the union of a fracture of the clavicle, 6 to 8 weeks for the humeral shaft, 10 to 12 weeks for the tibial shaft, and 12 to 14 weeks for the femoral shaft.
- However, in a young child a femoral shaft fracture may heal within a month, and fractures at other sites may heal more quickly.

Factors Influencing the Rate of Repair

- Not all fractures heal at the same rate.
- Many factors influence the time required for healing. Chief among them are the degree of local trauma, age of the patient, and vascularity of the fracture fragments.
- The capacity for healing decreases with age.
- A fracture of the shaft of the femur in an infant unites in 1 month, in an adolescent in 2 months, and in a 50-year-old man in 3 to 4 months.
- Healing varies in direct proportion to the degree of vascularity of the fracture fragments.
- In general, a greater blood supply exists in the metaphysis than in the diaphysis. Therefore healing is usually faster near the end of the bone than in the shaft.
- The loss of bone or separation of fragments, creating a gap in the fracture, results in significantly slower healing because the gap must be refilled with new bone.
- Gaps created by continued excessive traction also result in retardation of healing.
- A principal cause of slow fracture healing is inadequate immobilization.
- Motion injures the tissues involved in the reparative process and prolongs the time required to achieve a union.
- The motion may be caused by inadequate external immobilization, such as a short or loose cast.

COMPLICATIONS OF FRACTURE

- Complications include nonunion, osteomyelitis, reflex sympathetic dystrophy syndrome, and premature joint disease.

Nonunion

- Nonunion is a failure to complete osseous fusion across the fracture site (Fig. 6-23).
- Contributing factors of nonunion include distraction, inadequate immobilization, infection, and impaired circulation.
- The most common adult sites for nonunion are the midclavicle, ulna, and tibia.
- The radiographic signs of nonunion require many months to develop. These signs include

fracture rounding, lack of callus, sclerosis, and pseudarthrosis.

ROUNDING OF THE FRACTURE MARGINS

◆ Fractures that do not unite often become smooth at their margins, losing the roughened and irregular appearance.
◆ Later, the fractured ends become rounded and sclerotic.

LACK OF CALCIFIED CALLUS

◆ The failure to demonstrate callus formation across the fracture site is a sure sign of nonunion.

SCLEROSIS OF THE FRACTURE FRAGMENT MARGINS

◆ The fragment ends of the fracture may undergo increasing sclerosis when bony union fails to occur.

PSEUDARTHROSIS

◆ If the fracture is not adequately immobilized, motion between the fractured bone ends persists and small vessels that grow into the fracture site are constantly sheared. The callus is thus poorly vascularized and tends to produce cartilage instead of bone.
◆ An established nonunion requires operative intervention to reinitiate the healing process.
◆ A combination of internal fixation, bone grafting, and resection of the fracture line, including the pseudarthrosis, is usually necessitated.

Malunion

◆ Malunion is the healing of fragments of a fracture in a faulty position (Fig. 6-24).
◆ Usually this refers to an excessive rotatory or angular deformity.

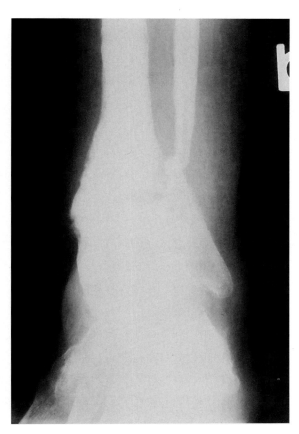

FIG. 6-23 The failure of complete osseous fusion traversing a fracture site may result in a state known as *nonunion*.

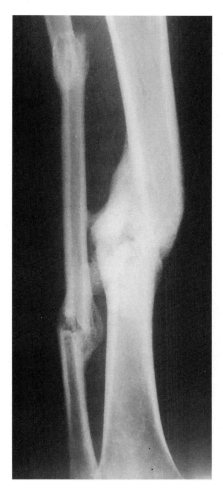

FIG. 6-24 Malunion, as observed here in the fibula and tibia, occurs subsequent to the healing of fracture fragments in a faulty position.

Osteomyelitis

- Fractures that become complicated by osteomyelitis are usually open (or compound) or require surgical reduction.
- The most common infecting organism is *Staphylococcus aureus.*
- Most cases manifest within a month of the occurrence of an open fracture or open surgical reduction.
- The dominant symptom is pain, and the radiologic features are a destructive "moth-eaten" matrix, sequestra formation, and periosteal response near the fracture site.

Reflex Sympathetic Dystrophy Syndrome (Sudeck's Atrophy)

- Severe and painful regional osteoporosis after trauma is referred to as *reflex sympathetic dystrophy syndrome (RSDS),* or *Sudeck's atrophy* (Fig. 6-25, *A* and *B*).
- This is a relatively rare complication of trauma to a limb.

Premature Osteoarthritis

- If a fracture is intraarticular, damage to the articular cartilage often occurs, yielding the worst prognosis.
- This is seen most commonly in weight-bearing joints such as the hip, knee, and ankle.
- The arthritic changes represent secondary degenerative joint disease (posttraumatic osteoarthritis).

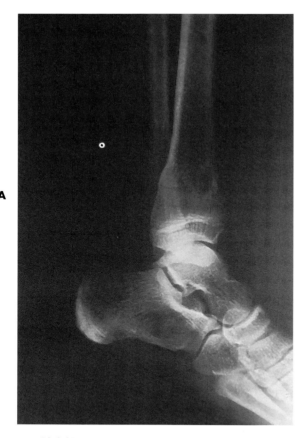
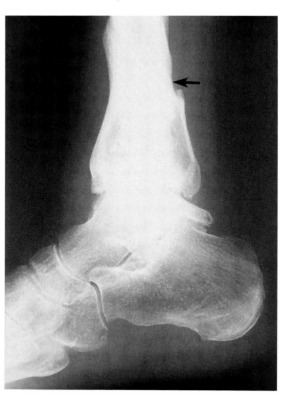

FIG. 6-25 A, Severe and painful regional osteoporosis after trauma is referred to as *reflex sympathetic dystrophy syndrome (RSDS),* or *Sudeck's atrophy.* **B,** Note the healed fracture of the lower leg (*arrow*), with regional osteopenia noted distal to the fracture site.

INTERPRETATION OF RADIOGRAPHS IN THE EVALUATION OF FRACTURE HEALING

- The determination of healing or union of a fracture is principally a clinical decision aided by the radiographic findings.
- Clinical union may occur while the fracture line is still radiographically apparent.
- Clinical union is usually present before there is radiographic consolidation with solid ensheathing bony callus and complete obliteration of the fracture line by bony trabeculae.
- The callus should be completely described as to its presence or absence, its nature (i.e., fluffy or mature), its position (i.e., unilateral or encircling), and whether it completely bridges the fracture line.
- The appearance of the fracture line should be stated in qualitative terms such as the following: *readily apparent, partially obliterated,* or *barely perceptible.*
- The alignment of the principal fragments should be fully described similar to the method of describing the original fracture.

Is the Fracture Old or New?

- Whether a fracture is old or recent may be difficult to distinguish. The following is a guideline to assist in this determination:
  - Determine the pertinent historical events.
  - Examine the injury site for signs of lacerations, contusion, or edema.
  - Conduct a physical examination, including percussion, vibration, and ultrasound over a suspected fracture site.
  - Perform serial studies to observe for reactionary periostitis and/or osseous callus formation.
  - Use a bone scan to assess the metabolic activity of an injured site.
  - Be aware that pain usually dissipates in 6 to 8 weeks.
  - Observe the cortical margins for continuity, smoothness, or eburnation.

FRACTURES OF THE SKULL

- Because of the complexity of anatomic structures and the difficulty in interpretation of skull fractures, they are visualized in less than 10% of plain film radiographs.

- Many skull series are performed for medicolegal reasons only.
- Intracranial soft tissue lesions such as intracerebral or subdural hematomas are found in the absence of a fracture in 15% of patients.
- The minimum routine radiographic study of the skull includes the posteroanterior (PA), Caldwell, anteroposterior (AP), Towne, Waters, and right and left lateral views.
- More specialized projections such as the tangential or submentovertex views may be helpful, along with tomography and computed tomograms, as clinically warranted.
- Paranasal sunus and mastoid process studies may complement a routine skull assessment.

Linear

- Linear fractures represent 80% of all skull fractures.
- These fractures are observed radiographically as sharp, radiolucent, irregular lines without sclerotic margination.
- They are usually several centimeters in length.
- Because its course may be straight, angular, or curvilinear, the linear fracture must be differentiated from vascular grooves or sutures.
- The fracture line is more radiolucent than a vascular groove because it incorporates the inner *and* outer tables of the skull, whereas the vascular groove represents only an impression of varying depth on the inner *or* outer table, rendering it less sharp in appearance.
- Fractures cross a suture, whereas vascular grooves do not.
- The most common bones involved are those in the temporal or parietal area, but all skull bones may be subject to linear fracture.

Depressed

- Depressed fractures occur as a result of an impact by a small mass at a high velocity, such as a direct blow with a small object.
- These represent 15% of all skull fractures.
- The depression usually comprises several fragments of bone that are angulated inward.
- This type of fracture may appear stellate (star-shaped) as a result of the radiating pattern of the multiple fragments, and it will appear extremely radiopaque when viewed en face as a result of the overlap of the fractured fragments.

TRAUMA

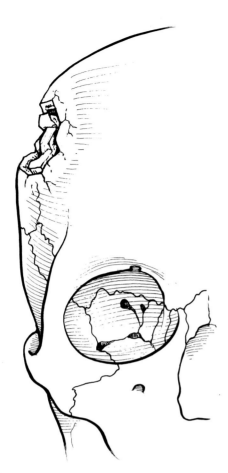

FIG. 6-26 A depressed fracture of the skull. This particular example is comminuted.

- Depressed fractures must be seen in profile to determine the depth of displacement of the fracture fragments (Fig. 6-26).
- Approximately one third of depressed fragments are associated with dural tears that require surgical repair.
- Displacement by 5 mm or more of depression beyond the inner table suggests a high probability of dural tear.

Ping Pong

- This fracture represents a variation of the depressed fracture and is seen most often in the young child whose skull is extremely soft and pliable.
- The skull sustains a deep and broad depression without an associated overt fracture, much like the indentation produced by fingers being pushed into a ping pong ball.

- This trauma is best seen on frontal radiographs because most of these lesions occur in the lateral surface of the skull.

SPINAL TRAUMA

- Fractures of the spine may involve the vertebral bodies, neural arch, or transverse and spinous processes.
- Injuries that involve compression with or without flexion or rotation injure the vertebral bodies, whereas the posterior elements are injured through direct violence or secondarily via disease.
- Distinguishing whether fractures and dislocations are stable is important.
- Stable fractures do not pose additional danger to the patient, whereas unstable fractures may result in potential complicating injury.
- Radiographic and neurologic examinations are invaluable in assessing the condition of the patient and the stability of a fracture.
- Most spinal injuries, if stable, are treated by conservative management.
- Unstable injuries, or major vertebral fractures or dislocations, in which the spinal cord is injured are grave and may result in permanent paralysis.
- Unstable fractures must be immobilized until bone and soft tissues heal.
- The application of traction ensures proper alignment and inhibits further injury.
- Possible clinical features of spinal injury may include the following:
  - Weakness or paralysis below the level of the injury
  - Loss of function in the lower or upper extremities
  - Loss of bowel and/or bladder control
  - Loss of pain or sensation to stimula
  - Painful movement
  - Tenderness
  - Lacerations or contusion
  - Deformity
  - Impaired respiration

CERVICAL SPINE

- Cervical spinal injuries are more serious than thoracic and lumbar injuries and account for a greater risk of harm to the spinal cord, with resultant disability.
- The most common type of injury to this area occurs in automobile accidents, resulting in whiplash, in which the head is suddenly oscillated.
- With trauma to the head, injury to the cervical spine must be suspected.

- The trauma may be direct or indirect and involve excessive ranges of motion of the head and neck extending beyond the physiologic limitations.
- The injuries are usually generated by forces in a combination of planes and not by one particular force in any particular direction.
- Initially, the direction of the force and extent of the injury may be somewhat difficult to assess. Therefore taking a complete history, including the position of the head at the moment of injury, is important.
- Injuries in the cervical spine are classified as flexion, flexion with rotation, hyperextension, hyperextension with rotation, and vertical compression.

Flexion

- Flexion usually results in a stable wedge-type compression fracture of the vertebral body.

Flexion with Rotation

- The facet joints of the cervical region possess small, smooth, flat articular surfaces. Thus they are vulnerable to dislocation and subluxation.

- The posterior ligaments are also susceptible to injury.
- A flexion or flexion-rotation force may also produce disc alteration without accompanying osseous injury.

Hyperextension

- A hyperextension force may produce a fracture of the neural arch or a comminuted-type fracture of the posterior elements, especially of the atlas or axis.
- The odontoid is also susceptible to fracture.
- This type of motion may also load the lower portion of the cervical spine, approximate the posterior joints, and stress the anterior longitudinal ligament, resulting in its rupture.

Hyperextension with Rotation

- This can produce fracture and dislocation of the articular pillars in the lower cervical spine (Fig. 6-27, *A-E*).

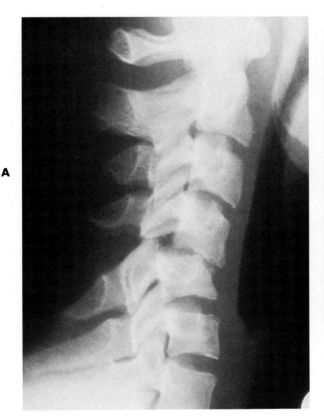 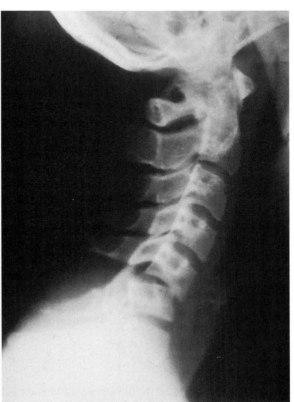

FIG. 6-27 A, A fracture-dislocation of the C4-C5 intervertebral motor segment. **B,** Bilateral facet joint dislocation at C5-C6. *Continued.*

TRAUMA

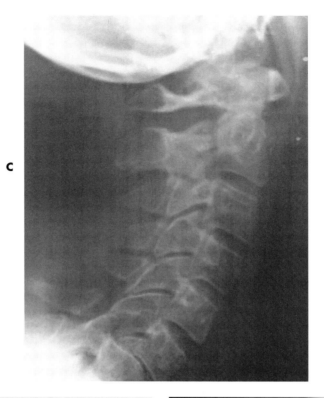

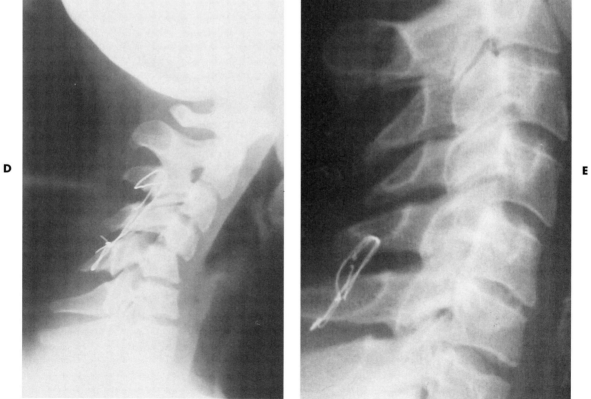

FIG. 6-27, cont'd. **C,** Bilateral inferior C6 facet dislocation, resulting in a Grade 3 anterolisthesis. **D,** Surgical wire stabilization of a C4-C5 facet dislocation. **E,** Surgical wire stabilization of a C5-C6 facet dislocation.

Vertical Compression

◆ Vertical compression acting through the skull may result in a fracture of the atlas (Jefferson fracture), or a burst fracture of a vertebral body in the lower cervical spine.

◆ The mechanism of a burst fracture is created by the force of the disc's nucleus being driven into the vertebral body, causing it to "explode."

Significant Indirect Signs of Cervical Spine Trauma

ABNORMAL SOFT TISSUE

◆ Hemorrhage caused by injury of the paracervical soft tissues displaces certain physiologic spaces that are appreciated radiographically, representing a "space-occupying lesion."
- Widened retropharyngeal space (in excess of 7 mm)
- Widened retrotracheal space (in excess of 21 mm)
- Displacement of the prevertebral fat stripe
- Tracheal deviation and laryngeal dislocation

ABNORMAL VERTEBRAL ALIGNMENT

◆ Injury of soft tissues (a strain or sprain of muscle, tendon, ligament, and capsule) reflexively produces spasm and may be identified by the following:
- Loss of lordosis
- Acute kyphotic hyperangulation
- Torticollis
- Widened interspinous space
- Rotation of vertebral bodies
- Widened middle atlantoaxial joint (the *atlantodental interspace,* or ADI) (in excess of 3 mm in adults or 5 mm in children)
- Abnormal intervertebral disc
- Widening of apophyseal joints

CERVICAL SPINE FRACTURES

Jefferson

◆ The atlas is most commonly fractured by a compression or vertical force directed axially through a straight cervical spine.

◆ The force is transmitted through the atlanto-occipital articulations. This tends to spread the lateral masses outwardly.

◆ The fracture usually occurs through the junctions of the lateral masses and the lamina of bone that connects them (posterior and anterior arches).

◆ The fragments appear to burst out peripherally in all directions.

◆ Posterior arch fractures of the atlas may be unilateral or bilateral and arise through the weakest point of the ring, where the vertebral artery forms a groove in the ring.

◆ The mechanism involved in this type of fracture is a combination of axial compression and/or a hyperextension force, with the posterior arch being compressed between the occiput and posterior arch of axis.

◆ With a bilateral fracture the posterior arch is displaced superiorly as a result of the pull of the rectus capitis posticus minor muscle.

◆ A burst-type fracture with fragmentation may produce compression of the cord, resulting in neurologic signs.

◆ The fracture may radiographically appear similar to a "butterfly" vertebra.

◆ Without displacement, no fracture line is demonstrated and the fracture may be easily missed.

TRAUMA

A

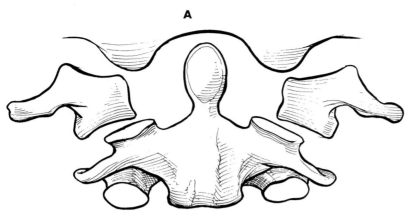

B

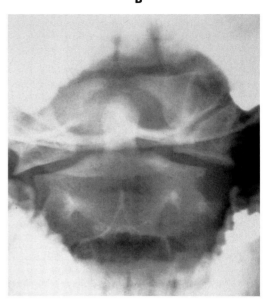

FIG. 6-28 A, Bilateral atlas lateral mass migration, as seen in a Jefferson's fracture. **B,** Jefferson fracture. Note that the lateral masses of the atlas extend bilaterally beyond the lateral margins of the facets of axis bilaterally. (Courtesy Ron Collett, DC, DACBR, Winnipeg, Manitoba.)

- Lateral migration of the lateral masses (beyond the C2 facet margins) may be the only radiographic feature of this condition (Fig. 6-28, *A* and *B*).
- Computed tomography is the optimal method of visualizing atlas ring fractures.
- This particular type of fracture is usually not life-threatening.
- The spinal canal is not compromised because the fracture usually results in an increase of its diameter.
- The mechanism of injury (compression) may produce diffuse bleeding, with a resultant space-occupying defect.

Odontoid

- Odontoid fractures are classified as follows:
  - Fracture through the upper portion of the odontoid, possibly confused with os odontoidium
  - Fracture at the base of the odontoid (Fig. 6-29, *A-C*) (most common site)
  - Fracture that extends into the body of C2 (Fig. 6-30, *A* and *B*)
- Observing the anatomic relationship of the dens and its association with the anterior tubercle of the atlas is important.
- The posterior surface of the dens should be contiguous with the posterior surface of the axis body.
- An undisplaced fracture of the dens may be subtle and easily overlooked.

- The fracture is obvious when the dens fragment is displaced along with the atlas.
- Radiographically, displacement is anterior in flexion injuries and retrograde in extension injuries.
- Odontoid fractures are common.
- The odontoid usually fractures before the rupture of the transverse ligament.
- In the event of dens fracture, healing is often delayed or entirely absent as a result of poor vascular supply.
- There is an extremely high incidence of odontoid nonunion after fractures (50% to 60% of the cases), and this type of fracture should not be confused with an os odontoideum.

Hangman's

- Hangman's fracture is featured by a bilateral fracture of the axis pedicles adjacent to the body.
- This injury is produced in automobile accidents as a consequence of the chin or forehead striking the steering wheel or dashboard, forcing severe hyperextension of the skull against the cervical spine.
- This fracture has also been referred to as a *traumatic spondylolisthesis of C2.*
- This is a bipedicular fracture of the axis, not a fracture of the laminae.
- When C2 is positioned anterior to C3, the pedicles should be examined for evidence of a healed or ununited hangman's fracture.

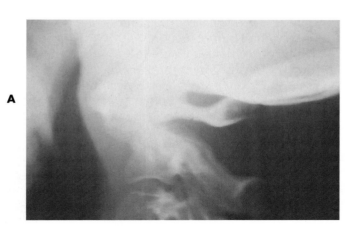

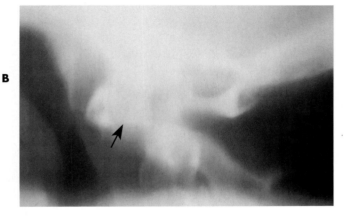

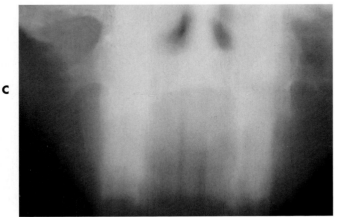

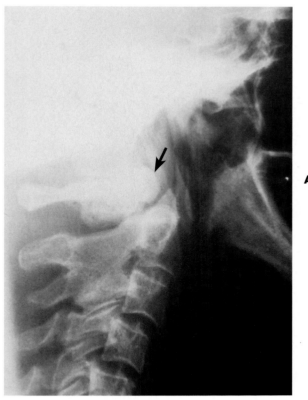

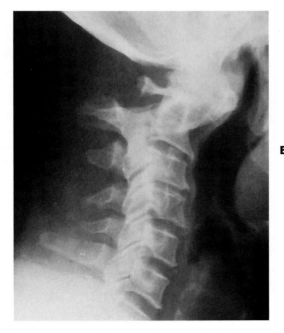

FIG. 6-29 A, Transverse fracture at the base of the odontoid process. Marked anterior atlas translation is evident. **B,** From the same patient, this tomogram clearly exhibits a transverse fracture at the base of the dens (*arrow*). **C,** Anteroposterior tomogram demonstrating the separation of the odontoid process. The body of C2 is not seen in this image. (Courtesy Don Henderson, DC, DACBR, FCCR[C], FCCS[C] Etobicoke, Ontario.)

FIG. 6-30 A, An odontoid process fracture including a small portion of the axis is visualized. Note the posterior displacement of the atlas, as indicated by the position of the anterior tubercle (*arrow*), situated just superior to the body of C2. **B,** Severe anterior displacement of the atlas is indicated by the anterior position of the C1 tubercle, the increased atlantodental interspace, and the marked interruption of the spinolaminar junction line.

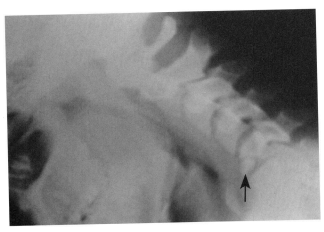

FIG. 6-31 A chip fracture of the anteroinferior body of C5 (*arrow*).

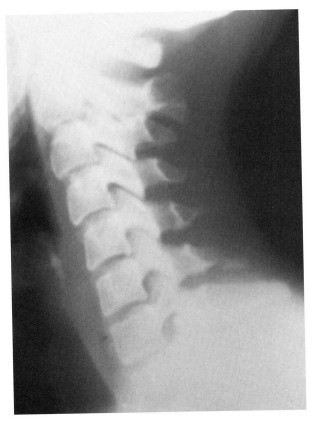

FIG. 6-32 An avulsion fracture of the terminal end of the C6 spinous process.

◆ Generally, severe trauma is required to produce this entity.

Chip (Margin, Teardrop)

◆ Chip fractures occur at the anterior margins of the vertebral end plates.
◆ This fracture is most commonly found in the lower cervical segments and occurs at the anteroinferior (Fig. 6-31) or anterosuperior aspects of the vertebral body.
◆ The mechanism of injury is usually attributable to a hyperflexion or hyperextension force, with resultant avulsion.
◆ The teardrop fracture is misleading because it appears quite small and benign; yet for the patients, it may be the most serious as a result of the insufficiency of the attachment of the anterior longitudinal ligament.
◆ A chip fracture most commonly occurs at the anteroinferior corner of a lower cervical vertebral body, usually with fragment displacement, after a whiplash flexion-extension–type injury.
◆ There may be an extremely large increase in retropharyngeal and retrolaryngeal interspaces secondary to hemorrhage.
◆ Caution should be observed because this fracture may be life-threatening.

Uncinate Process

◆ This is a transverse fracture across the uncus, with some displacement of the fragment.
◆ The mechanism of injury is lateral hyperflexion.
◆ The clinical presentation may consist of neck pain, upper limb weakness, and radiculopathy as a result of intervertebral foraminal compromise.

Spinous Process

◆ This fracture usually involves the seventh cervical or first thoracic spinous process (Fig. 6-32).
◆ It is usually produced by extreme muscular activity (trapezius and rhomboid muscles), such as occurs with shovelling, and has become termed *clay-shoveller's fracture* (also *root-puller's, gold-digger's, coal-shoveller's,* and *snow-shoveller's fracture*).
◆ A spinous process fracture can result from direct or indirect trauma and usually presents as an oblique fracture of the proximal portion of the spinous process.
◆ The fragment is displaced downward, with the opposing margins appearing serrated and sharp (Fig. 6-33).

Vertebral Body Compression (Wedge)

◆ Severe flexion forces may crush the cancellous bone of one or more vertebral bodies.

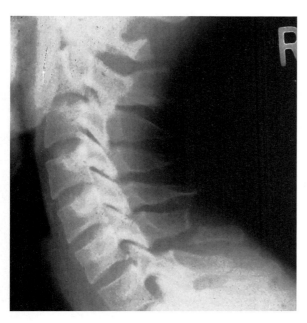

FIG. 6-33 C6 and C7 manifest inferior displacement of the terminal ends of their respective spinous processes. The opposing surfaces of the fracture fragments exhibit serrated margins.

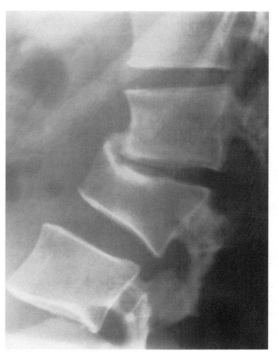

FIG. 6-34 A typical wedge-shaped compression fracture of a thoracolumbar vertebral body.

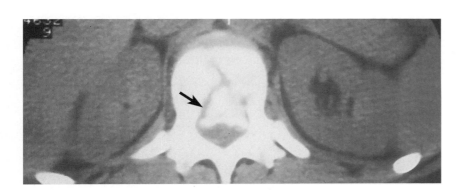

FIG. 6-35 A computed axial tomographic scan demonstrating fragmentation of a lumbar vertebral body (*arrow*).

◆ The compression is always most marked at the anterior aspect of the vertebral body, resulting in a wedge-shaped deformity (Fig. 6-34).

◆ The posterior elements remain intact.

◆ Cervical compression fractures generally occur in the mid- or lower cervical region.

◆ An x-ray examination is vital for a patient who incurs head or neck injury after an automobile, diving, or sport accident.

◆ Radiographically, visualizing the neck from the occiput to the level of T1 is important.

◆ The lateral view is most important to examine for fractures, followed by the anteroposterior, open-mouth, oblique, and pillar views.

◆ Other special views such as flexion-extension studies may be helpful in disclosing cervical spinal injury and instability.

◆ Fractures may be so obscure that tomographs or computed tomographic scans may be necessary to view the fracture sites, (Fig. 6-35) especially at the level of C1.

♦ Abnormal soft tissue signs are also extremely important indicators of areas of fracture and dislocation in the lateral projection.

♦ Anterior displacement by 25% of the body width occurs with unilateral facet dislocation, and displacement by 50% indicates bilateral facet dislocation ("bow-tie" sign).

♦ A horizontal translation greater than 3.5 mm of one vertebra on another may be indicative of a site of instability.

♦ Flexion-extension studies provide much information in assessing the relative hypermobility and hypomobility of each respective vertebral segment, especially at the level of C1-2.

THORACIC AND LUMBOPELVIC FRACTURES

♦ Vertebral body size and shape, intervertebral disc thickness, posterior facet orientation, and integrity of spinal ligaments are features that determine the vulnerability of each spinal region.

♦ The paraspinal muscles, curvatures, and ranges of motion of each spinal region are other factors that may predispose to a higher incidence of traumatic vulnerability.

Flexion Compression Fractures

♦ Most injuries involving the thoracic and lumbar spines are sustained in flexion.

♦ Structural factors may play an important role in injuries of the spine.

♦ The cancellous bone is compressible and spongy.

♦ The tendency toward flexion injury is enhanced by the normal kyphosis of the thoracic spine.

Roentgenographic Findings in Anterior Compression Fractures

♦ Buckling of the anterior vertebral body cortex

♦ Wedge deformity of the fractured vertebral body, with loss of the vertebral body height anteriorly compared with its posterior height (Fig. 6-36)

♦ Possibility of some focal increase in kyphosis (Fig. 6-37)

♦ A zone of condensation, caused by compaction of the trabecular elements of the spongiosa, appearing as a band of increased osseous density through the medullary bone beneath the affected end plate

♦ Vertebral end-plate fractures occur more frequently in the lower thoracic and upper lumbar spines (Fig. 6-38, *A* and *B*).

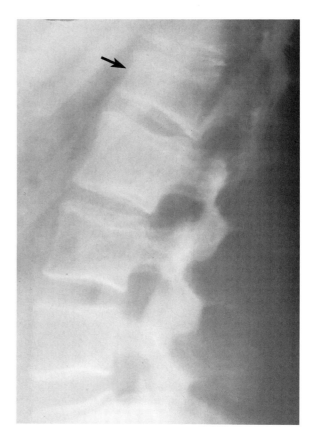

FIG. 6-36 Wedge deformity of the anterior vertebral body height may be indicative of a compression fracture (*arrow*).

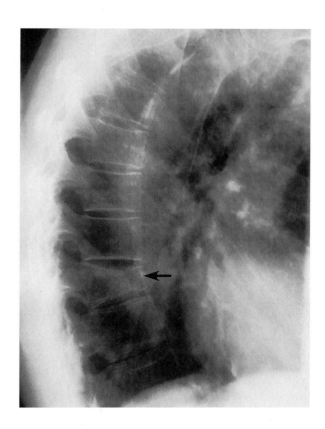

FIG. 6-37 Anterior vertebral body fractures may result in focal or generalized hyperkyphotic angulation of the spine (*arrow*).

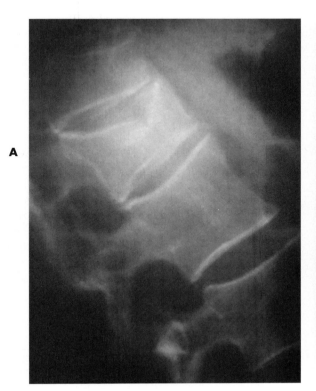

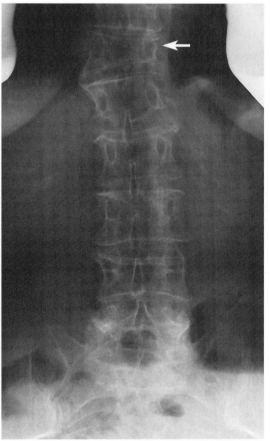

A

B

FIG. 6-38 A and **B,** Vertebral body compression fractures occur more frequently in the upper lumbar or lower thoracic spine (*arrow*). (Courtesy Jerry Cott, DC, Toronto, Ontario.)

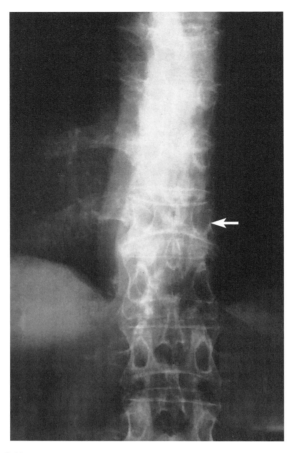

FIG. 6-39 A "frog-face" sign observed on an anteroposterior radiograph suggests the presence of a vertebral body compression fracture (*arrow*).

- Vertebral body compression fractures may be suspected when a "frog-face" sign is exhibited on the anteroposterior study (Fig. 6-39).
- Paraspinal soft tissue injury is frequently observed with spinal compression fractures.

Axial Compression Injuries

- When an axial load is placed on a vertebra with minimal flexion or extension, collapse of the vertebral body may occur.
- Extensive herniation of the nucleus pulposus into the fractured vertebral body is common in this type of injury, and the body may be vertically cleaved into two or more fragments by extruded nuclear material (Fig. 6-40, *A* and *B*).
- The fragments may be forced anteriorly, posteriorly, or laterally.

- The smaller upper lumbar vertebrae are without the stability of the rib cage to absorb these forces, and as a result, L1 or L2 may be fractured.
- Collapsed or burst fractures are usually stable in that they are not associated with ligamentous disruption.
- Many of these fractures present with significant neurologic damage as a result of rapid retropulsion of the vertebral body into the neural canal, with potential subsequent anterior cord complications.

Radiographic Findings

- Enlargement of the vertebral body diameter with posterior margin displacement into the spinal canal may be evident.

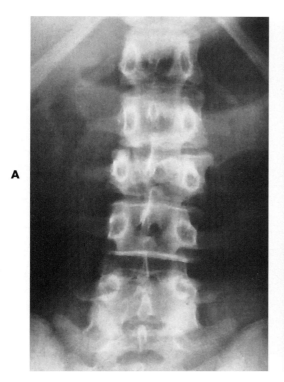 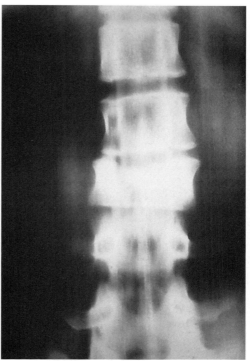

FIG. 6-40 A, Axial compressive loading forces may produce extensive nuclear herniation into a vertebral body, resulting in its vertical cleavage. **B,** Tomogram of the same spine, demonstrating the vertical cleavage of the vertebral body.

Flexion of the Body with Distraction Rorce or Seat-Belt Injuries

◆ These injuries are sustained by rapid deceleration while a person is wearing a lap seat belt.
◆ Seat-belt injuries pivot around a fulcrum situated at the anterior abdominal wall.
◆ When the trunk forcibly flexes, a distraction force is exerted on the posterior elements of the vertebrae.
◆ The injury usually arises in the upper to midlumbar spine (L2, L3, or L4) as a result of the position in which lap constraints are customarily used.
◆ Any injury in which the body is projected against a horizontal object may produce a similar result.
◆ Compression fractures of the vertebrae anteriorly are minimal or absent because the axis of flexion is completely anterior to the vertebral column.
◆ Posterior ligament tearing may occur in which the posterior ligament complex (supraspinous, interspinous, flavum, and capsular) becomes insufficient.

Chance Fracture

◆ A horizontal line may extend through the spinous process, splitting the neural arch (through the laminae, articular pillars, and pedicles) and extending into the posterior body surface.
◆ The fracture line divides the vertebra into upper and lower halves.
◆ Significant abdominal soft tissue injuries, as well as spinal neurologic injury, have been noted in 15% of all patients who have injuries as a result of seat belts.
◆ The intraabdominal injuries may include intestinal contusions, intramuscular tears, and visceral perforation.

Radiographic Features

◆ Horizontal fracture lines may extend from the spinous process anteriorly into the laminae, articular pillars, and pedicles.
◆ The fracture line divides the vertebrae into upper and lower parts.

◆ Other forms of spinal fractures may include the following:
  · Lateral body compression-type fractures
  · Pillar fractures
  · Lamina-pedicle fractures
  · Transverse process fractures (Fig. 6-41)

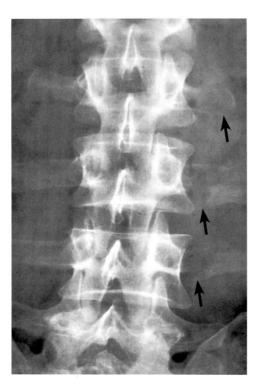

FIG. 6-41 Note the transverse process fractures at L2, L3, and L4 on the reading right (*arrows*). The distal fragments are displaced inferiorly, and the opposing end surfaces manifest serrated margins.

SACRAL INJURIES

◆ Sacral injuries occur often as the result of trauma transmitted through one leg or one side of the pelvis.
◆ Anterior pelvic fractures of the pubic and ischial rami are frequently associated.
◆ The sacroiliac joint resists rupture or dislocation as a result of its oblique orientation and the great tensile strength of the fibers that hold it together.
◆ The first and second sacral nerve root foraminae, which perforate the sacral ala medial to the sacroiliac joint, structurally weaken the bone in this vicinity.
◆ Sacral fractures may arise in any orientation.
◆ Isolated fractures of the sacrum are uncommon (only 1% of all fractures).
◆ Sacral fractures are usually associated with fractures involving other parts of the pelvis.
◆ Visceral and neurologic injuries are often associated with sacral fractures.
◆ Complications may be vascular, resulting in presacral or retroperitoreal hematoma.
◆ Cauda equina lesions, particularly of the sacral nerves, may produce urinary incontinence.
◆ With a vertical fracture the space between each transverse process of L5 and the sacrum may reveal asymmetry.
◆ Avulsion fractures from excessive traction of the sacrospinous and sacrotuberous ligaments may be observed.

COCCYGEAL INJURIES

◆ In approximately 6% of all pelvic fractures, there is an associated coccygeal fracture.
◆ These injuries are most often produced by a direct blow to the coccygeal region, such as a fall on the buttocks.
◆ Fracture of the coccyx may result in severe pain, particularly when the fracture fragments are displaced, exerting pressure on the rectum or adjacent soft tissue structures (Figs. 6-42, *A* and *B*).

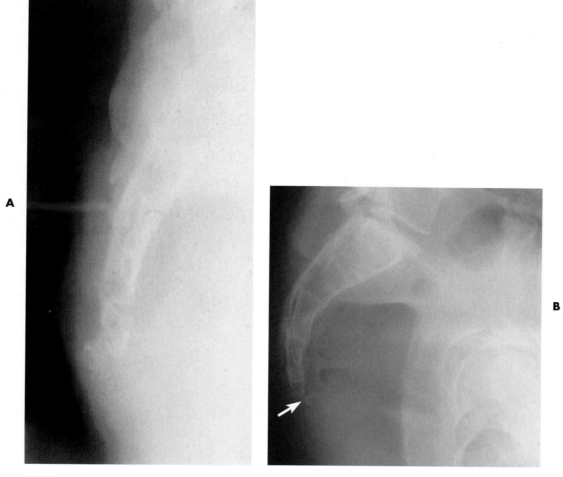

FIG. 6-42 A, Observe the posterior displacement of the fractured coccygeal apex. **B,** Anterior displacement is seen at the level of the sacrococcygeal junction (*arrow*).

FRACTURES AND DISLOCATIONS OF THE APPENDICULAR SKELETON
Epiphyseal Fractures
SALTER-HARRIS CLASSIFICATION
- This is a classification system of growth-plate injuries based on the radiologic findings proposed by Salter and Harris in 1963.
- This system has gained widespread acceptance and is a standard in the description of these injuries, allowing certain prognostic predictions.
- Essentially, the components involved in the fracture determine its type.

SALTER-HARRIS TYPE 1
- This represents a fracture along the growth plate (Fig. 6-43).
- A clinical diagnosis is frequently necessary because the radiographs may be unremarkable.
- It is helpful to compare x-ray films of the affected limb with radiographs of the normal limb to assist in discerning any subtle epiphyseal displacement.

SALTER-HARRIS TYPE II
- This is a fracture through the displaced growth plate, which carries with it a corner of the metaphysis (Fig. 6-44).
- The metaphyseal fragment has been called the *Thurston-Holland sign.*
- This is the most common epiphyseal injury, comprising approximately 75% of cases.

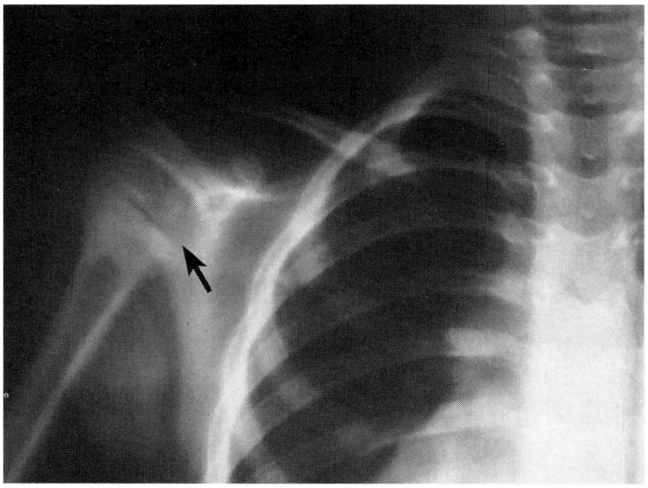

- The most common sites of involvement are the distal radius (50%), as well as the distal tibia, fibula, femur, and ulna.
- The epiphyseal separation is usually easily reduced, and the prognosis is generally favorable.

SALTER-HARRIS TYPE III
- This fracture is directed along the growth plate and then traverses the epiphysis (Fig. 6-45).
- This is an intraarticular fracture that may require open reduction treatment.

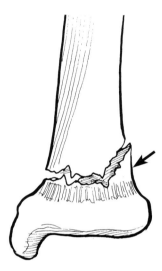

FIG. 6-44 Salter-Harris Type 2 fracture. The fracture line has resulted in the separation of a portion of the metaphysis (Thurston-Holland fragment) (*arrow*), as well as the entire epiphysis.

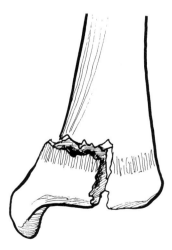

FIG. 6-45 Type 3 Salter-Harris fracture along the physeal plate and continuing through the epiphysis to include the articular surface.

![Figure 6-43 radiograph]

FIG. 6-43 Salter-Harris Type 1 fracture seen along the proximal humeral physeal growth plate (*arrow*) in a 3-year-old girl.

SALTER-HARRIS TYPE IV

- This is an obliquely oriented fracture, consisting of portions of the metaphysis, growth plate, and epiphysis (Fig. 6-46).
- The prognosis is poor without expedient open reduction and internal fixation, with a potential for permanent deformity.

SALTER-HARRIS TYPE V

- This fracture involves a crushing of the physeal growth plate, resulting from axial compression forces (Fig. 6-47).

- This injury is the least common of all Salter-Harris epiphyseal lesions.
- Initially, radiographs often appear normal until the cessation of growth, creating bone shortening as a result of partial arrest.
- A comparison with the contralateral limb may be required to assess the relative symmetry of the physeal plate width.

Upper Extremity

SHOULDER

- Bankart lesion
  - Avulsion of a small fragment of the glenoid rim at the site of the triceps insertion (Fig. 6-48)
- Flap fracture
  - Avulsion of the greater tuberosity (Fig. 6-49, *A-D*)
- Hill-Sachs ("hatchet") deformity
  - An impaction fracture of the posterosuperior surface of the humeral head produced by repetitive traumatization by the inferior glenoid rim after recurrent anterior glenohumeral joint dislocation

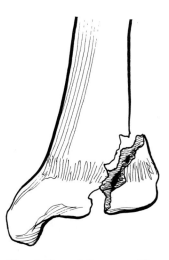

FIG. 6-46 Salter-Harris Type 4 fracture. The oblique fracture line has sheared off a portion of the epiphysis and metaphysis.

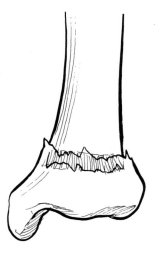

FIG. 6-47 An impaction fracture along the physeal plate. This fracture constitutes a Salter-Harris Type 5 fracture.

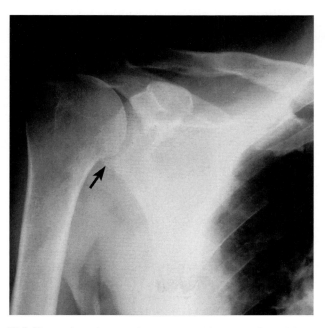

FIG. 6-48 Bankart lesion characterized by a small avulsion fragment of the inferior glenoid rim at the site of the triceps insertion (*arrow*).

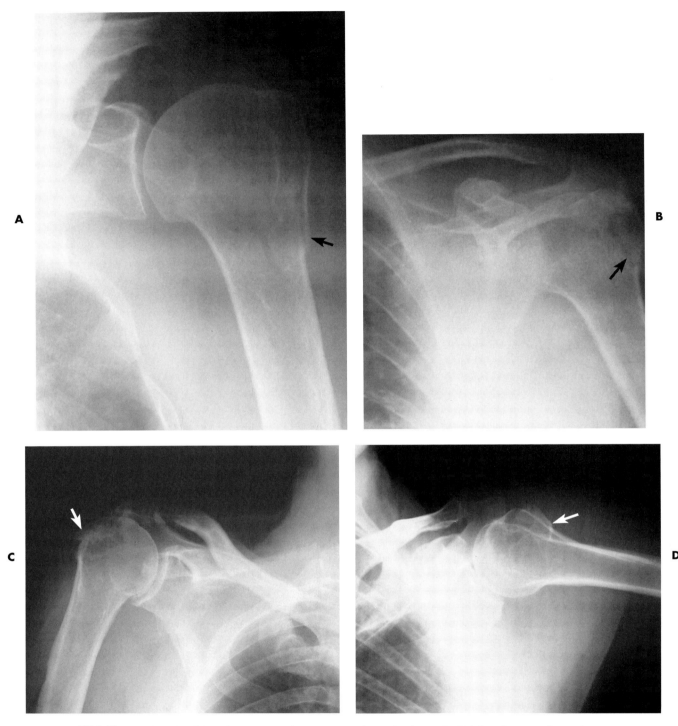

FIG. 6-49 **A** and **B,** Avulsion fracture of the greater tuberosity (*arrow*). **C,** Flap fracture featuring an avulsion of the greater tuberosity (*arrow*). **D,** The greater tuberosity demonstrates avulsion (*arrow*). (**C,** Courtesy Shahbahram Mavandadi, MD, Amol, Iran; **D,** Courtesy Susan DeWolfe, DC, Toronto, Ontario.)

- ◆ Shoulder dislocation
  - • A loss of anatomic continuity between the opposing surfaces of the glenohumeral articulation (Figs. 6-50 and 6-51)
- ◆ Shoulder separation
  - • A loss of anatomic continuity between the opposing surfaces of the acromioclavicular articulation (Fig. 6-52, *A* and *B*)
- ◆ Miscellaneous shoulder girdle trauma
  - • Clavicular fracture (Fig. 6-53)
  - • Scapular fracture (Fig. 6-54)

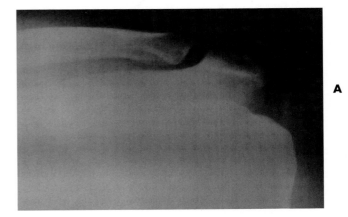

A

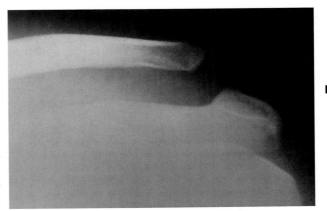

B

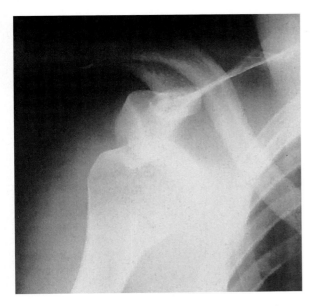

FIG. 6-50 Anteroinferior dislocation of the proximal humerus.

FIG. 6-52 **A,** Acromioclavicular joint evaluated without weight-bearing. **B,** The same acromioclavicular joint with weight-bearing exhibiting severe separation.

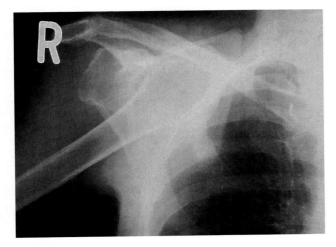

FIG. 6-51 Subclavicular dislocation of the humeral head.

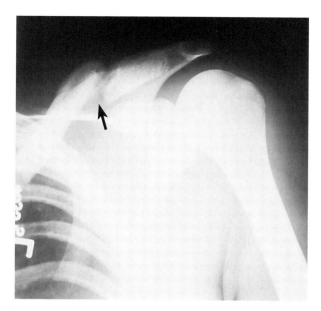

FIG. 6-53 Fracture of the distal portion of the clavicle (*arrow*).

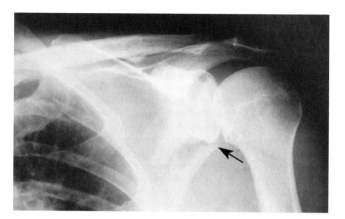

FIG. 6-54 Fracture of the axial scapular border inferior to the glenoid labrum (*arrow*).

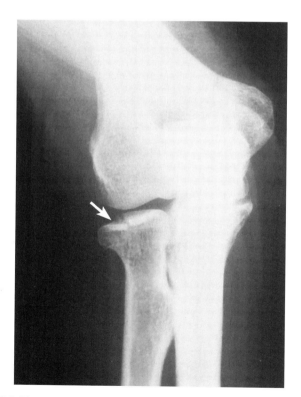

FIG. 6-55 Chisel fracture of the lateral radial head (*arrow*). Note the slight inferior displacement of the fracture fragment.

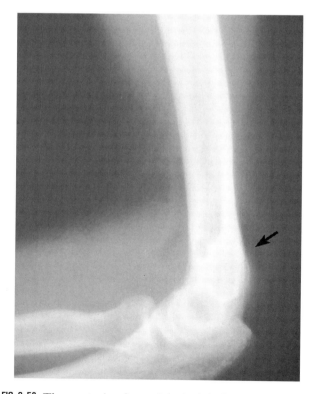

FIG. 6-56 The posterior fat pad (*arrow*) is depicted as a lucent stripe immediately posterior to the humerus.

ELBOW

- Chisel fracture
  - Vertical fracture through the radial head, with mild depression (Fig. 6-55)
- Fat pad sign
  - Visualization of the posterior fat pad on a lateral elbow view associated with intraarticular fractures, most commonly of the radial head (Fig. 6-56)
- Little Leaguer's elbow
  - Avulsion of the medial epicondyle

- Sail sign
  - Triangular enlargement of the normally visualized anterior fat pad (Fig. 6-57, *A* and *B*) (not as reliable a diagnostic indicator as the posterior fat pad sign)
- Sideswipe (traffic, baby car) fracture
  - Fracture of the distal humerus, proximal radius, and ulna when an elbow protruding from a car window is struck by an object

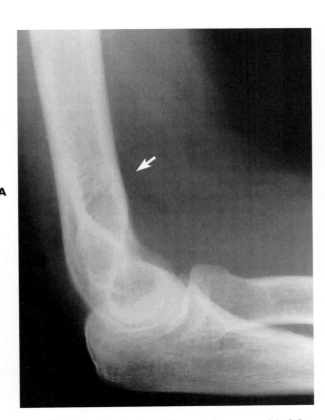
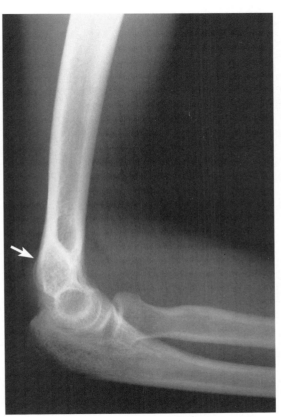

FIG. 6-57 A, Sail sign. Observe the antecubital fat pad seen as a lucency (*arrow*). **B,** Elevation of the anterior fat pad in a triangular pattern gives rise to the sail sign. Note the posterior fat pad as well (*arrow*).

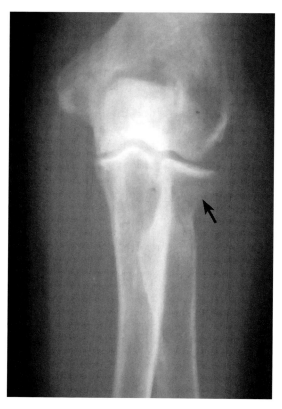

FIG. 6-58 Impaction fracture of the radial head (*arrow*).

- Miscellaneous elbow trauma
  - Impaction of lateral portion of radial head (Fig. 6-58)
  - Prosthetic radial head (Fig. 6-59)
  - Old fracture of lateral humeral condyle with nonunion (Fig. 6-60)

FOREARM

- Galeazzi (Piedmont) fracture
  - Fracture at the junction of the distal and middle thirds of the radial shaft, with associated dislocation of the inferior radioulnar joint (Fig. 6-61)
- Monteggia fracture
  - Fracture of the proximal ulnar shaft, with associated radial head dislocation (Fig. 6-62)
- Nightstick (Parry) fracture
  - Fracture of the ulnar shaft when the arm is raised to protect the head from a blow

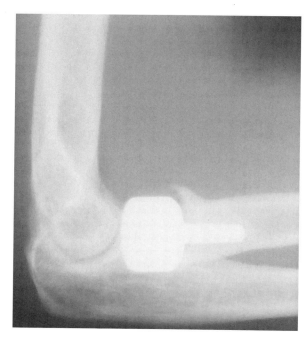

FIG. 6-59 Prosthetic radial head. (Courtesy Joseph D'Ippolito, DC, Toronto, Ontario.)

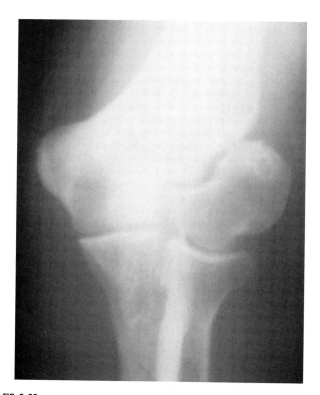

FIG. 6-60 Nonunion of the lateral humeral condyle.

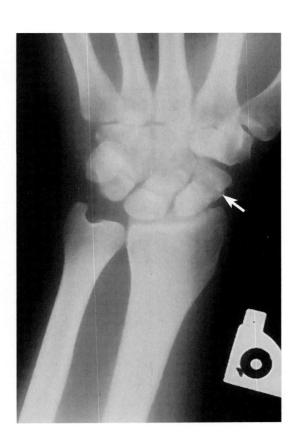

FIG. 6-70 Fracture of the waist of the scaphoid (*arrow*).

- Terry Thomas sign
  - Widened scaphoid-lunate interspace (greater than 4 mm) caused by scapholunate disassociation (Fig. 6-66)

HAND

- Bar room fracture
  - Fracture of the fourth or fifth metacarpal neck, with anterior displacement of the head (Fig. 6-67)
- Baseball (mallet) fracture
  - Intraarticular avulsion or chip fracture of the base of a distal phalanx (Fig. 6-68)
- Bennett's fracture
  - Intraarticular fracture through the base of the first metacarpal, with dorsal and radial displacement of the shaft
- Boxer's fracture
  - Fracture of the second or third metacarpal neck, with associated anterior head displacement
- Gamekeeper's fracture
  - Triangular avulsion of the ulnar aspect of the base of the first proximal phalanx, with disruption of the ulnar collateral ligament (Fig. 6-69)

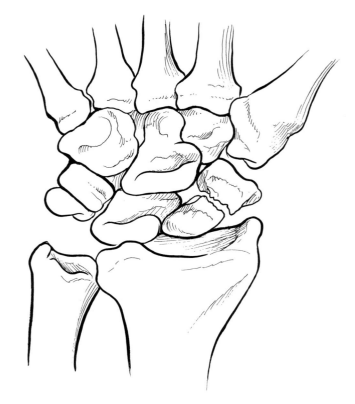

FIG. 6-71 A fracture through the waist of the scaphoid.

- Rolando's (comminuted Bennett's) fracture
  - Intraarticular, comminuted fracture at the first metacarpal base
- Miscellaneous wrist and hand trauma
  - Scaphoid fracture (Figs. 6-70 and 6-71)
  - Fracture-dislocation (old) of the fifth proximal interphalangeal joint (Fig. 6-72)

TRAUMA

Lower Extremity

PELVIS

- Bucket handle fracture
  - Fracture of the superior *and* inferior pubic rami, with associated dislocation of the contralateral sacroiliac articulation (Fig. 6-73)
- Dashboard fracture
  - Fracture of the posterior acetabular rim
- Duverney's fracture
  - Fracture of the iliac region of the innominate (Fig. 6-74)

- Explosion fracture
  - Bursting comminution of the central portion of the acetabulum
- Malgaigne's fracture
  - Fracture of the superior and inferior pubic rami, with associated dislocation of the ipsilateral sacroiliac articulation (Fig. 6-75)
- Rider's bone fracture
  - Exuberant enlargement of an ununited secondary apophysis of the ischial tuberosity, secondary to avulsion (Fig. 6-76)
- Sprung (open book) pelvis fracture
  - Diastasis of the symphysis pubis and sacroiliac articulations bilaterally

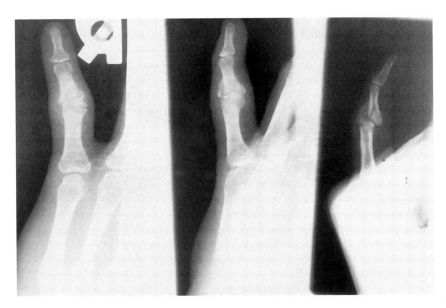

FIG. 6-72 Old fracture-dislocation of the fifth proximal interphalangeal joint.

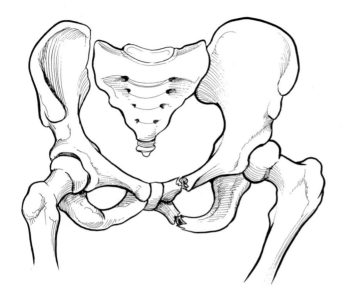

FIG. 6-73 A bucket handle fracture.

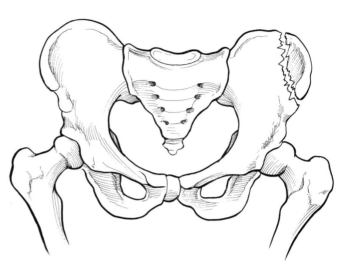

FIG. 6-74 A Duverney's fracture of the iliac wing.

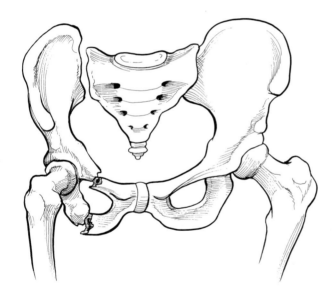

FIG. 6-75 Malgaigne's pelvic fracture.

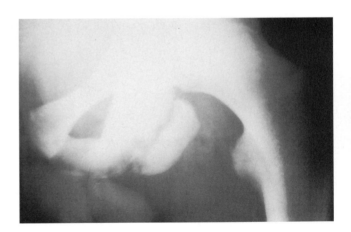

FIG. 6-76 Rider's bone. Exuberant enlargement of the ununited apophysis of the ischial tuberosity secondary to an avulsion fracture.

TRAUMA

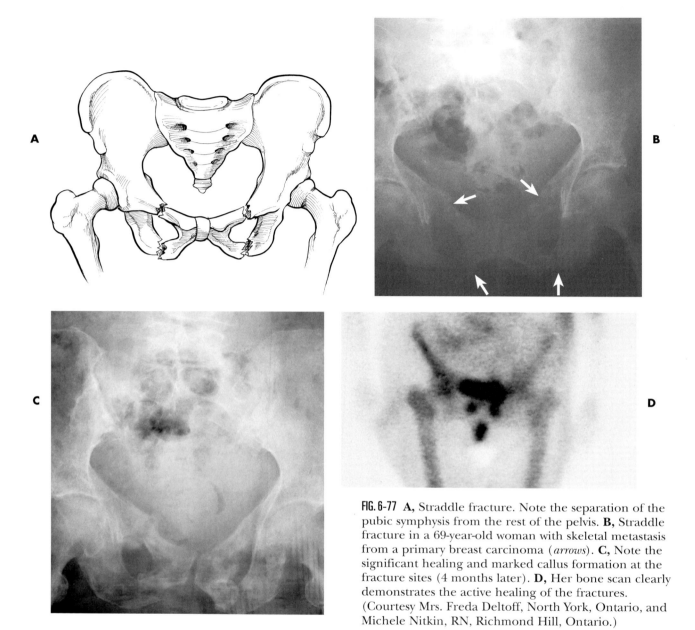

FIG. 6-77 **A,** Straddle fracture. Note the separation of the pubic symphysis from the rest of the pelvis. **B,** Straddle fracture in a 69-year-old woman with skeletal metastasis from a primary breast carcinoma (*arrows*). **C,** Note the significant healing and marked callus formation at the fracture sites (4 months later). **D,** Her bone scan clearly demonstrates the active healing of the fractures. (Courtesy Mrs. Freda Deltoff, North York, Ontario, and Michele Nitkin, RN, Richmond Hill, Ontario.)

- ◆ Straddle (saddle) fracture
  - • Complete fracture through the bilateral superior pubic rami and ischiopubic junction, effectively resulting in a "floating" pubic symphysis (Fig. 6-77)
- ◆ Miscellaneous pelvic trauma
  - • Iliopubic junction fracture (Fig. 6-78)
  - • Ischial tuberosity fracture (Fig. 6-79)
  - • Femoral neck fracture (Fig. 6-80)
  - • Femoral head dislocation (Fig. 6-81)

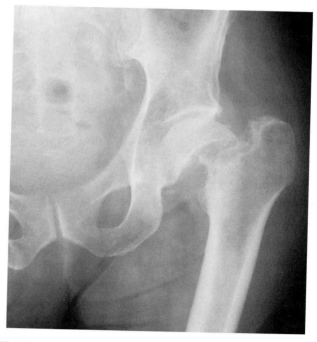

FIG. 6-80 Femoral neck (subcapital) fracture. Note the superolateral migration of the femoral shaft. (Courtesy Bryan Sher, DC, Toronto, Ontario.)

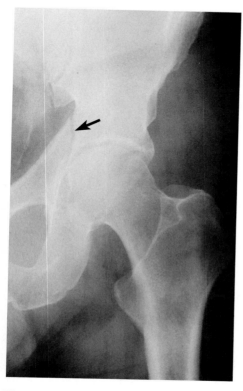

FIG. 6-78 Iliopubic junction fracture (*arrow*).

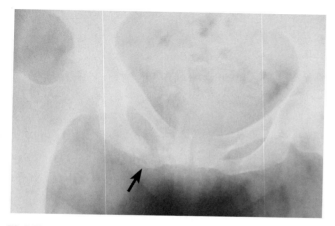

FIG. 6-79 Ischial tuberosity fracture (*arrow*).

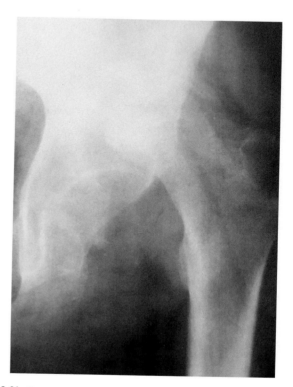

FIG. 6-81 Superior dislocation of the femoral head. Observe the empty acetabulum.

KNEE

- Bumper (fender) fracture
  - Fracture of the medial or lateral tibial plateau, as a result of a severe varus or valgus force (Figs. 6-82 and 6-83)

ANKLE

- Bimalleolar fracture
  - Fractures of the medial *and* lateral malleoli (Fig. 6-84)
- Boot-top (skier's) fracture
  - Spiral fracture of the distal diametaphyseal portions of the tibia and fibula
- Maissoneuve fracture
  - Fracture of the proximal fibula, as a result of severe inversion and external rotation of the ankle

- Frequently unobserved because of the severity of the ankle injury
- Pott's fracture
  - Fracture of the metadiaphyseal region of the distal fibula, with associated rupture of the distal tibiofibular ligament (Fig. 6-85, *A* and *B*)
- Toddler's fracture
  - Spiral fracture of the distal diametaphyseal region of the tibia in a toddler
- Trimalleolar (Cotton's) fracture
  - Fracture of the medial and lateral malleoli, in addition to the posterior tibial lip
  - Often with tibiotalar dislocation

FOOT

- Aviator's fracture
  - Fracture through the neck of the talus

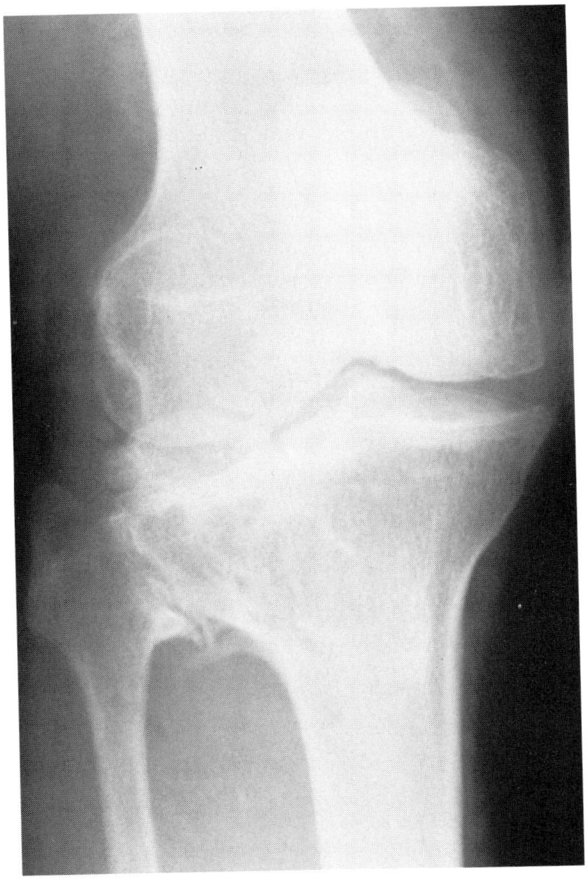

FIG. 6-82 Fracture of the lateral tibial plateau as a consequence of a severe valgus force. (Courtesy Zachary Rivietz, DC, Toronto, Ontario.)

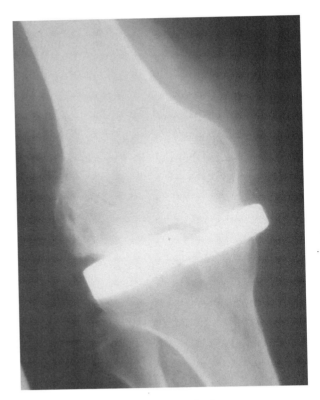

FIG. 6-83 Prosthetic tibial articular devices.

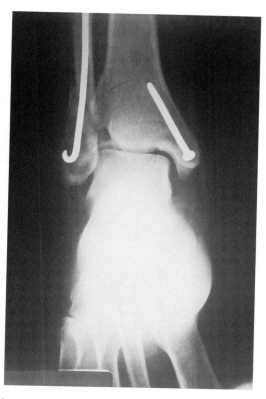

FIG. 6-84 Bimalleolar fracture with a surgical screw in the
medial malleolus and an intramedullary Rush pin in the
lateral malleolus.

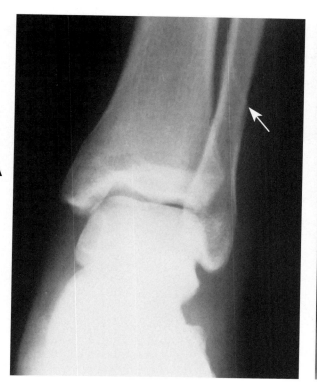

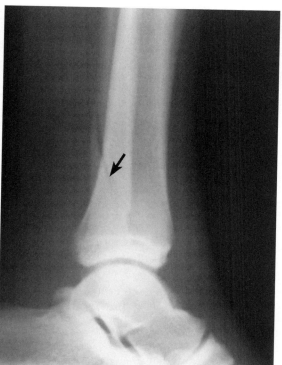

FIG. 6-85 A and **B,** Pott's fracture (*arrows*).

FIG. 6-86 A comminuted fracture of the fifth proximal pha-lanx is referred to as a *bedroom fracture.*

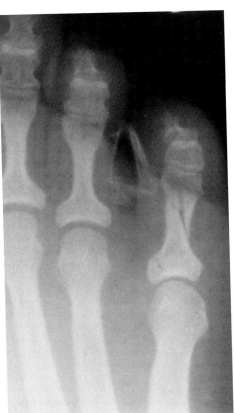

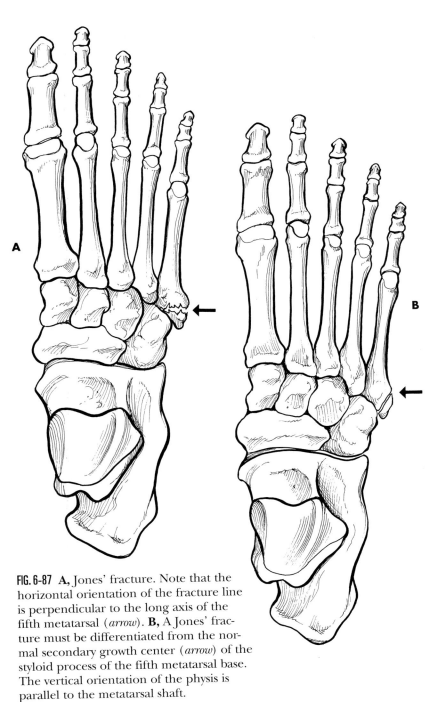

FIG. 6-87 A, Jones' fracture. Note that the horizontal orientation of the fracture line is perpendicular to the long axis of the fifth metatarsal (*arrow*). **B,** A Jones' fracture must be differentiated from the normal secondary growth center (*arrow*) of the styloid process of the fifth metatarsal base. The vertical orientation of the physis is parallel to the metatarsal shaft.

- ◆ Bedroom fracture
  - Oblique fracture of any toe phalanx secondary to striking the foot on an object (Fig. 6-86)
- ◆ Jones' (dancer's) fracture
  - Avulsion fracture of the fifth metatarsal base styloid, depicted as a transverse lucency

- Must be differentiated from the vertically oriented, unfused apophysis observed in children (Fig. 6-87, *A* and *B*)
- ◆ March fracture
  - Stress or insufficiency fracture of the second or third metatarsals (Fig. 6-88, *A* and *B*)
- ◆ Chopart's dislocation (Fig. 6-89)

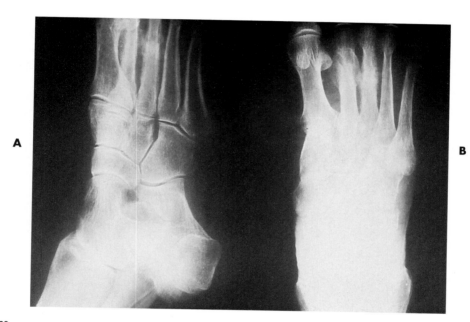

FIG. 6-88 **A** and **B,** Stress, or insufficiency, fractures of the second and third metatarsal shafts. These are also known as *March fractures*. Note the onset of osseous callus formation.

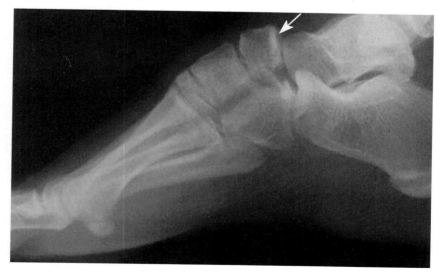

FIG. 6-89 Chopart's dislocation demonstrates separation at the talonavicular (*arrow*) and calcaneocuboid articulations.

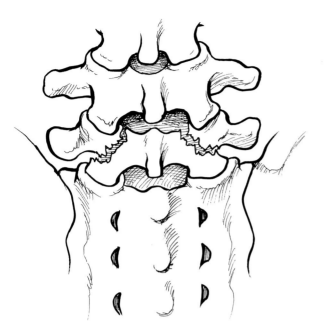

FIG. 6-90 Bilateral pars defects of L5, as seen in the coronal plane.

SPONDYLOLISTHESIS

SPONDYLOLISTHESIS
- ◆ Displacement of one vertebral body on another
- ◆ Involves a forward slippage of the superior vertebra on the inferior vertebra
- ◆ Anterolisthesis
  - A chiropractically adopted term denoting the anterior slippage of one vertebral segment on another
  - Disruption (usually) of the pars interarticularis, permitting forward slippage of the superior vertebra (Figs. 6-90, 6-91, and 6-92)

SPONDYLOLYSIS (SPONDYLOSCHISIS)
- ◆ Splitting of a vertebra
  - A cleft in the pars interarticularis, without any displacement of the vertebral body (Fig. 6-93)
- ◆ Sites of predilection
  - 90% at L5 (Fig. 6-94)
  - 5% at L4 (Figs. 6-95, 6-96, and 6-97)
  - 3% at L1-3 (Figs. 6-98 and 6-99)
  - 3% at C5-7

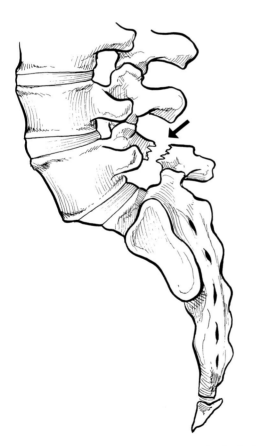

FIG. 6-91 Disruption in the L5 pars interarticularis (*arrow*), as seen in the sagittal plane.

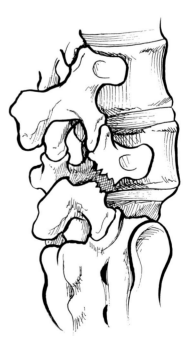

FIG. 6-92 A lucent collar on the neck of the L5 scotty dog denotes a pars defect, as seen on a diagram of an oblique projection.

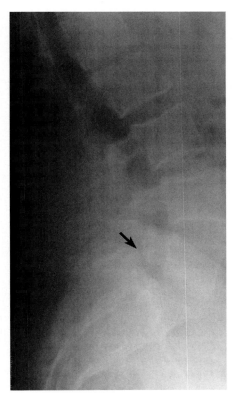

FIG. 6-93 A radiolucent cleft (*arrow*) traversing the pars interarticularis in the absence of anterior vertebral body displacement is termed *spondylolysis*. (Courtesy Lynette Nissen, DC, Toronto, Ontario.)

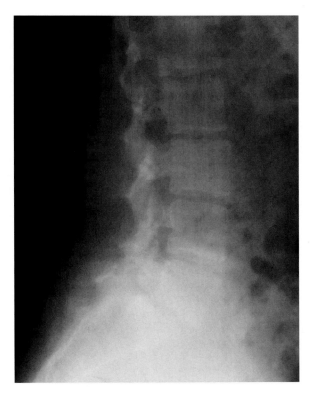

FIG. 6-94 About 90% of spondylolistheses occur at the L5 level.

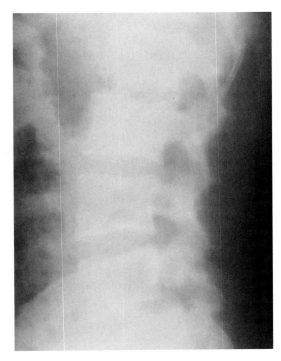

FIG. 6-95 About 5% of spondylolistheses arise at the L4 level.

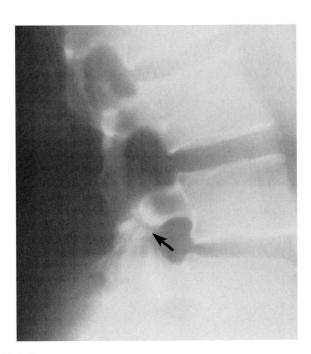

FIG. 6-96 L4 spondylolysis (*arrow*).

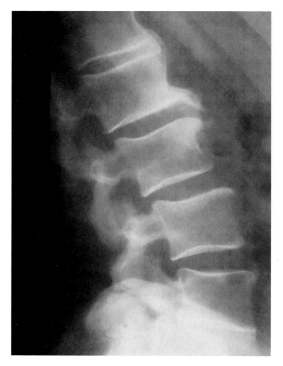

FIG. 6-97 L4 spondylolisthesis.

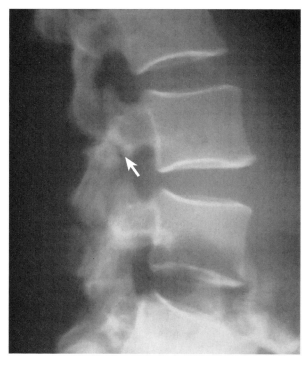

FIG. 6-99 L3 spondylolysis (*arrow*).

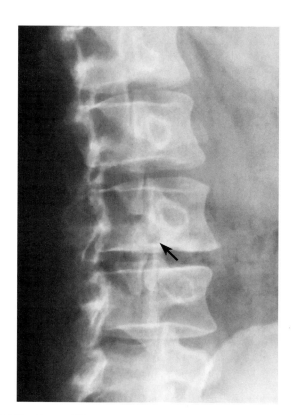

FIG. 6-98 About 3% of spondylolistheses arise at the levels of L1 to L3. Note the L3 spondylolysis (*arrow*).

SPONDYLOLYTIC SPONDYLOLISTHESIS

- Spondylolytic spondylolisthesis arises as a consequence of complete bilateral defects in the pars interarticularis.

NONSPONDYLOLYTIC SPONDYLOLISTHESIS (PSEUDOSPONDYLOLISTHESIS)

- This represents an anterior slippage of a superior vertebra as a consequence of any other cause, while retaining intact partes interarticulares.

RETROLISTHESIS

- Posterior displacement of the superior vertebra (Fig. 6-100, *A* and *B*)
- More frequent occurrence at L4 and L3
- Frequent association with disc degeneration

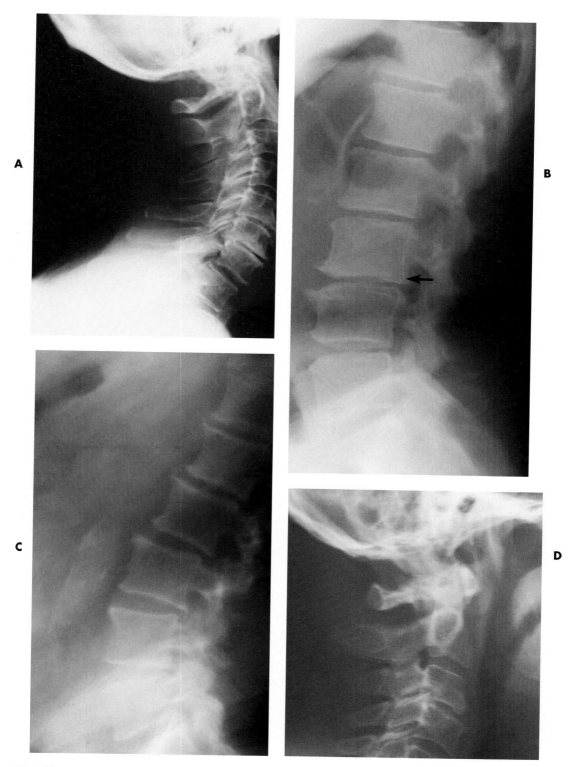

FIG. 6-100 A, Degenerative disc disease and facet arthrosis in this 75-year-old man have contributed to Grade 1 retrolistheses at C3 and C5. **B,** The L3 vertebral body of this 45-year-old woman demonstrates a Grade 1 retrolisthesis that occurred as a result of marked degenerative disc disease at L3-L4 (*arrow*). **C,** A Grade 1 degenerative retrolisthesis at L2. Degenerative disc disease is also noted at multiple levels. Observe the moderate calcification in the abdominal aorta. **D,** C3 demonstrates a Grade 1 retrolisthesis secondary to degenerative disc disease in this 50-year-old man. (**A** and **B,** Courtesy Robert Cannon, DC, Toronto, Ontario; **C,** Courtesy Lisette Logan, MRT, Brampton, Ontario; **D,** Courtesy Katrina Kulhay, DC, Toronto, Ontario.)

TRAUMA

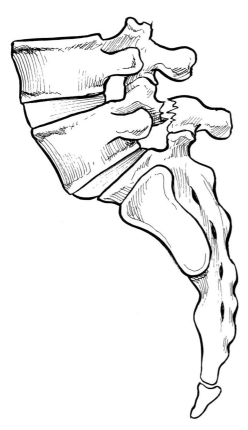

FIG. 6-101 A Grade 1 spondylolytic spondylolisthesis of L5.

Meyerding Classification

◆ The categorization of spondylolisthesis into five grades, based on the division of the superior surface of the subjacent vertebral body into quadrants
  · Grade 1: a slip of less than 25% (Figs. 6-101 and 6-102)
  · Grade 2: a slip of 25% to 50% (Figs. 6-103, 6-104, and 6-105)
  · Grade 3: a slip of up to 75% (Fig. 6-106 and 6-107)

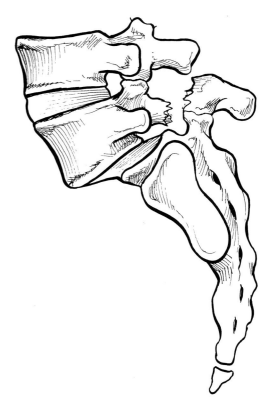

FIG. 6-103 A Grade 2 L5 spondylolisthesis.

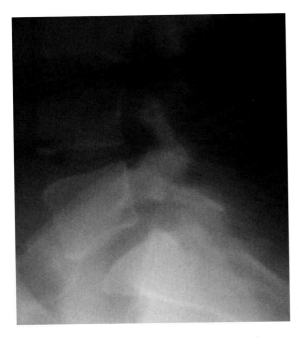

FIG. 6-102 A Grade 1 spondylolisthesis accompanies pars defects at L5.

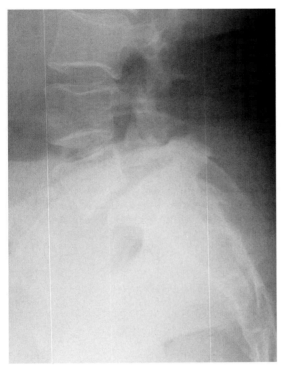

FIG. 6-104 Grade 2 spondylolisthesis of L5.

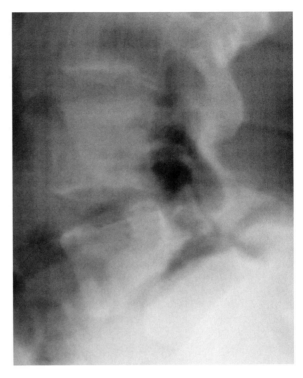

FIG. 6-105 A 50% anterior translation of the L5 body denotes a Grade 2 spondylolisthesis.

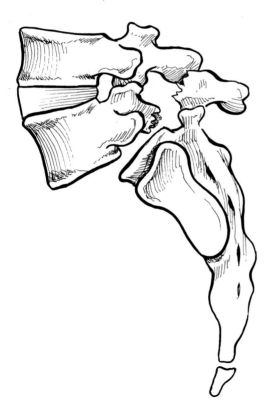

FIG. 6-106 A Grade 3 spondylolisthesis of L5.

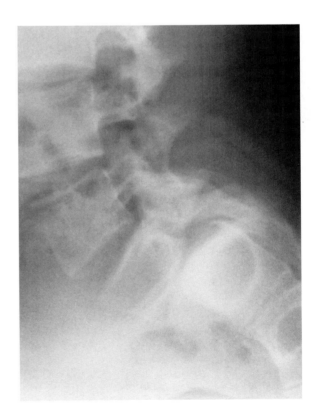

FIG. 6-107 L5 has slipped anteriorly over 50% in this Grade 3 spondylolisthesis.

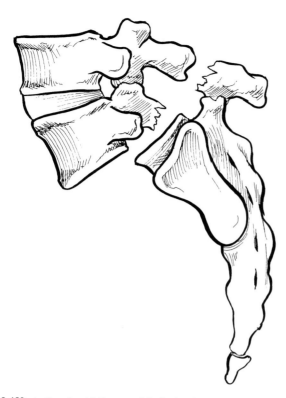

FIG. 6-108 A Grade 4 L5 spondylolisthesis.

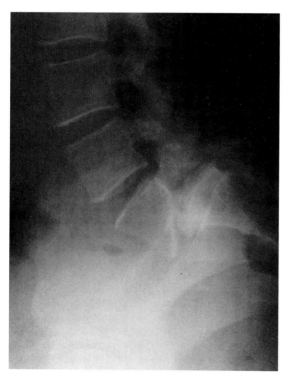

FIG. 6-109 The trapezoidal L5 vertebral body has almost completely slipped off of the sacral base in this Grade 4 spondylolisthesis.

- Grade 4: a slip of over 75% (Figs. 6-108, 6-109, 6-110, and 6-111)
- Grade 5: a slip of over 100% (Figs. 6-112 and 6-113, **A**).

SPONDYLOPTOSIS

- Spondyloptosis arises when the vertebral body of the superior segment slips completely anterior to the vertebral body of the segment below (Grade 5).
- The inverted "Napolean hat" sign (Fig. 6-113, **B**) is observed on the anteroposterior view, by which the vertebral body and transverse processes of the slipped vertebra superimpose over the subjacent segment.

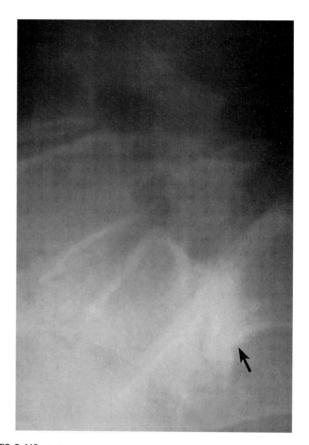

FIG. 6-110 A Grade 4 spondylolisthesis of L5 is depicted. Note the marked sclerosis and buttressing of the anterior sacral base (*arrow*) in an attempt to stabilize L5.

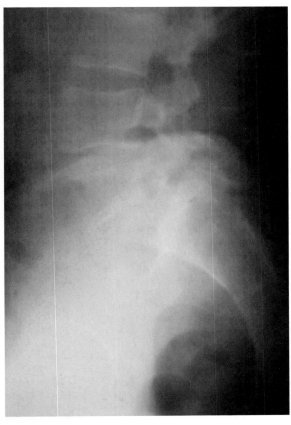

FIG. 6-111 Marked anterior slippage of L5 in a Grade 4 spondylolisthesis.

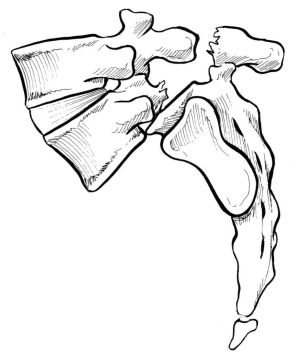

FIG. 6-112 Spondyloptosis with complete anterior slippage of L5 beyond the sacral promontory.

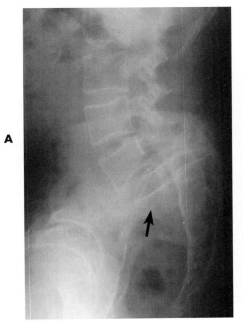

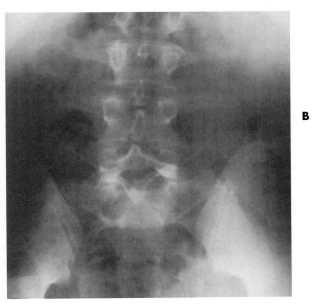

FIG. 6-113 A, Spondyloptosis. Observe the marked inferior position of the L5 vertebral body (arrow) in this Grade 5 spondylolisthesis. **B,** A severe spondylolisthesis of L5 results in the inverted "Napoleon hat" sign visualized through the sacrum on an anteroposterior radiograph. (**A,** Courtesy Catherine Owens, Lakefield, Ontario.)

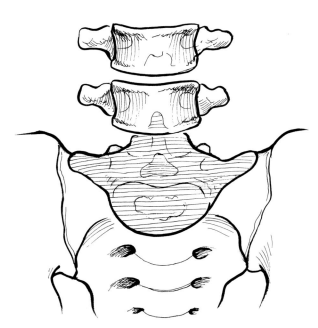

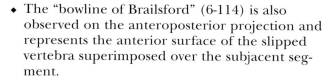

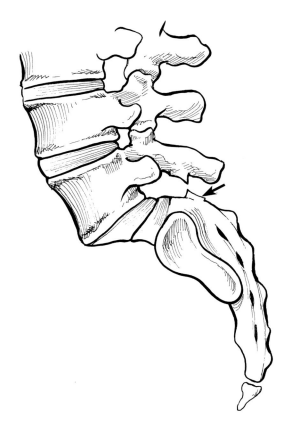

FIG. 6-114 The shaded area depicts an inverted "Napoleon hat" in this L5 spondyloptosis. The lower margin of the hat, representing the anterior aspect of the L5 body, has been referred to as the *bowline of Brailsford*.

FIG. 6-115 Dysplastic spondylolisthesis. The superior articular facets of S1 are hypoplastic (*arrow*), permitting an anterolisthesis of L5.

◆ The "bowline of Brailsford" (6-114) is also observed on the anteroposterior projection and represents the anterior surface of the slipped vertebra superimposed over the subjacent segment.

Newman Classification
◆ Dysplastic (formerly called *congenital*)
◆ Isthmic (spondylolytic)
◆ Degenerative
◆ Traumatic
◆ Pathologic

DYSPLASTIC
◆ It results from the structural abnormalities of the articular processes that allow forward slippage to occur.
◆ It is associated with deficient congenital development of the sacrum, particularly the S1 vertebral arch, and hypoplasia or absence of the S1 articular processes.

◆ Aplasia or hypoplasia of the S1 articular processes allows L5 to slip forward and downward over the top of the sacrum (Fig. 6-115).
◆ Eventually, the L5 spinous abuts against the fibrous defect in the neural arch of S1, preventing further slippage.
◆ An L5 spina bifida occulta is usually present. This may allow more severe, progressive displacement.
◆ Spina bifida at S1 and S2 are also common.
◆ The term *congenital* did not imply the presence of spondylolisthesis at birth, but rather the presence of the sacral articular deficiency at birth.
◆ Stretching and elongation of the lower lumbar vertebral arches results in response to increased mechanical traction on the pars and pedicles.
◆ The oblique lumbars present a "greyhound" configuration (Fig. 6-116), rather than the classical "scotty dog" appearance.
◆ This type may produce severe symptoms and deformity, such as S1 nerve root signs, even moreso than the spondylolytic type.

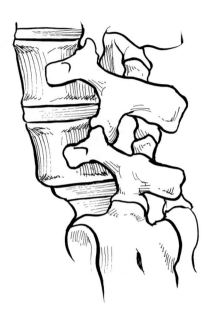

FIG. 6-116 "Greyhound" appearance on an oblique lumbar view results from the thinning and elongation of the neck (pars interarticularis) of the "scotty dog." This is a response to increased mechanical forces on the posterior arch.

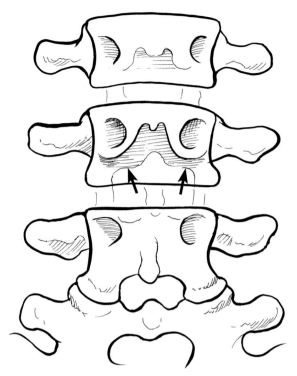

FIG. 6-117 The "baggy-eye" sign at (*arrows*). The relative radiolucencies immediately under the pedicles in the anteroposterior projection represent bilateral defects of the pars interarticularis.

ISTHMIC (SPONDYLOLYTIC)

- This type involves forward slippage as a result of bilateral defects in the pars.
- Several observations support the currently accepted theory of an acquired origin.
  - Pars defects are unknown in fetuses or stillborns.
  - These defects are rarely seen before the usual walking age (1 year).
  - No case of spondylolysis or spondylolisthesis has ever been reported in life-long nonambulatory patients, although these people have the same prevalence of other spinal anomalies as the general population.
- Isthmic spondylolisthesis is considered a type of fatigue or stress fracture caused by the repeated mechanical stress or microtraumas that are placed on the vertebral arch by an upright-walking posture.
- The incidence is higher in female gymnasts and sport divers than in their nonathletic female peers.

- Families of affected individuals have a 30% incidence. This evidence suggests a possible genetic predisposition.

Radiographic Features

- The oblique projection demonstrates a lucent collar around the neck of the "scotty dog."
- The defect may be seen on a lateral or an anteroposterior projection, but the oblique film is the definitive view.
- Isthmic defects, when observed in the anteroposterior view, may be identified by the "baggy-eye" vertebral sign (Figs. 6-117 and 6-118), which represents the lucent defect demonstrated immediately inferior to the pedicles.
- The affected vertebral body acquires a trapezoidal shape, with the posterior height being less than the anterior height (Fig. 6-119).
- An increased lordosis is common.
- The presence of slippage may be evaluated by Ullmann's line (Fig. 6-120).

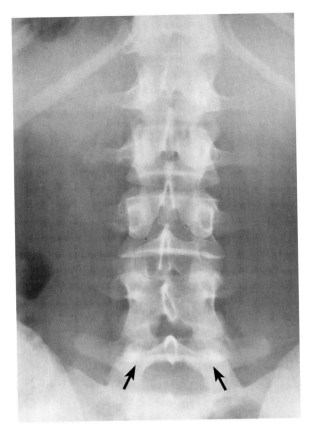

FIG. 6-118 Radiograph of a "baggy-eye" sign at L5 (*arrows*).

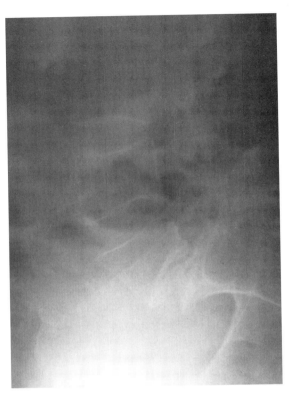

FIG. 6-119 Isthmic spondylolisthesis of L5. Note the characteristic trapezoid shape of the vertebral body, with its posterior height less than its anterior height. This is fairly reliable evidence of the presence of pars defects at this level.

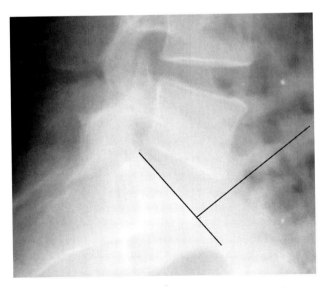

FIG. 6-120 Ullman's line. A line is drawn perpendicular to the sacral base at the sacral promontory. Spondylolisthesis exists if the anteroinferior corner of the L5 vertebral body protrudes beyond this line. This patient demonstrates no spondylolisthesis.

- With buttressing the hypertrophic spurring of the anterosuperior margin of the end plate of the inferior body develops to support the anteriorly slipped upper segment (Fig. 6-121).

Clinical Features

- Patients may have low back pain (deep-seated, dull, local).
- It is not usually the cause of pain itself.
- Patients may have a history of recent trauma and relate it to such.
- Patients cannot stoop or lift.
- Half of patients with radiographic signs of spondylolisthesis never develop symptoms.
- No correlation exists between the degree of displacement and the severity of symptoms.
- There is no displacement or fetal risk in pregnant patients with spondylolisthesis.
- Lesser degrees of spondylolisthesis can go undetected.
- In more severe cases, hyperlordosis is noted.
- Prominent buttocks and sacrum may be featured.
- Nonspecific muscle spasm may be seen paraspinally, and hamstring tightness is often encountered.

- Midline prominence is palpable as a result of the spinous process (differentiate with the depression palpated with the nonspondylolytic variety).
- Few cases of isthmic spondylolysis progress after 18 years of age.
- A unilateral spondylolisthesis may exist, demonstrating no vertebral slippage.
- Reactive sclerosis of the opposite pars and pedicle is often seen as a result of increased mechanical stress and an altered weight-bearing pattern (compensatory stress hypertrophy).
- This increased stress can result in a fatigue fracture of the pars opposite the defect. Thus unilateral spondylolysis may progress to a bilateral involvement.

DEGENERATIVE

- May occur with degenerative changes in the zygapophyseal joints, discs, or even the soft tissue–holding elements (Fig. 6-122).
- This type tends not to appear in people less than 40 years of age.
- The ratio of females to males is 3:1 and increases to 6:1 after the age of 60 years.

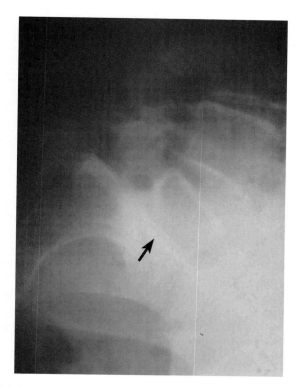

FIG. 6-121 Hypertrophic spurring, or buttressing, of the anterosuperior end plate of the lower segment develops to support the anterior-slipping upper segment (*arrow*).

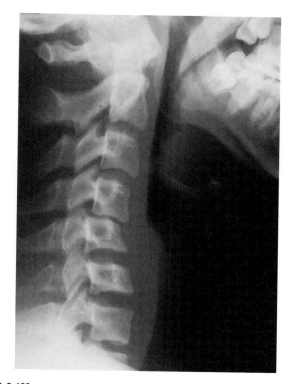

FIG. 6-122 Degenerative changes in the facet joints, discs, and soft tissue–holding elements may result in modest degrees of spondylolisthesis. Note the disc degeneration at C4-C5.

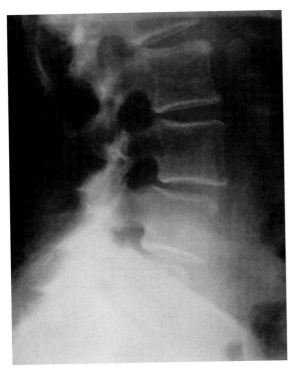

FIG. 6-123 Facet articular surfaces frequently exhibit sclerotic, irregular, and proliferative degenerative alterations, as observed at the L4-L5 level in this patient.

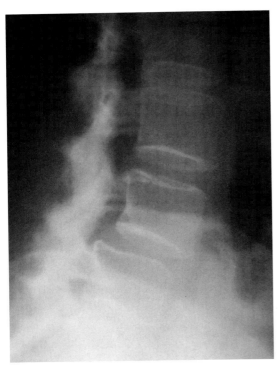

FIG. 6-124 L4 degenerative spondylolisthesis secondary to facet osteoarthritis.

- The ratio of blacks to whites is 3:1.
- It is four times more likely to occur if L5 is sacralized.
- The extent of vertebral slippage does not exceed 25%.
- It usually progresses at a rate of 2 mm per year.
- Degenerative retrolisthesis can often be seen.

Radiographic Features

- Forward slippage of the vertebra occurs with an intact neural arch.
- It is 10 times more frequent at L4 than at L5 or L3.
- Proliferative degeneration of zygapophyseal joints occurs. The articular facets are frequently sclerotic and irregular (Figs. 6-123 and 6-124).
- Osteophytic spurring may encroach on the spinal canal, and anterior slippage may result in spinal stenosis, which may compress the nerve roots of the cauda equina.
- Overriding of the articular surfaces occurs after degenerative arthritis weakens the supporting soft tissue structures.
- The bodies of L4 and L5 assume a more rectangular morphology than normal, resulting in greater mechanical stability.
- A buttressing effect may be observed.

Clinical Presentation

- Patients tend to have a long history of low back pain, often radiating into the buttocks and thighs.
- There is increased rigidity of the lumbar spine and tenderness to deep palpation at L4-L5.
- Up to 50% of patients have nerve root symptoms, usually L5. (A common finding is decreased sensation to skin pricking of the lateral thigh.)

TRAUMATIC

- Although most spondylolyses probably represent a fatigue fracture of the pars (the result of continual, repeated mechanical weight-bearing stress on the neural arch), there remains a small role for an acute traumatic episode in the acquisition of spondylolysis.
- An isolated fracture of the vertebral arch resulting from direct injury is extremely rare and usually involves the laminae rather than the pars when it does occur.

Radiographic Features

* Sharp, irregular margins of the opposing fragments are characteristic. No sclerosis of the bone at the fracture site is seen on initial presentation.
* Callous formation occurs with healing.
* Noting a history of trauma is important.
* An acute traumatic fracture of the normal pars is almost always accompanied by severe spinal injury.
* A common example is the C2 hangman's fracture (Fig. 6-125).
* Thoracic spondylolisthesis is usually due to trauma.

PATHOLOGIC

* This spondylolisthesis arises in a spine already weakened by preexisting bone disease.
* Examples of osteopathology
  * Osteogenesis inperfecta
  * Achondroplasia
  * Paget's disease (Fig. 6-126)
  * Tuberculous spondylitis
  * Metastatic malignant deposits (Fig. 6-127)
  * Osteopetrosis

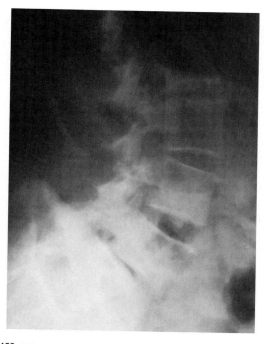

FIG. 6-126 This patient demonstrates an L5 spondylolisthesis caused by a pathologic fracture of the pars interarticularis secondary to Paget's disease.

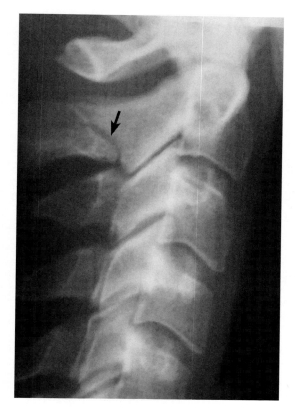

FIG. 6-125 This hangman's fracture (*arrow*) consists of a traumatic spondylolysis of the axis. No anterior slippage is observed in this patient.

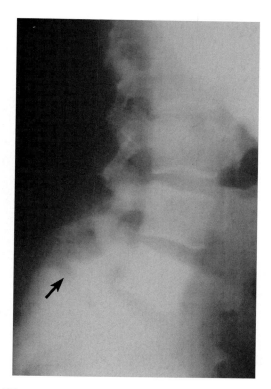

FIG. 6-127 Pathologic spondylolisthesis secondary to a fracture through a metastatic malignant deposit in the L5 pars interarticularis (*arrow*).

TRAUMA

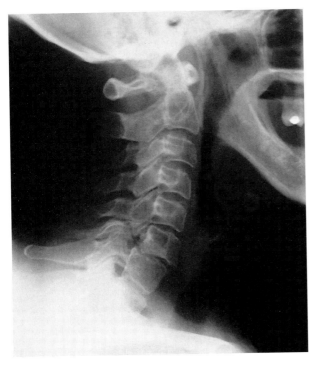

FIG. 6-128 Cervical spondylolisthesis, although rare, is most commonly observed at the C6 level.

Cervical Spondylolisthesis

- This type of spondylolisthesis is rare.
- It is most common at C6 (Figs. 6-128 and 6-129).
- It occurs mostly in males.
- It is likely due to a congenital dysplasia. Therefore bilateral hypoplasia of the articular processes and pedicles, or even unilateral pedicular agenesis, may be seen.
- About 50% of the patients have accompanying spina bifida occulta of the affected vertebra.
- A flexion-extension study is performed to assess possible segmental instability.

Treatment

- Children over 10 years of age should be allowed to enjoy normal activities, with no fear of progressive displacement or disabling pain.
- Children under 10 years of age in whom spondylolisthesis has been detected should have limitation of gymnastics and other sports until serial flexion-extension lumbar views performed 6 months apart demonstrate no evidence of progressive displacement.

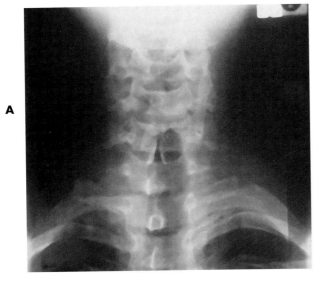

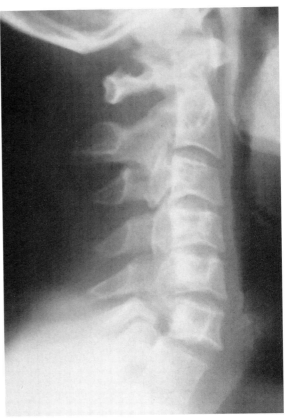

FIG. 6-129 C6 spondylolisthesis. **A,** Note the accompanying C6 spina bifida. **B,** Observe the pars defects and Grade 1 anterolisthesis.

- When patients exhibit back pain of several years duration, after the development of spondylolisthesis, this is unlikely to be the cause of their discomfort.
- No evidence supports the idea that cessation of sports in spondylolytic adults prevents the development of more serious complications.
- A conservative approach should be pursued.
- Abdominal and back muscle–strengthening exercises should be implemented.
- Low back bracing may be used.
- Chiropractic manipulation is helpful in managing with the commonly associated facet syndrome and sacroiliac fixations.

INSTABILITY EVALUATION

- Flexion-extension radiographs of the lumbar spine should be performed.
- Controversy exists, but vertebral movement (forward or backward) of 4 mm or greater on flexion-extension radiographs is felt to suggest a poor prognosis and will likely be symptomatic.
- Few patients demonstrate instability.

SURGERY

- Surgical arthrodesis, either bilateral vertebral body fusion or transverse process fusion, is performed only in patients with instability or progressive neurologic deficits.

TRAUMA

Endocrine and Metabolic Bone Disease

Human bone is living tissue that constantly undergoes dynamic alteration. While older bone is resorbed, new bone is produced, resulting in a constant state of osseous remodelling. This state, or homeostatic continuum, relies largely on the normal functioning of cellular elements, normal concentrations of such elements, adequate nutrition, healthy metabolic and endocrine balances, adequate stress levels and neurologic function, and normal digestive and renal performance.

In certain conditions, these balances may become altered, resulting in decreased production of the osteoid matrix, diminished mineralization of such, and increased or decreased production of bone. Several metabolic conditions may produce generalized, diffuse loss of bone substance. Three states include osteoporosis, osteomalacia, and hyperparathyroidism. Neoplasia, such as multiple myeloma, must also be considered as a differential diagnostic possibility. Attempting to categorize bone disease processes producing diffuse radiolucency on plain film is important because they may all present with similar radiographic appearances.

Bone loss occurs naturally after the ages of 25 to 30 years and progresses until 20% to 40% loss of organic and mineral content occurs by age 65 years. This transition is accelerated in the postmenopausal state.

The following presentations display some of the more frequently occurring endocrine and metabolic disturbances of the skeletal system.

OSTEOPOROSIS

- Osteoporosis is the most commonly encountered metabolic disease of bone.
- There is diminished bone quantity. The bone is otherwise normal. Therefore this is a situation of normal bone quality and decreased bone quantity.

(Osteomalacia involves normal bone quantity, but the bone itself is abnormal in that it is not well-mineralized. Osteomalacia results in excess nonmineralized osteoid.)

- It is not possible in the vast majority of cases to distinguish between osteoporosis and osteomalacia on plain films.

Biconcave deformities ("fish" vertebrae, "codfish" vertebrae, "hourglass" vertebrae, "biconcave lens" vertebrae, Kummel's deformity)

- This type of deformity is described as a central biconcave depression of the superior and inferior vertebral body end plates, which may be seen at multiple contiguous levels (Figs. 7-6, and 7-7).
- This depression is due to the direct mechanical force of the nucleus pulposus on the weakened end plate.
- This deformity is characteristic of disorders producing diffuse weakening of bone, including osteoporosis, osteomalacia, sickle cell anemia, hyperparathyroidism, and Paget's disease.
- The deformity resembles a fish's normal vertebral body contour.

Isolated end-plate deformities

- These deformities are infractions that represent tiny microfractures.
- They are often depicted only on one view, usually the lateral.
- The end plate may exhibit a sharp offset in continuity ("step off"), resulting in increased density adjacent to the fracture site.

Schmorl's nodes

- These nodes are localized intrabody disc herniations frequently seen in an osteoporotic spine.
- They are most commonly observed in the thoracic and upper lumbar regions.

- The pelvis and femora possess areas that are normally anatomically thin and distinctively reflect diminished bone mass, including the iliac fossa, pubis, supraacetabular area, femoral neck, and greater trochanter.
- With accentuation of weight-bearing trabeculae in the proximal femur, analysis of the trabecular pattern (Ward's triangle) is an indicator of osteoporotic severity.

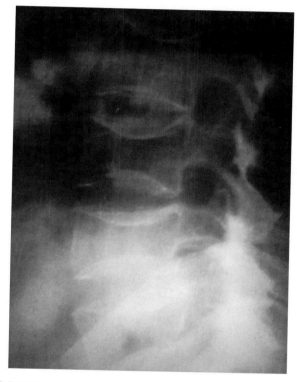

FIG. 7-7 Multiple "codfish" vertebral presentation.

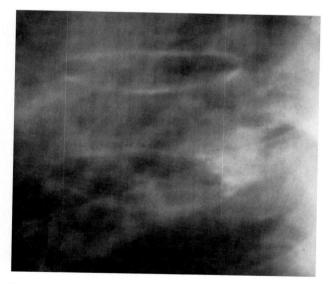

FIG. 7-6 Biconcave vertebral end-plate deformity producing a "codfish" vertebral configuration.

ENDOCRINE

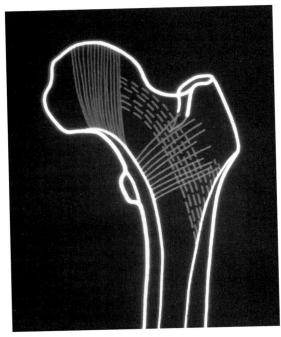

FIG. 7-8 The three principal trabecular distributions observed in the proximal femur (Ward's triangle).

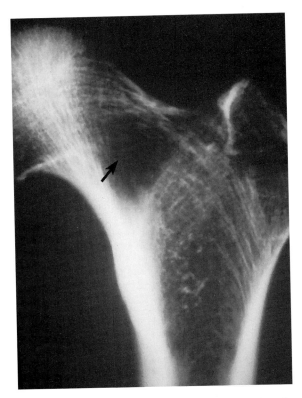

FIG. 7-9 Radiographic demonstration of Ward's triangle (*arrow*) in the proximal femur.

◆ Three main patterns of trabeculae have been distinguished (Figs. 7-8 and 7-9).
  • Principal compressive group
    From the medial metaphyseal cortex to the superior femoral head
    Represent the major weight-bearing trabeculae
  • Secondary compressive group
    From the medial cortex next to the lesser trochanter, curving upward and laterally toward the greater trochanter
    Characteristically thin and widely separated
  • Principal tensile group
    From the lateral cortex, inferior to the greater trochanter, extending in an arch to the mid-femoral head

OSTEOMALACIA

◆ Osteomalacia is a disorder characterized by a lack of osteoid mineralization, resulting in generalized bone softening. Therefore this is a disorder of bone quality.
◆ There is an insufficient deposit of inorganic salts in normal osteoid.
◆ Osteomalacia has been referred to as *adult rickets* and was formerly known as *osteitis fibrosa cystica*.
◆ There are many etiologies, most commonly involving alterations in calcium, phosphorus, or vitamin D metabolism (vitamin D aids in the gastrointestinal absorption of calcium).
◆ Other etiologies include the following:
  • Deficiencies in vitamin D, calcium, and phosphorus
  • Malabsorption from gastric, biliary, and enteric disease (i.e., sprue, Crohn's disease, diverticulosis)
  • Renal tubular disease (primary, secondary), including patients on renal dialysis
◆ The most common cause today is renal osteodystrophy.
◆ Osteomalacia may be radiographically indistinguishable from osteoporosis (unless pseudofractures are seen).

Clinical Presentation

◆ Muscle weakness, bone pain, and bone deformities are present.
◆ Symptoms of the etiology often mask the manifestations of osteomalacia itself (e.g., enteric malabsorption [sprue]), resulting in abdominal pain, bloating, and diarrhea.

Laboratory Analysis

◆ Inconsistent
◆ Elevated parathormone, alkaline phosphatase
◆ Normal to decreased serum phosphorus and calcium

Pathophysiology

◆ Increased amounts of uncalcified osteoid tissue (osteoid seams)
◆ Pseudofractures, Looser's lines, Milkman's lines, umbauzonen: likely insufficiency fractures, which heal with uncalcified osteoid
◆ Additional occurrence of pseudofractures in other bone-softening diseases, such as Paget's disease, fibrous dysplasia, and rickets

Radiographic Features

◆ Frequently not an x-ray diagnosis; requires clinical and laboratory correlation
◆ Decreased bone density
  • All bones are more radiolucent than normal and secondary to diminished bone mineral content.
◆ Loss of cortical definition
  • The cortex is thinner than normal and may appear smudged.
  • The endosteal surface is usually blurred and indistinct (Fig. 7-10).
  • An ill-defined cortex is a distinguishing feature. This may aid in the differentiation of osteomalacia from osteoporosis.
◆ Pseudofractures (linear radiolucencies, usually bilateral and symmetric, possessing sclerotic margins)
  • The most common sites of pseudofractures are the femora (Fig. 7-11), pubic rami, ischial rami, ribs, and axillary margins of the scapula.
  • Pseudofractures may heal with vitamin D administration and a high-calcium diet.
  • Deformities in weight-bearing bones (Fig. 7-12)

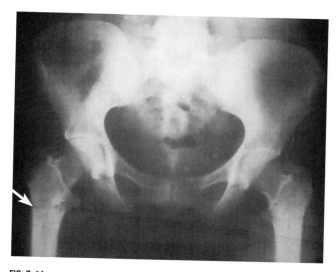

FIG. 7-11 Pseudofractures (*arrow*) of the proximal femora associated with advanced osteomalacia.

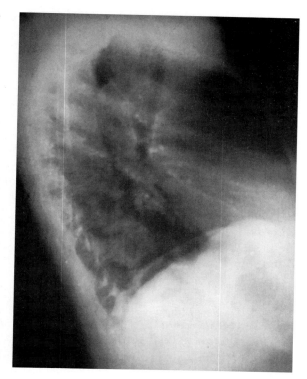

FIG. 7-10 Loss of vertebral cortical definition, as seen in advanced osteomalacia.

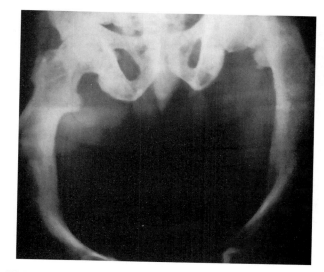

FIG. 7-12 Bone softening resulting in marked bilateral femoral bowing deformities.

- These deformities include protrusio acetabulae, bowing of the femur and tibia, kyphoscoliosis, and increased end-plate concavity.
- Residual bone deformities may require corrective surgery (osteotomies).

RICKETS

- ◆ Rickets is a systemic disease affecting infants and children.
- ◆ It classically develops between 6 months and 1 year.
- ◆ Three forms of rickets (childhood osteomalacia) are recognized.
  - Vitamin D–deficiency rickets
    Lack of dietary vitamin D or, especially, natural sunlight, which induces lack of mineralization of the osteoid matrix
  - Renal osteodystrophy (renal rickets)
    Chronic renal disease, which produces rickets and secondary hyperparathyroidism simultaneously
  - Renal tubular–defect rickets
    Failure to reabsorb phosphate from the urine, which prevents proper osteoid mineralization as a result of a lack of phosphorus
- ◆ The most common cause is renal disease, although other causes such as biliary disease and dietary insufficiencies are also responsible.

Clinical Presentation

- ◆ Muscle tetany, irritability, weakness, delayed development, small stature, and bone deformities occur.
- ◆ Clinically palpable soft tissue swellings occurring around growth plates ("rachitic rosary") are due to hypertrophied cartilage.
- ◆ Upper and lower extremities may be selectively involved, depending on whether the child has assumed an upright posture.
- ◆ The upper extremities become deformed (bowed) as the child begins to crawl.
- ◆ Anterior bowing of the tibial diaphysis usually occurs before the child is upright.
- ◆ Lateral bowing is characteristically seen in children who have begun to walk (Fig. 7-13).

Laboratory Analysis

- ◆ Elevated alkaline phosphatase
- ◆ Normal to slightly decreased serum calcium and phosphorus

Pathophysiology

- ◆ The most important changes occur at the growth plates.

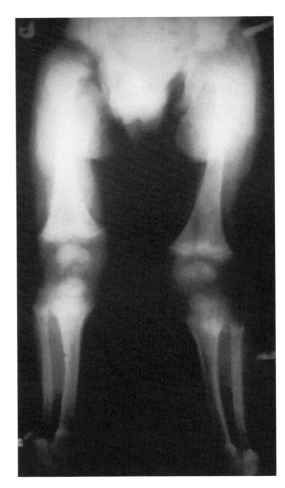

FIG. 7-13 Rickets with resultant mild bowing of the weight-bearing long bones in the lower extremities of a child.

- ◆ Cartilage cells in the physis grow normally, but they fail to calcify and subsequently degenerate.
- ◆ Consequently, the growth plate is occupied by large masses of overgrown cartilage. This widens the physeal plate, as seen on x-ray.
- ◆ Because of a lack of osteoid mineralization, the metaphyseal zone of provisional calcification is absent radiographically.

Radiographic Features

- ◆ The entire skeleton appears more radiolucent (generalized osteopenia).
- ◆ The most conspicuous abnormalities occur at the growth plates.
  - Widened growth plates; late epiphyseal closure
  - "Paintbrush" metaphysis: irregular, frayed metaphyseal margins

- Metaphyseal abnormalities (area of greatest metabolic activity) (e.g., widened, frayed, irregular, and cupped)
- Metaphyses, widened and splayed as a result of weight-bearing on softened bone; bending of long bones after softening
- Distinct white line of provisional calcification not visible (reappears on healing, useful indicator of sufficient therapeutic response)
- Fractures and pseudofractures are possible.
- In the spine, biconcave lens vertebrae may be seen.
- The initial sign of healing rickets features mineralization of the wide zone of provisional calcification (in physeal plate). This is seen as a reestablishment of the radiopaque metaphyseal band.

HYPERPARATHYROIDISM

- Overactivity of the parathyroid glands
- A variety of etiologies
- Glands release parathormone, a strong osteoclastic hormone
- Skeletal effects, widespread and frequently specific enough for a definitive radiologic diagnosis

Primary Hyperparathyroidism

- Possibly due to a parathyroid adenoma, carcinoma, or hyperplasia, producing an abnormally high titre of parathormone

Secondary Hyperparathyroidism

- Most commonly due to chronic renal glomerular disease, which creates a negative feedback as a result of persistent hypocalcemia

Clinical Presentation

- Patients are typically female, 30 to 50 years of age.
- The female-male ratio is 3:1.
- Weakness, lethargy, polydypsia, and polyuria are present.
- As a result of hypercalcemia, muscles are hypotonic and weak, and kidney calculus formation may be the reason a patient presents to practice.

Laboratory Analysis

- Primary disease is featured by intermittent hypercalcemia.
- Secondary disease features normal to low serum calcium and elevated parathormone.

Pathophysiology

PRIMARY DISEASE

- Elevated parathormone stimulates osteoclastic resorption of bone, liberating calcium and phosphorus into the bloodstream.
- Phosphorus is more readily excreted, and calcium tends to be retained.
- The net result is hypercalcemia and hypophosphatemia.

SECONDARY DISEASE

- A combination of calcium loss and abnormal renal vitamin D formation creates continuous hypocalcemia, which increases the release of parathormone, with subsequent bone resorption.
- The histopathology essentially consists of osteoclastic activity, with osteolytic resorption and fibrous tissue replacement (osteitis fibrosis cystica).
- Bone becomes soft and fragile.
- Brown tumors: Occasionally, the accumulations of fibrous tissue containing numerous osteoclastic giant cells produce local cystlike destructive bone lesions that appear brown on gross examination. These lesions may contain hemorrhagic debris.
- Subperiosteal resorption is a pathologic hallmark, arising at the interface of the outer cortex and insertional points of ligaments and tendons.

Radiographic Features

- Radiologic differentiation between primary and secondary hyperparathyroidism is usually not possible. One notable difference is the greater tendency to initiate osteosclerosis in the secondary form (Table 7-1).
- There is decreased density and diffuse skeletal rarefaction.

TABLE 7-1
Classic Differential Diagnosis:
Primary Versus Secondary Hyperparathyroidism

Primary	Secondary
Subperiosteal resorption	Subperiosteal resorption
Osteopenia	Osteosclerosis
Widened sacroiliac joint	"Rugger jersey" spine
Brown tumors	Soft tissue calcifications
Lamina dura resorption	
"Salt and pepper" skull	

ENDOCRINE

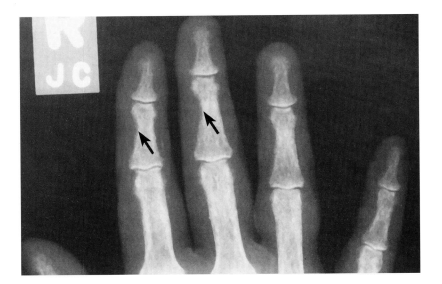

FIG. 7-14 Hyperparathyroidism. Subperiosteal resorption is observed on the radial aspects of the proximal and intermediate (*arrows*) phalanges.

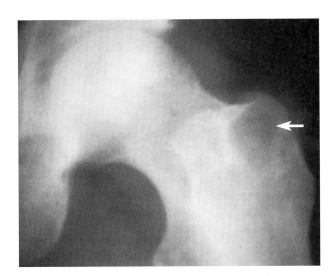

FIG. 7-15 Hyperparathyroidism manifesting as a brown tumor (*arrow*) in the greater trochanter.

- A loss of cortical definition occurs. The outer surface appears blurred and irregular, producing a frayed, lacelike appearance of the external cortical surface.
- With subperiosteal resorption the most characteristic sites include the radial margins of the middle and proximal phalanges of the second and third digits of the hand (Fig. 7-14), the medial proximal metaphysis of the humerus and tibia, the undersurface of the distal clavicle, the trochanters and tuberosities, and the lamina dura of the teeth.
- Brown tumors are distinct central geographic lucencies that may be slightly expansile and lightly septated.

- A brown tumor may mimic a benign cystic neoplasm.
- A brown tumor is composed of fibrous tissue, giant cells, and sanguinous fluid, including congealed blood from intraosseous hemorrhages.
- Brown tumors may heal with sclerosis.
- A brown tumor can affect any bone, but favors the mandible, pelvis, and proximal femur (Fig. 7-15).
- A brown tumor is potentially complicated by pathologic fracture.
- At one time, brown tumors were common in primary hyperparathyroidism. However, the majority today are seen most commonly in secondary hyperparathyroidism because there is an overwhelming preponderance of patients with the secondary form of the disease, compared with the primary form.
- A brown tumor is not included in the differential diagnosis of a cystic lesion if the remainder of the skeleton is normal.

SITES OF INVOLVEMENT OF HYPERPARATHYROIDISM
Hands
- Demonstration of subperiosteal resorption is the hallmark of hyperparathyroidism and is first identified in the hands.
- The second and third proximal and middle phalanges are most conspicuously involved.

Skull
- Diffuse granular deossification produces a mottled appearance to the calvarium ("salt and pepper" skull) (Fig. 7-16).

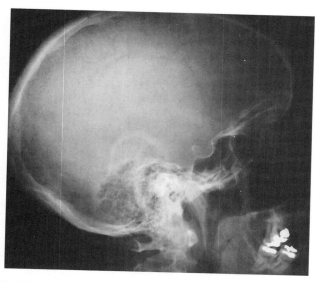

FIG. 7-16 Hyperparathyroidism: granular deossification appearance of the calvarium, resulting in a "salt and pepper" skull.

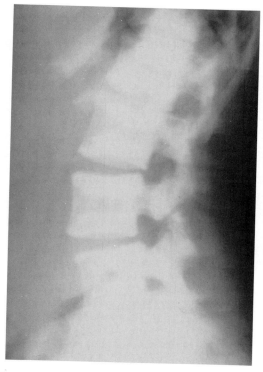

FIG. 7-17 Typical "rugger jersey" spine, as observed in advanced hyperparathyroidism.

♦ A characteristic sign is resorption of the cortical bone surrounding the tooth sockets (lamina dura).

Spine
♦ Universal generalized deossification (osteopenia) occurs.
♦ Frequent accentuation of end-plate concavities arise as a consequence of bone softening.
♦ In the secondary form, during attempted healing, a characteristic alteration is the uniform condensation-sclerosis of the sub-endplate areas of the vertebral bodies ("rugger jersey" spine, resembling the horizontal bands on a rugby jersey) (Fig. 7-17).
♦ Osteosclerosis observed in secondary hyperparathyroidism is of an undetermined etiology.

Pelvis
♦ Bilateral, symmetric cartilage fibrillation and erosion of the articular margins is more prominent on the iliac side of the sacroiliac joint and may produce hazy surfaces and pseudowidening.
♦ Similar changes may also arise in the symphysis pubis.

Soft tissues
♦ Urinary tract
  • Manifestations of hypercalcemia result in nephrocalcinosis and renal calculi in up to 75% of patients (Fig. 7-18).

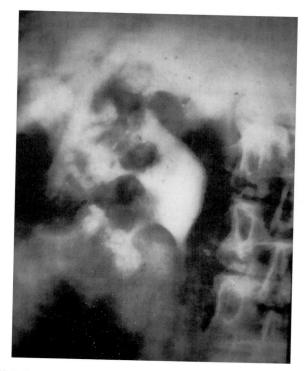

FIG. 7-18 Renal staghorn calculus associated with hyperparathyroidism. Note the involvement of the entire renal pelvis, as well as the major and minor calyceal-collecting system.

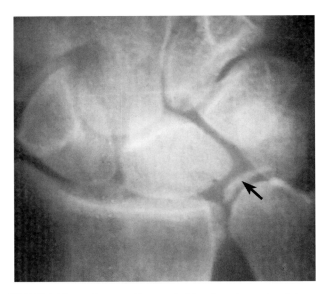

FIG. 7-19 Triangular cartilage calcification (*arrow*) of the wrist, as observed in hyperparathyroidism.

- ◆ Articulations
  - • Chondrocalcinosis, calcification of joint cartilages, occurs in 20% of patients with primary disease.
  - • It is common in knee menisci, triangular wrist cartilage (Fig. 7-19), shoulders, and hips.
- ◆ Miscellaneous
  - • Blood vessels (Fig. 7-20), ligaments, tendons, and subcutaneous tissues (Fig. 7-21) may calcify, especially in secondary disease.
  - • Calcification in the salivary glands, pancreas, lung, and prostate is possible.

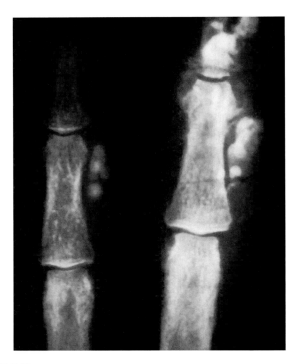

FIG. 7-21 Subcutaneous calcifications of the digits as a consequence of hyperparathyroidism.

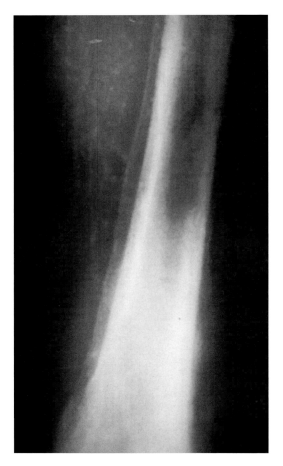

FIG. 7-20 Hyperparathyroidism manifesting as calcification of the vascular components of the thigh.

CUSHING'S DISEASE AND STEROID-INDUCED OSTEONECROSIS

- Produced by excessive quantities of glucocorticoid steroids released by the adrenal cortex

Clinical Presentation

- Obesity, especially in the thorax and face ("moon facies")
- Accelerated hair growth (hirsutism)
- Hypertension
- Deposition of fat over upper thoracic spine, producing a distinct soft tissue protuberance known as the *buffalo hump*
- Purple striae on abdominal and axillary surfaces
- Possible precipitation of identical clinical and radiologic presentation by long-term administration of therapeutic corticosteroids

Radiographic Features

- The osteoporosis of Cushing's disease and iatrogenic osteoporosis is no different radiographically than the more common postmenopausal variety.
- Diminished density, pencil-thin cortices, and fracture deformities are evident.
- Fractures tend to heal with excess callus formation.
- In the spine, biconcave lens, or "fish" vertebrae may be seen.
- An intravertebral vacuum cleft sign may be seen in corticosteroid-induced vertebral collapse, which assists in the differentiation from multiple myeloma, or metastatic disease.
- Osteonecrosis is rare in Cushing's disease but commonly induced by the therapeutic use or abuse of corticosteroids.
- Common sites of osteonecrotic involvement include the femoral head, humeral head, vertebral body, distal femora, and talus.

PAGET'S DISEASE

- Unknown etiology
- Initially characterized by destruction of bone, followed by abnormal attempt at repair
- Concurrent osteoblastic and osteoclastic activity
- Results in architectural distortion, with loss of normal bone pattern, referred to as *mosaic bone*

Clinical Presentation

- Paget's disease is most common in middle life (usually over age 50 years).
- The male-female ratio is 2:1.
- Lesions are seldom painful, unless pathologic fracture occurs.
- Every bone in the skeleton has been known to be affected by Paget's disease.
- Less commonly affected sites include the clavicle and scapula.
- Rare sites of involvement include the sternum, calcaneus, talus, patella, phalanx, metatarsal, hand, and sesamoids.
- The skull demonstrates basilar invagination, which may result in severe neurologic disturbances.
- Skull expansion manifests clinically with the patient complaining of having to buy increasingly larger hats.
- Paget's disease can be monostotic or polyostotic.
- The end result is a weakened, deformed, and thickened skeleton.
- Cardiovascular sequelae may ensue (hypertension, arterosclerosis) as a result of increased shunting of blood through the increased bone volume.
- Malignant degeneration can occur (usually in the seventh or eighth decades).

Laboratory Analysis

- Serum calcium and phosphorus levels are normal.
- There is marked elevation of serum alkaline phosphatase (up to 20 times normal) with polyostotic involvement.
- A sudden rise in an already elevated alkaline phosphatase may signify degeneration into osteosarcoma.

Radiographic Features

- Stage 1: destructive phase
- Stage 2: combined (mixed destruction and regeneration) phase
  - This is the most commonly encountered phase.
  - Radiographic findings in the combined (mixed) phase are pathognomonic.
- Stage 3: sclerotic phase
  - This phase is less frequent and is characteristically uniform bone sclerosis.
- Stage 4: malignant degeneration into Paget's sarcoma (osteosarcoma) in 10% of instances

ENDOCRINE

Pelvis

- The pelvis is involved in two thirds of cases (Fig. 7-22).
- Cortical thickening with universal innominate enlargement occurs (Fig. 7-23).
- There are coarsened trabeculae (Fig. 7-24).
- A thickened pelvic rim results in the "brim," or "rim," sign (Fig. 7-25).

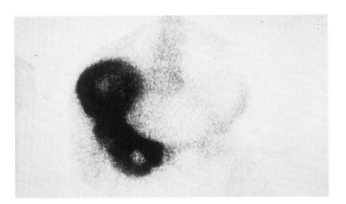

FIG. 7-22 Paget's disease. The right innominate exhibits universal increased radioisotope uptake, which is characteristic of monostotic pelvic involvement.

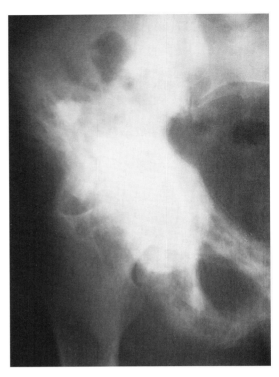

FIG. 7-24 Paget's disease. The innominate demonstrates a coarse trabecular pattern with "mosaic" architecture.

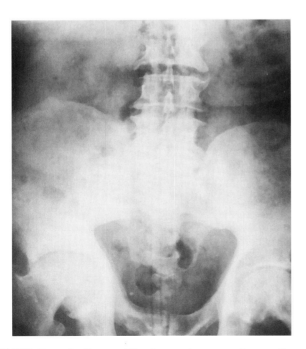

FIG. 7-23 Paget's disease. The innominate on the reading left demonstrates cortical thickening with universal enlargement.

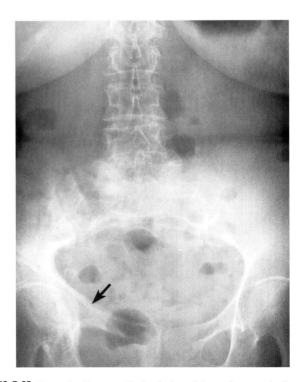

FIG. 7-25 Paget's disease: "brim" sign. Note the cortical thickening and expansion of the iliopubic junction (*arrow*). (Courtesy Richard Collis, DC, Toronto, Ontario.)

◆ Irregular patches of bony sclerosis are seen in the combined phase, and this appearance must be differentiated from osteoblastic metastasis (Fig. 7-26).

◆ Deformity and protrusion of the acetabulum (protrusio acetabulum) may be seen (Figs. 7-27, 7-28, and 7-29).

◆ The iliofemoral joint is predisposed to degenerative joint disease.

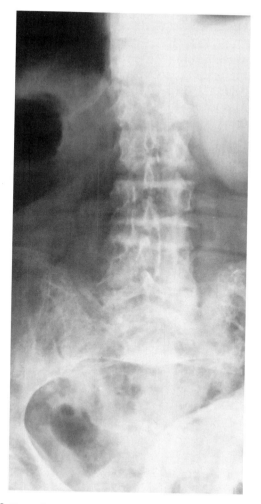

FIG. 7-28 Paget's disease: protrusio acetabulum. Marked unilateral deformity is seen secondary to pelvic bone softening.

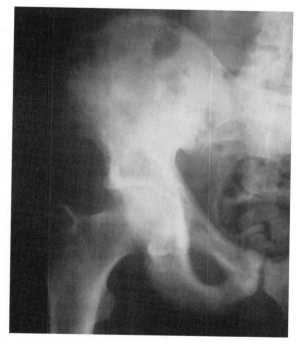

FIG. 7-26 Paget's disease of the innominate. Observe the focal areas of patchy sclerosis, which are noted in the combined phase.

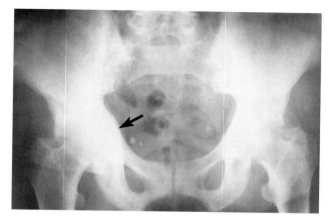

FIG. 7-27 Paget's disease: protrusio acetabulum. Observe the unilateral axial migration of the femoral head into the acetabular fossa, resulting in a convex distortion of the pelvic rim (*arrow*).

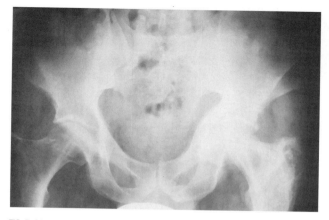

FIG. 7-29 Paget's disease. Mild unilateral protrusio acetabulum is observed.

Spine

- Vertebral involvement in the combined phase is most commonly monostotic but may be polyostotic.
- The vertebral body is enlarged in all planes and exhibits a loss of its normal anterior concavity ("squaring") (Fig. 7-30).
- The rim of the thickened body cortex gives rise to a "picture frame" appearance (Fig. 7-31).
- There is a coarsened, irregular trabecular pattern.
- The vertebral body may be observed in the sclerotic phase. It is usually monostotic and homogenously dense, giving rise to the "ivory" vertebra (Fig. 7-32). This must be differentiated from the ivory vertebral formation of osteoblastic metastasis and Hodgkin's lymphoma.

- Paget's disease demonstrates the enlargement of the body and squaring of the anterior body surface, whereas malignant metastasis retains normal body contour and size. Hodgkin's lymphoma is frequently associated with erosion of the anterior vertebral body surface by localized hypertrophied lymph nodes, but normal body size is retained.
- The cervical spine is rarely involved, but when it is, serious neurologic sequelae may result consequent to spinal stenosis.
- The destructive phase may lead to vertebral body collapse, with the disc spaces remaining intact.
- Neural arches are likely to be involved.
- Uncommonly, the atlas and axis are involved with accompanying neural canal narrowing.

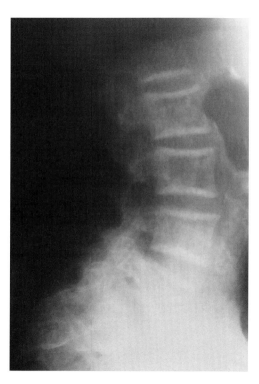

FIG. 7-30 Paget's disease: lumbar spine. Early vertebral body involvement manifests as squaring of its normally concave anterior surface.

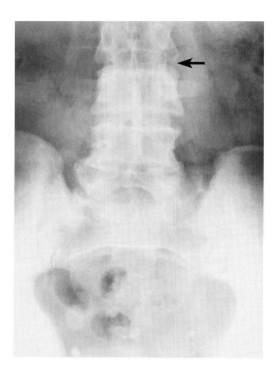

FIG. 7-31 Paget's disease: "picture frame" vertebra. Observe the thickened vertebral body cortex at L3 (*arrow*). In addition, note the minimal protrusio acetabulum on the reading left, denoting a measure of innominate bone softening.

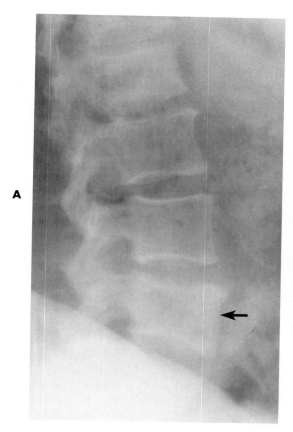

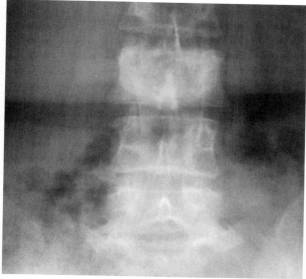

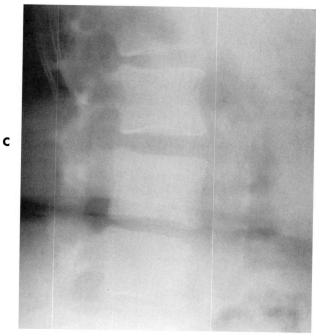

FIG. 7-32 Paget's disease: spine. **A,** An "ivory" vertebra at L5 may be observed in the sclerotic phase (*arrow*). **B** and **C,** L3 demonstrates sclerosis, expansion, and mild squaring in this 60-year-old woman. Also, note the abdominal aortic sclerosis. (Courtesy Mario Poirier, DC, Ile Perrot, Québec.)

Skull

◆ The disease begins as a rarefied area (osteoporosis circumscripta), which has been described as a maplike or geographic resorption of bone, commonly including frontal and occipital regions, with gradual progression to encompass the entire calvarium (Fig. 7-33).

◆ This lesion is well-demarcated and represents the destructive phase of the disease.

◆ The outer table is destroyed, whereas the inner table is spared (Fig. 7-34, *A* and *B*).

◆ The reparative process is characterized by irregular areas of sclerosis in the thickened diploe, which assumes a "cotton wool" appearance (Figs. 7-35, 7-36, 7-37, and 7-38).

◆ Basilar invagination may arise as a consequence of occipital bone softening (dens penetrates foramen magnum as a result of weight-bearing of the skull, resulting in positive Chamberlain's and McGregor's lines).

◆ Paranasal sinuses may be obliterated as a result of bone expansion.

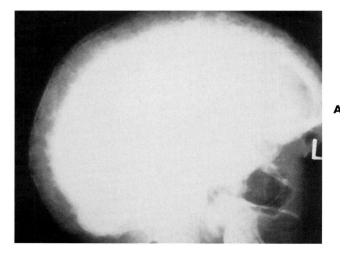

A

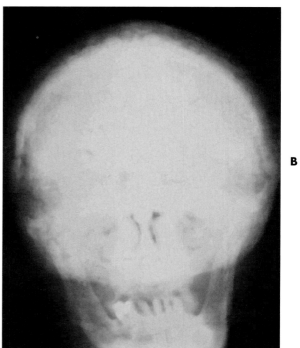

B

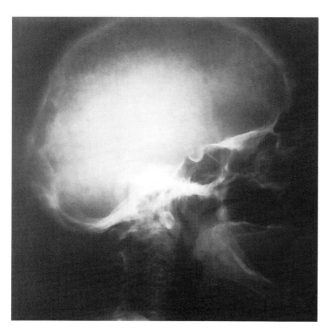

FIG. 7-33 Paget's disease: osteoporosis circumscripta. A geographic resorption of the calvarium is demonstrated.

FIG. 7-34 Paget's disease of the skull. **A,** Lateral. **B,** Anteroposterior. Expansion of the outer skull table is seen, whereas the inner table is spared. Note that involvement of the occipital bone may give rise to a platybasia deformity.

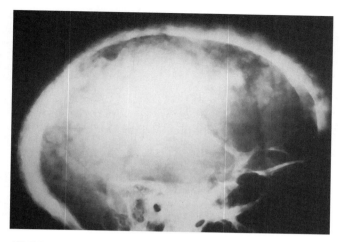

FIG. 7-35 Paget's disease. The expanded skull may demonstrate irregular areas of sclerosis, resulting in a "cotton wool" appearance.

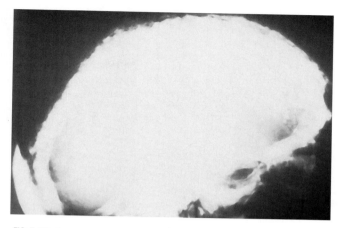

FIG. 7-36 Paget's disease: "cotton wool" effect.

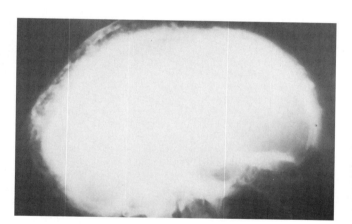

FIG. 7-37 "Cotton wool" appearance of the skull in the mixed phase of Paget's disease.

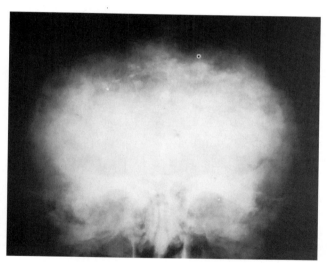

FIG. 7-38 Paget's disease. An anteroposterior view of the skull exhibits the classic "cotton wool" appearance.

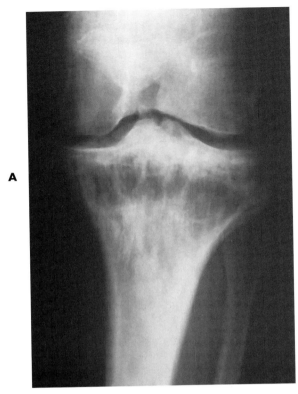

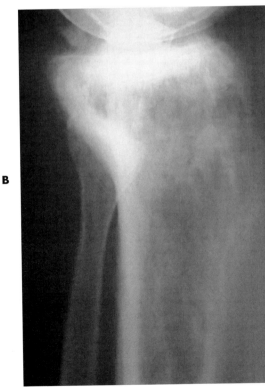

FIG. 7-39 Paget's disease: tibia. **A,** Anteroposterior. **B,** Lateral. Observe the marked expansion of the proximal tibia, with subarticular cortical thickening and coarsened internal trabeculae.

Long bones

- Long bones are occasionally observed while undergoing the destructive phase but are more frequently seen radiographically during the combined phase.
- Destructive phase
  - The lesion begins in the subarticular region of bone or at an apophysis (Figs. 7-39, *A* and *B,* and 7-40).
  - An advancing front of radiolucency extends along the diaphysis and terminates in a typically sharply demarcated, angulated configuration, rendering the appearance of a "blade of grass" or "flame" sign (Fig. 7-41).
- Combined phase
  - Widening of the bone diameter and thickening of the cortex are exhibited (Figs. 7-42 and 7-43).
  - The architectural pattern is disrupted (Figs. 7-44 and 7-45).

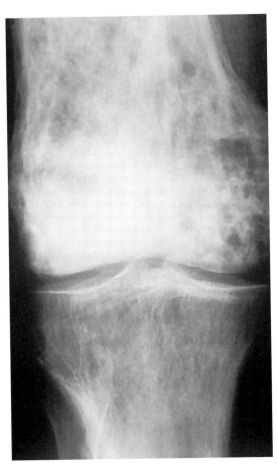

FIG. 7-40 Paget's disease: femur. Irregular, coarsened subarticular trabeculae are exhibited in the expanded terminal portion of the femur.

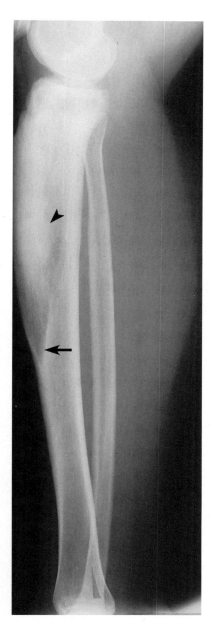

FIG. 7-41 Paget's disease: "blade of grass," or "flame," sign. The tapered advancing front (*arrow*) of the lytic phase in this tibia is closely followed by the thickened cortex and expansion of the combined phase (*arrowhead*).

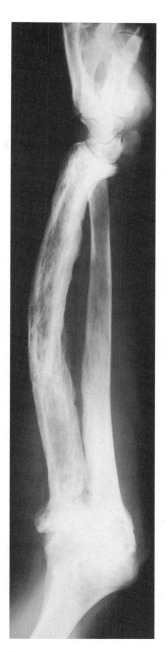

FIG. 7-42 Paget's disease: combined phase. Widening of the bone diameter, thickening of the cortex, "mosaic" internal architecture, and marked bowing of the softened radius are seen in this example.

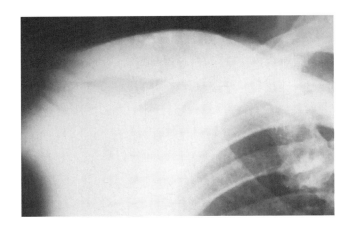

FIG. 7-43 Paget's disease: clavicle. Significant expansion and cortical thickening are characteristic of the combined phase.

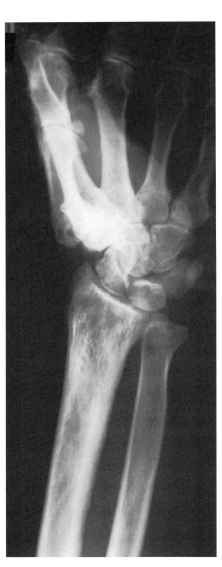

FIG. 7-44 Paget's disease: combined phase. Altered architectural pattern with thickened cortex is noted in the distal radius.

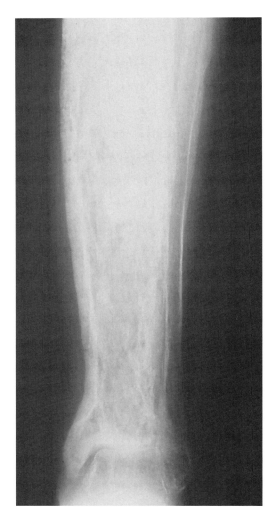

FIG. 7-45 Paget's disease of the tibia. Cortical thickening, coarsening of the trabeculae, and marked expansion are exhibited in this 71-year-old man. (Courtesy Cecil McQuoid, DC, Brighton, Ontario.)

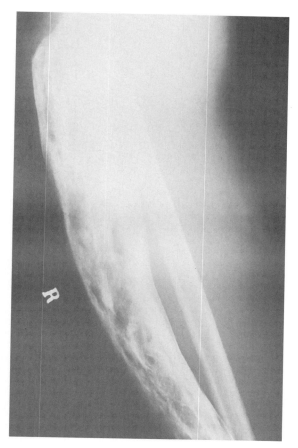

FIG. 7-46 The lateral projection of the same patient demonstrates moderate anterior bowing of the softened tibia.

- Bowing and deformity are the result of monostotic long-bone softening and expansion (Figs. 7-46, 7-47, 7-48, and 7-49).
- In the lower extremity, weight-bearing may exacerbate the bowing and deformity.
- Softening of the femur may produce a "shepherd's crook" deformity (Fig. 7-50).
- Softening of the tibia results in a "sabre shin" deformity (Fig. 7-51).
- Pseudofractures (Looser's zones, Milkman's fractures, umbauzonen) are radiolucent defects affecting the cortex on the convex surface of long bones (Figs. 7-52 and 7-53).
- These pseudofractures represent local areas of demineralization in the bone, which may predispose to complete pathologic transverse "banana" fractures (Figs. 7-54 and 7-55).

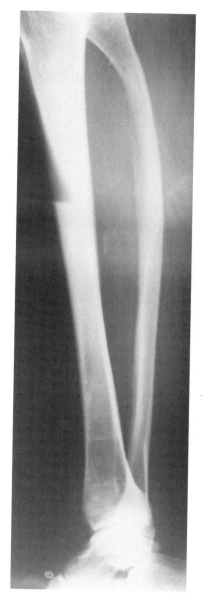

FIG. 7-47 Paget's disease of the fibula. A moderate bowing deformity may be seen in a softened long bone.

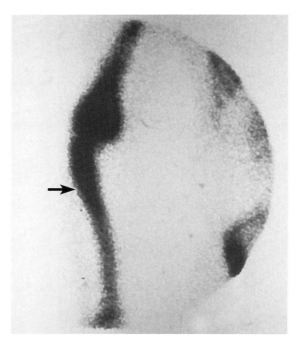

FIG. 7-48 Paget's disease of the upper extremity. Bone scintigraphy reveals increased uptake in the distal humerus and ulna. In addition, note the bowing of the ulna (*arrow*).

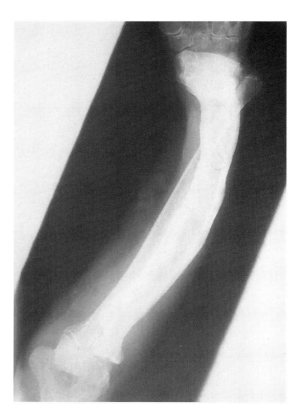

FIG. 7-49 Paget's disease: combined phase. Severe bowing deformity with universal expansion, cortical thickening, and trabecular coarsening is observed in the radius.

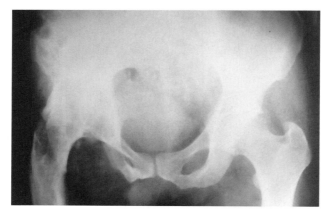

FIG. 7-50 Paget's disease. Softening of the proximal femur may manifest as a "shepherd's crook" deformity.

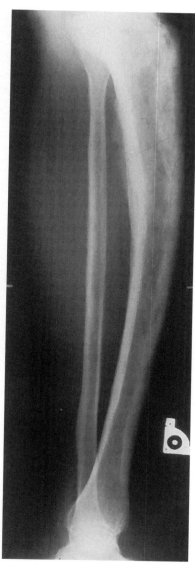

FIG. 7-51 Paget's disease. Marked anterior bowing of the tibia as a consequence of its softening may result in a typical "sabre shin" deformity.

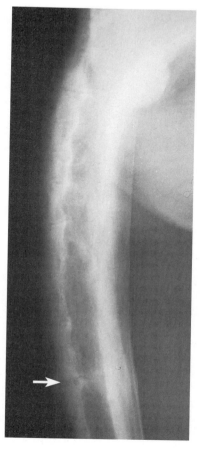

FIG. 7-52 Paget's disease. A linear radiolucent defect extending through the convex surface of a long bone is indicative of a pseudofracture (*arrow*).

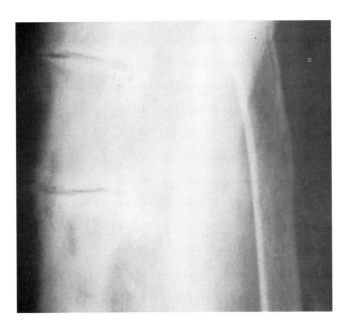

FIG. 7-53 Paget's disease. Typical pseudofractures are demonstrated in the tibia. These represent seams of uncalcified osteoid.

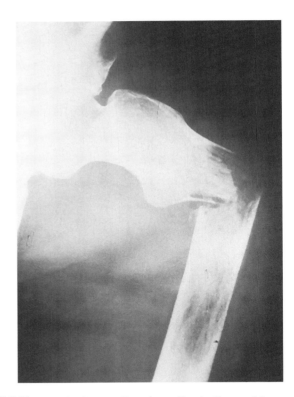

FIG. 7-54 Paget's disease. Demineralized, diseased bone may predispose it to complete pathologic transverse fracture. This condition has been termed a *banana fracture*.

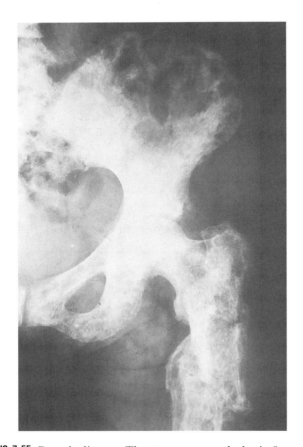

FIG. 7-55 Paget's disease. The transverse pathologic fracture in this proximal femur has healed with exuberant callus formation.

Soft Tissue

A variety of soft tissue lesions may be demonstrated by plain film radiography Figs. 8-1 to 8-95). Physical displacement of tissue planes or organs may be the earliest identification of an underlying disease state. More frequently, the observer is confronted by the presence of calcific infiltrations into various soft tissue components.

It is not uncommon, for example, to observe atherosclerotic plaquing of major abdominal vascular elements. Invariably, any human soft tissue anatomic structure can be the target of calcific infiltration. These include muscles, tendons, and bursae, as well as organs and neoplastic masses. Periodically, lesions in soft tissues or artifacts must also be identified. The art of soft tissue radiodiagnosis is frought with peril and frequently represents one of the most interesting, yet most challenging, subjects of diagnostic imaging. Soft tissue calcific depositions may be classified by various characterictic presentations.

CONCRETIONS

- Concretions are characterized by a calcified mass in a vascular lumen or hollow viscus.
- The most frequent sites of origin are the urinary tract, pelvic veins, and biliary vesicle.
- Calculi formation in other hollow viscera (e.g., appendicoliths) and parenchyma (e.g., pancreatic calculi) is not uncommon.
- They generally exhibit sharply defined external margins and may develop into any size.
- Some concretions may appear homogeneously dense, some exhibit laminations, others may manifest small eccentric radiolucencies, and still others may demonstrate a whorled or amorphous calcific pattern.

CONDUIT WALL CALCIFICATIONS

- Conduit wall calcifications are characterized by calcific infiltration of hollow tube structures.
- The calcium presents as parallel tracks or interrupted lines when observed in profile and ring-shaped when observed en face.
- Serpiginous patterns may be observed with calcific infiltration of the splenic artery or vas deferens.

CYST WALL CALCIFICATIONS

- Cyst wall calcifications are featured by calcific infiltration of the walls of fluid-filled cysts, for example.
- They generally appear larger than the ringlike calcifications of vascular walls.
- They are not usually perfectly round.

SOLID MASS CALCIFICATIONS

- Solid mass calcifications may be characterized by amorphous, whorled, "popcorn," or flecked appearances.
- Calcified lymph nodes and fibromyomas may manifest one of these patterns.

LOCATION OF ABDOMINAL CALCIFICATIONS

The site or location of a calcific lesion is often important in arriving at a reasonable differential diagnosis. A good rule of thumb when trying to determine whether a lesion is retroperitoneal is to carefully examine the lateral lumbar view. If the lesion is superimposed over the spine, it is probably retroperitoneal. If, on the other hand, it lies anterior to the spine, the lesion is likely intraperitoneal.

- Left upper quadrant
  - Retroperitoneal
    Left renal lithiasis
    Left renal artery calcification
    Renal and adrenal cysts
    Left adrenal calcification
  - Intraperitoneal
    Aortic arteriosclerosis
    Pancreatic calcification
    Splenic arteriosclerosis
    Splenic parenchymal calcification
    Costochondral cartilage calcification
- Left lower quadrant
    Mesenteric lymph node calcification
    Left common iliac artery arteriosclerosis
    Calcified iliac artery aneurysms
    Uterine fibromata
    Urethral calculi
- Right upper quadrant
  - Retroperitoneal
    Right renal lithiasis
    Right renal artery calcification
    Renal and adrenal cysts (less common)
    Right adrenal calcification
  - Intraperitoneal
    Cholelithiasis
    Porcelain gallbladder
    Hepatic calcifications (e.g., cysts, fungal infections)

    Calcifications of the pancreatic head
    Costochondral cartilage calcification
- Right lower quadrant
    Mesenteric lymph node calcification
    Right common iliac artery arteriosclerosis
    Calcified iliac artery aneurysms
    Uterine Fibromata
    Urethral calculi
    Appendicoliths
    Cholelithiasis with ptosis

Calcifications That May Cross the Midline

- Pancreatic calculi
- Aortic sclerosis
- Calcific pelvic tumors such as uterine fibromata

PELVIC CALCIFICATIONS

- Phleboliths (generally limited to the regions inferior to the iliac spines and adjacent to the pelvic rim)
- Calcification of the external iliac artery
- Appendicoliths
- Urinary vesicle calculi
- Prostatic calcification at the level of the symphysis pubis
- Vas deferens wall calcification
- Dermoid cysts that may contain a tooth-shaped inclusion
- Uterine fibromata
- Ovarian neoplasms (occasionally)
  Lesion movement may be influenced by gravity, peristalsis, respiration, or mass augmentation.
- Gravitational layering of milk of calcium bile can be influenced by postural alterations.
- Retroperitoneal masses are less likely to move with respiration than intraperitoneal masses.
- Costal cartilage calcifications generally move along with rib respiratory excursion.
- Urinary tract calculi migrate with the parastaltic activity of the ureters.
- Intraluminal gastrointestinal calcifications may similarly move with tract parastalsis.
- The size and location of calcification contained in a known mass may alter as the size or location of the mass in which it is contained changes.
- Enlarging pelvic masses may displace previously identified abdominal or pelvic calcifications.
  The following pages offer a selection of commonly presenting soft tissue lesions discovered during radiographic assessment.

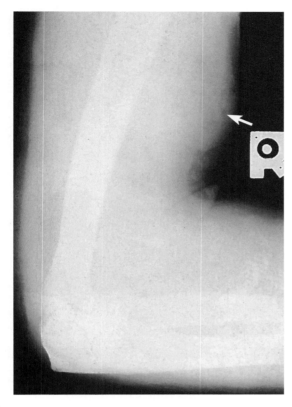

FIG. 8-1 Ruptured head of the biceps tendon gives rise to a "Popeye's" muscle (*arrow*).

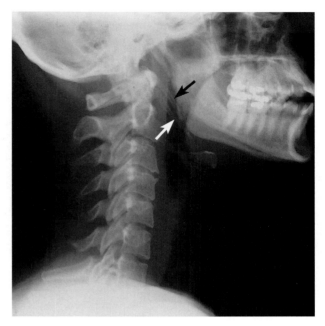

FIG. 8-2 Extensive calcification of the stylohyoid ligaments is exhibited (*arrows*).

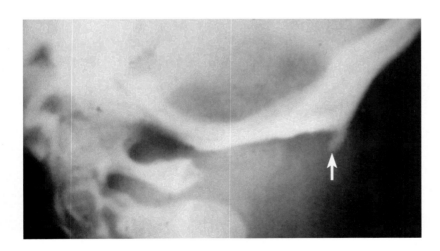

FIG. 8-3 Calcification of the origin of the nuchal ligament at the external occipital protuberance is evident (*arrow*).

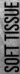

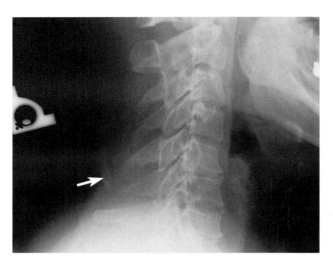

FIG. 8-4 A linear benign calcification of the nuchal ligament posterior to the C5 spinous process is observed (*arrow*). This appearance has been associated with the presence of degenerative disc disease.

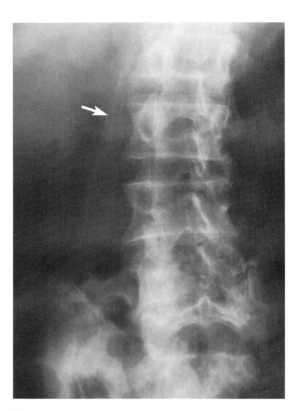

FIG. 8-5 Myositis ossificans of the psoas muscle is visualized (*arrow*).

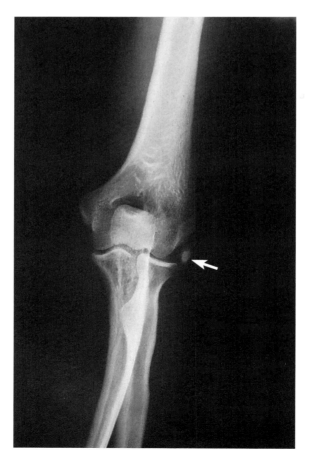

FIG. 8-6 Calcification of the common extensor tendon of the elbow is noted (*arrow*).

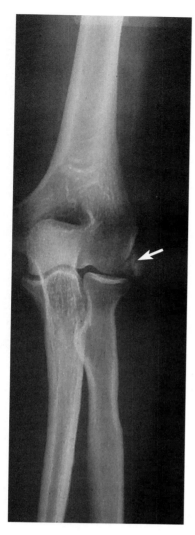

FIG. 8-7 The same common extensor tendon is seen at a 6-month interval (*arrow*).

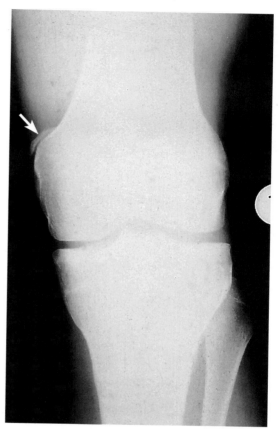

FIG. 8-8 Pellegrini-Stieda disease is characterized by calcification of the medial collateral ligament (*arrow*), adjacent to the medial femoral epicondyle.

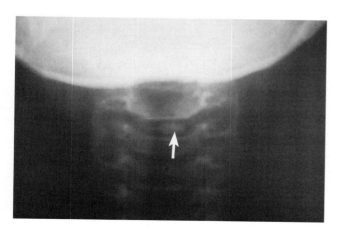

FIG. 8-9 Idiopathic nuclear calcification of the intervertebral disc (*arrow*) is observed at the C3-C4 level.

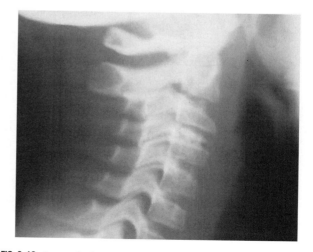

FIG. 8-10 Lateral view of idiopathic nuclear disc calcification at C3-C4.

SOFT TISSUE

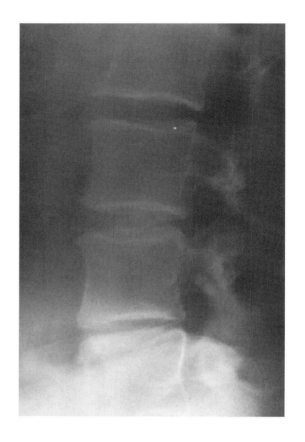

FIG. 8-11 Idiopathic calcification of the nuclear portion of a disc is noted at the L3-L4 intervertebral level. Nuclear calcification has also been associated with degenerative disc disease or may be idiopathic in origin.

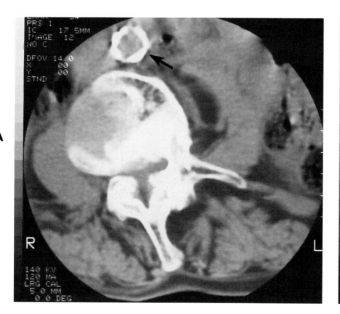

A

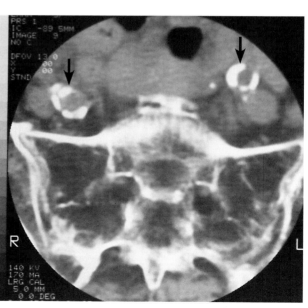

B

FIG. 8-12 A, Computed axial tomographic scan demonstrating a sclerotic abdominal aorta (*arrow*). **B,** Computed tomographic study depicting extensive bilateral plaquing of the common iliac arteries (*arrows*).

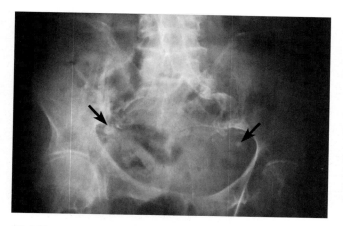

FIG. 8-13 Sclerosing of the internal iliac artery is noted (*arrows*).

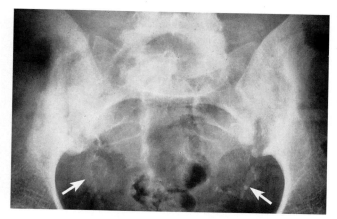

FIG. 8-14 Bilateral internal iliac arterial sclerosis is observed (*arrows*).

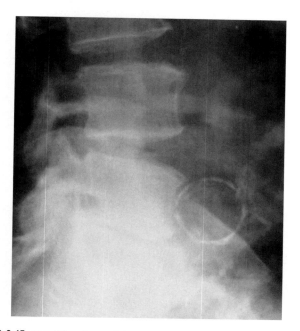

FIG. 8-15 Calcification of the aortic bifurcation is observed en face in this lateral projection.

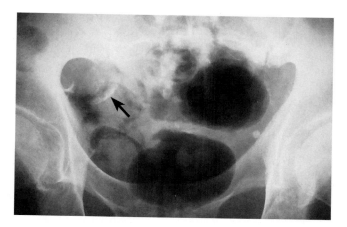

FIG. 8-16 An internal iliac artery aneurysm is demonstrated (*arrow*).

SOFT TISSUE

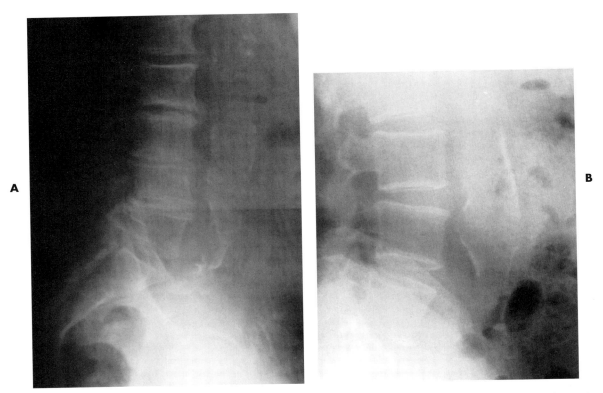

FIG. 8-17 **A,** A descending abdominal aortic aneurysm is observed, measuring 3.9 cm in its sagittal diameter. **B,** This 81-year-old man demonstrates a 4.3-cm abdominal aortic aneurysm. Note the characteristic curvilinear calcification denoting the posterior bulge of the vascular wall. (Courtesy Daniel Proctor, DC, Toronto, Ontario.)

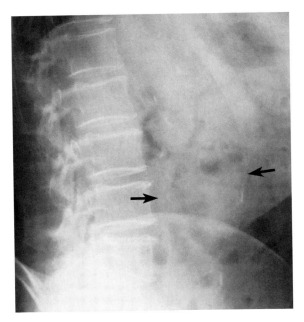

FIG. 8-18 A descending abdominal aortic aneurysm (*arrows*) measuring 7.5 cm in its sagittal diameter. (Courtesy Bryan Sher, DC, Toronto, Ontario.)

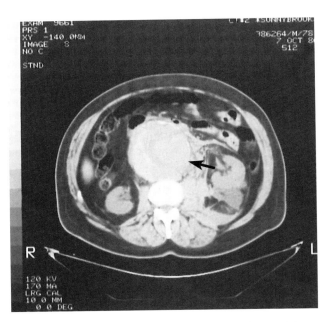

FIG. 8-19 A large aortic aneurysm (*arrow*) is observed in this computed tomographic scan.

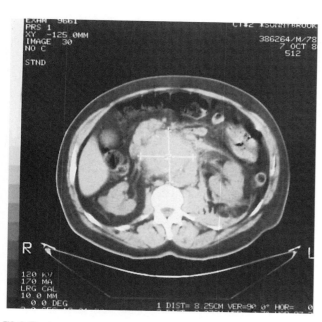

FIG. 8-20 A cursor measures the anteroposterior and lateral dimensions of this aortic aneurysm. At 5 cm the aneurysm is considered surgical, and at 9 cm, aneurysms rupture 90% of the time.

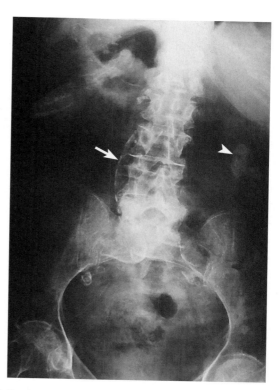

FIG. 8-21 Anteroposterior projection of an abdominal aortic aneurysm (*arrow*), with its typical interrupted curvilinear calcific appearance. A renal "staghorn" calculus is also exhibited (*arrowhead*).

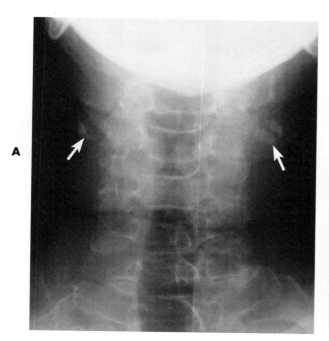

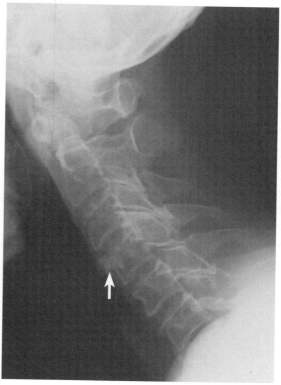

FIG. 8-22 Bilateral carotid artery sclerosis is observed (*arrows*). **A,** Anteroposterior. **B,** Lateral.

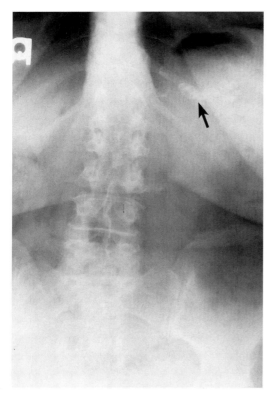

FIG. 8-23 Splenic artery sclerosis is noted on this antero-posterior radiograph (*arrow*).

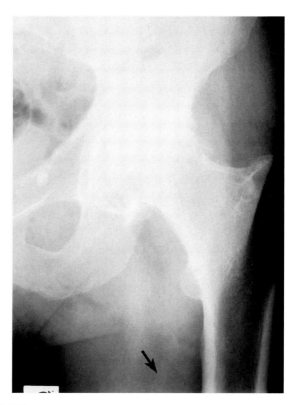

FIG. 8-24 Sclerosis of the femoral artery is noted (*arrow*).

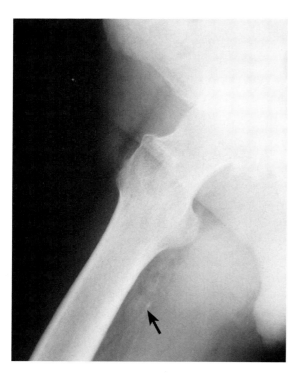

FIG. 8-25 Frog-leg projection demonstrates moderate sclerosing of the femoral artery (*arrow*).

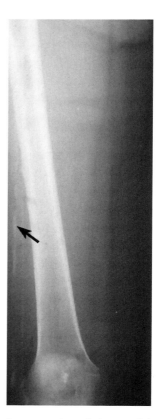

FIG. 8-26 Femoral artery sclerosis is noted in this study (*arrow*).

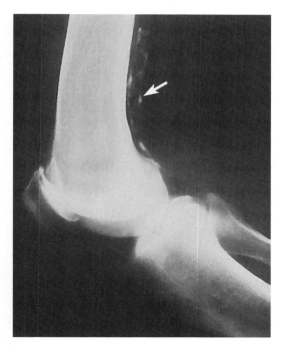

FIG. 8-27 Femoral arterial sclerosis is visualized in the distal thigh (*arrow*).

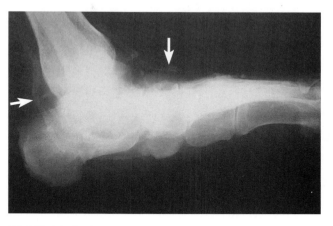

FIG. 8-28 Marked Monckeberg's medial sclerosis (*arrows*) is observed in the arteries of this diabetic patient's foot.

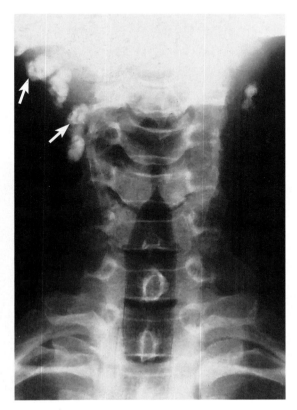

FIG. 8-29 Calcific lymphadenopathy is noted in the paracervical lymph node chain (*arrows*). Note the popcorn-shaped calcific appearance.

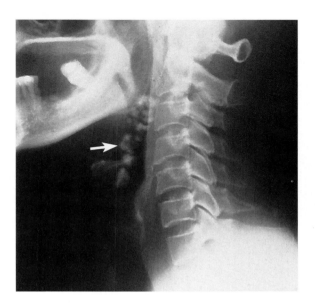

FIG. 8-30 A lateral view of the cervical spine reveals calcific lymphadenopathy (*arrow*).

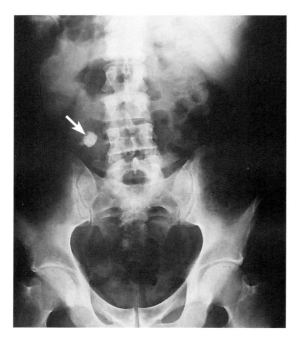

FIG. 8-31 A solitary calcified mesenteric lymph node (*arrow*) is demonstrated in this anteroposterior projection.

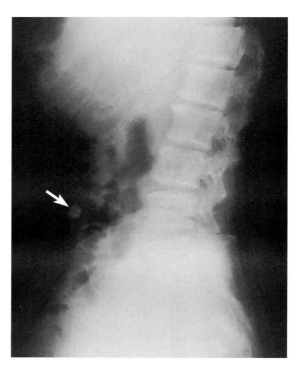

FIG. 8-32 A calcified mesenteric lymph node (*arrow*) is demonstrated in this lateral projection.

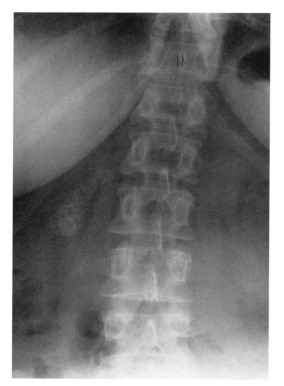

FIG. 8-33 A cluster of multiple mixed calcium and cholesterol cholelithiasis completely fills the biliary vesicle.

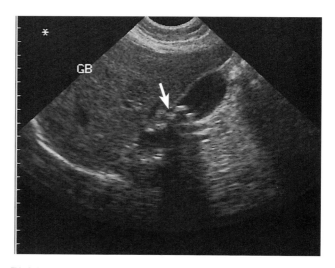

FIG. 8-34 An ultrasound study of a gallbladder demonstrating multiple cholelithiasis (*arrow*).

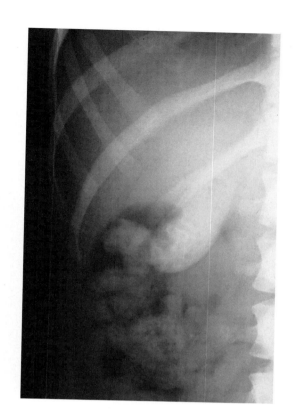

FIG. 8-35 Multiple mixed cholelithiasis.

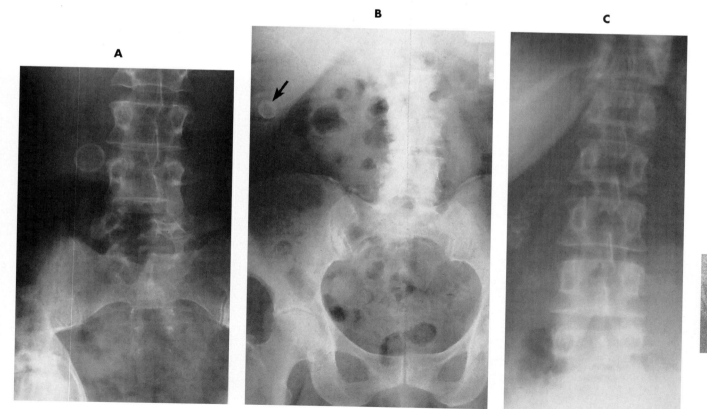

FIG. 8-36 **A,** A large solitary laminated gallstone. **B,** A solitary calcium gallstone (*arrow*).
C, Multiple mixed laminated gallstones.

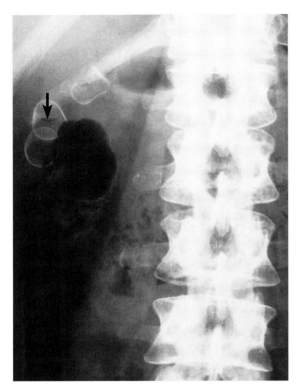

FIG. 8-37 "Mercedes-Benz" sign. Multiple large gallstones in this study demonstrate a characteristic trilinear central fissuring filled with nitrogen gas and resembling the logo of the Mercedes-Benz automobile company (*arrow*).

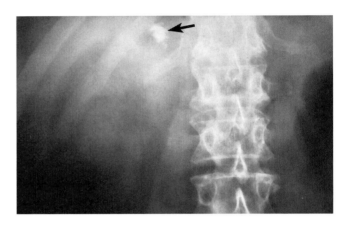

FIG. 8-38 A solitary calcium gallstone (*arrow*).

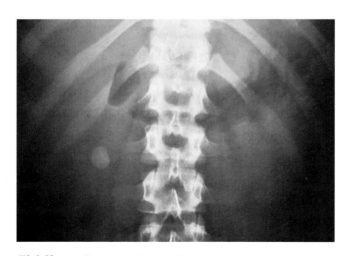

FIG. 8-39 A solitary calcium gallstone.

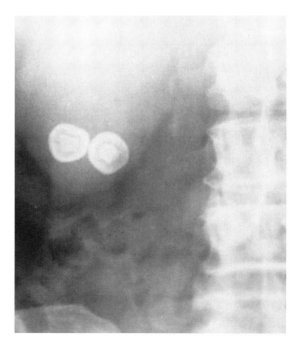

FIG. 8-40 Large concentrically laminated, faceted gallstones.

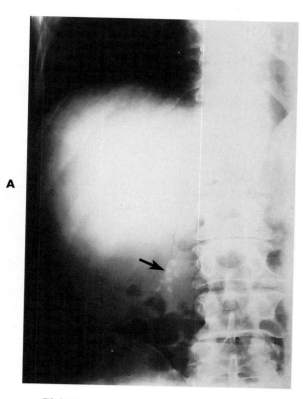

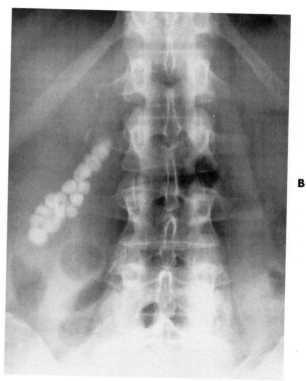

FIG. 8-41 A, Multiple calcium gallstones (*arrow*). **B,** Multiple calcium gallstones fill the entire gallbladder lumen.

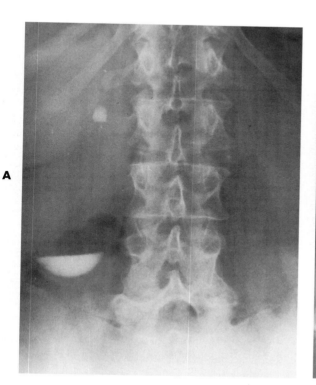

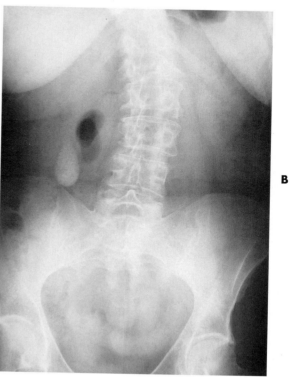

FIG. 8-42 A, Milk of calcium bile consists of hundreds of tiny gallstones forming a suspension. Note the air-fluid meniscus level, demonstrating the upright posture of the patient. Note the solitary calcium calculus in the cystic duct. **B,** Milk of calcium bile completely fills the biliary vesicle.

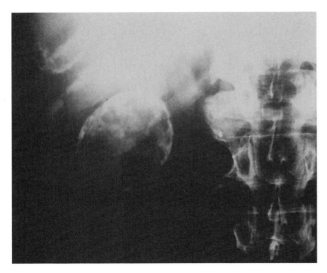

FIG. 8-43 Chronic gallbladder disease may result in a distended, calcified wall known as *porcelain gallbladder*.

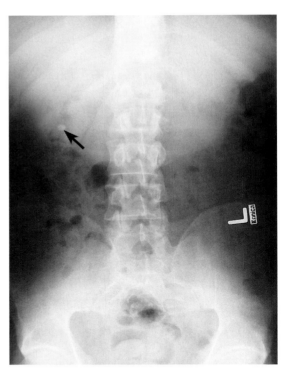

FIG. 8-44 A solitary renal calculus measuring 5 mm in diameter (*arrow*) is seen in the right renal silhouette.

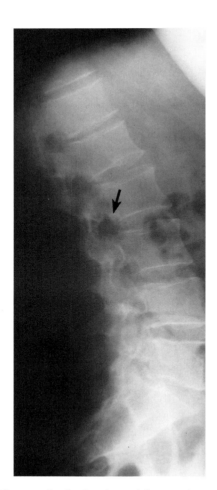

FIG. 8-45 The renal calculus (*arrow*) is superimposed over the posteroinferior margin of the L2 vertebral body. Its retroperitoneal location helps distinguish this stone from one that may exist in the gallbladder.

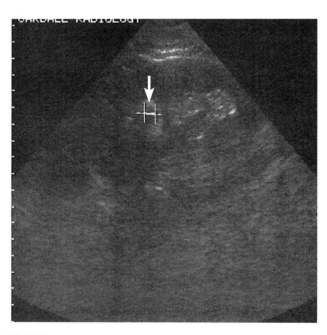

FIG. 8-46 An ultrasound study of the left kidney reveals the presence of a 7-mm renal stone (*arrow*).

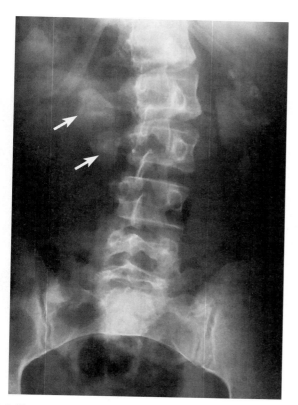

FIG. 8-47 This anteroposterior view of the abdomen demonstrates renal lithiasis (*arrows*).

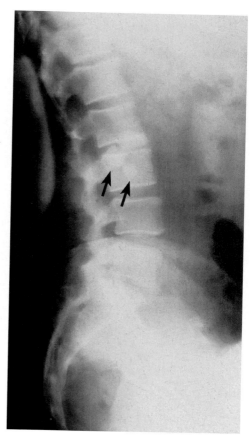

FIG. 8-48 Characteristic retroperitoneal location of renal lithiasis (*arrows*).

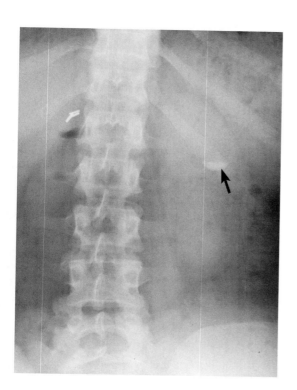

FIG. 8-49 A solitary major calyceal stone (*arrow*) is seen in this anteroposterior projection. Postcholecystectomy neurovascular clips are observed incidentally in the right upper quadrant.

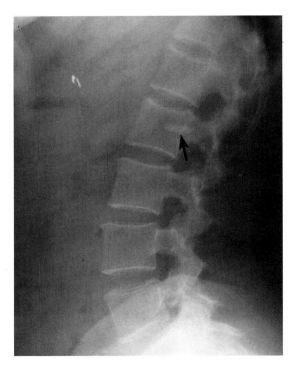

FIG. 8-50 A lateral view of a solitary retroperitoneal calyceal calculus (*arrow*).

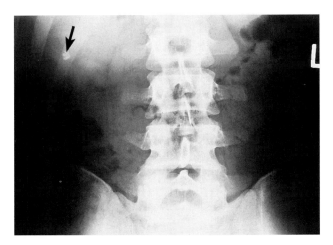

FIG. 8-51 A minor calyceal calculus (*arrow*) is seen on an inspiration view. Note the trident shape of the calculus conforming anatomically to the minor calyx in which it is contained.

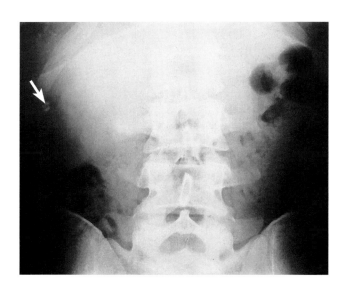

FIG. 8-52 The same minor calyceal calculus (*arrow*), as observed on an expiration film. Note the way the stone alters its position relative to the respective phases of respiration.

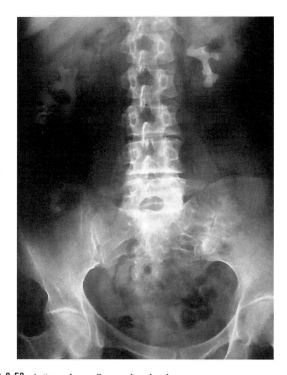

FIG. 8-53 A "staghorn" renal calculus.

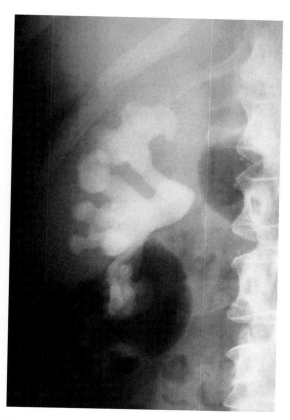

FIG. 8-54 A large "staghorn" renal calculus occupying the renal pelvis, as well as the major and minor calyces.

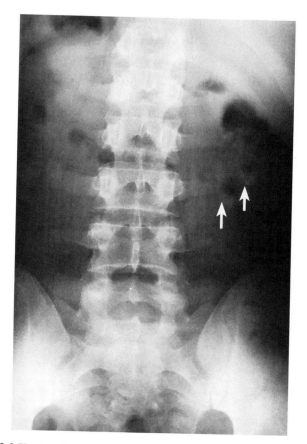

FIG. 8-55 Renal calcinosis (nephrocalcinosis) secondary to old, healed tuberculosis of the kidney (*arrows*).

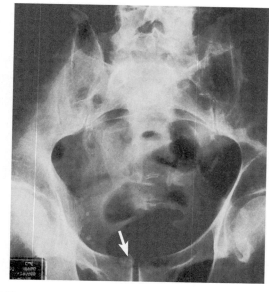

FIG. 8-56 Benign prostatic calcification (*arrow*) is observed superimposed over the superior symphysis pubis.

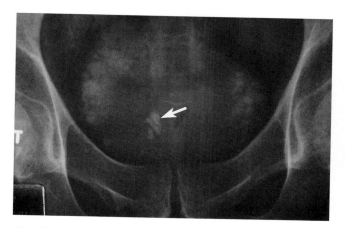

FIG. 8-57 A calculus (*arrow*) is noted in the urinary vesicle.

SOFT TISSUE

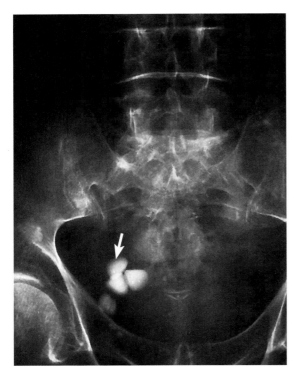

FIG. 8-58 Large radiopaque urinary vesicular calculi are observed (*arrow*).

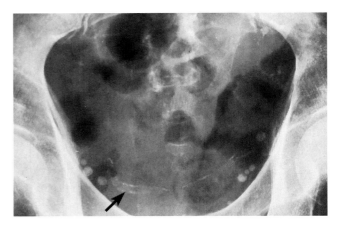

FIG. 8-59 Serpiginous calcification of the vas deferens (*arrow*) is noted. This condition has been linked to the presence of diabetes mellitus.

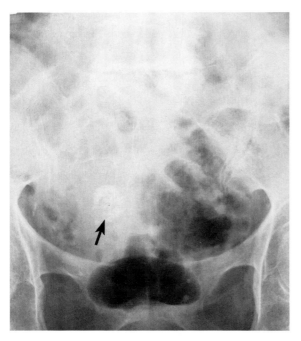

FIG. 8-60 A calcified uterine fibroma 2 cm in diameter is present (*arrow*).

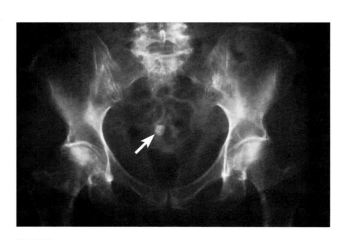

FIG. 8-61 A calcified uterine fibroma (*arrow*) is exhibited in the midline of the pelvic basin.

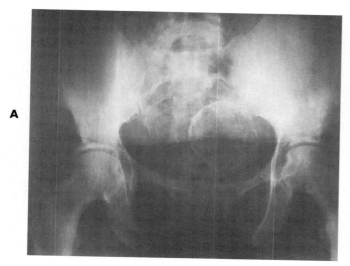

A

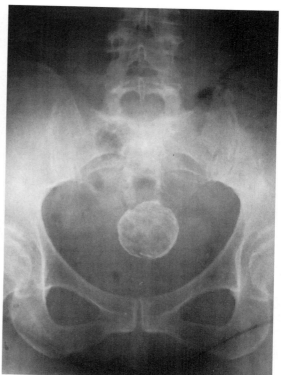

B

FIG. 8-62 A and **B,** A solitary massive calcified uterine fibroma is demonstrated in each of these women.

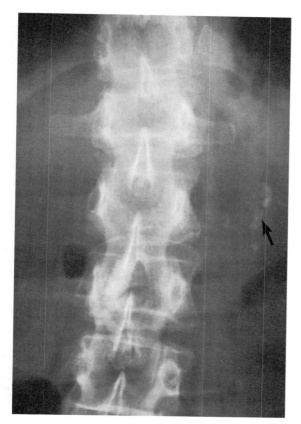

FIG. 8-63 Stippled calcification is noted throughout the parenchyma of the pancreas (*arrow*). This frequently arises as a consequence of chronic pancreatitis.

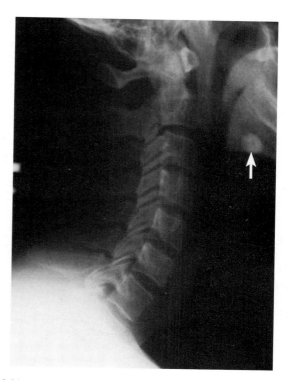

FIG. 8-64 A submandibular stone (sialolith) measuring 1 cm in diameter is visualized (*arrow*).

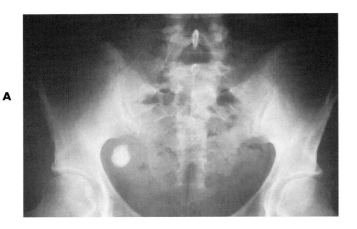

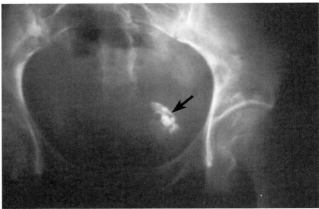

FIG. 8-66 A dermoid cyst with tooth formation (*arrow*) is contained in the matrix of the lesion.

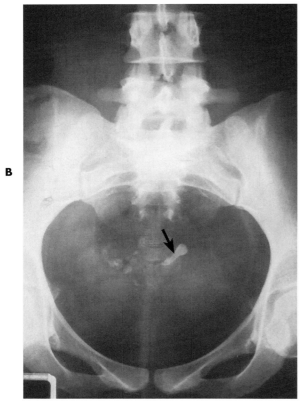

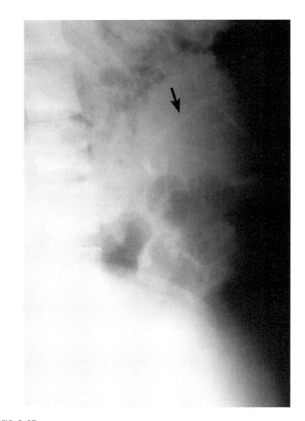

FIG. 8-65 **A,** A calcified ovarian cyst. **B,** A dermoid cyst with tooth formation (*arrow*) noted in the pelvis.

FIG. 8-67 A fetus in utero (*arrow*).

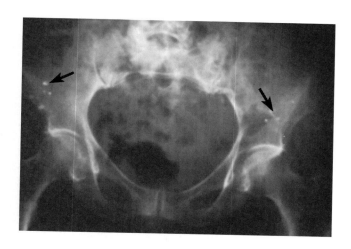

FIG. 8-68 Multiple injection granulomata (*arrows*) in the gluteal musculature.

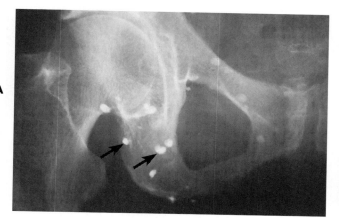

A

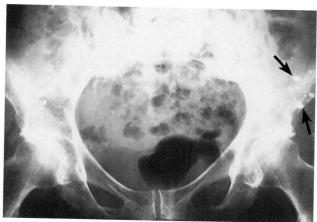

B

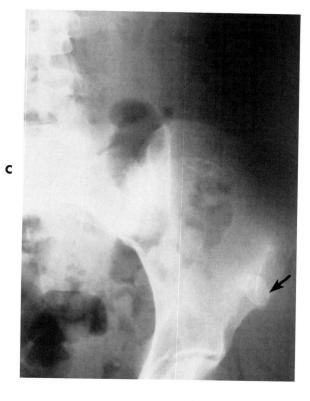

C

FIG. 8-69 **A,** Heavy metal injection sites (*arrows*). **B,** Heavy metal injection sites (*arrows*). **C,** Large injection granulomata (*arrow*) are observed in the gluteal musculature.

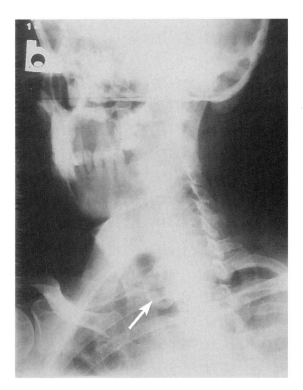

FIG. 8-70 A large calcified thyroid gland adenoma (*arrow*).

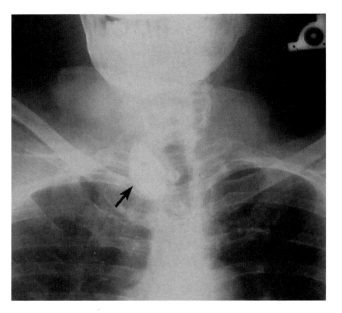

FIG. 8-71 Anteroposterior view of a large calcified thyroid gland adenoma (*arrow*).

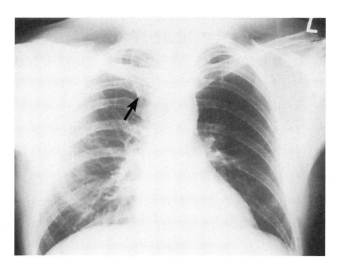

FIG. 8-72 An azygous fissure is noted in the apical portion of the right upper lobe. This represents a normal variant accessory fissure produced by the azygous vein (*arrow*).

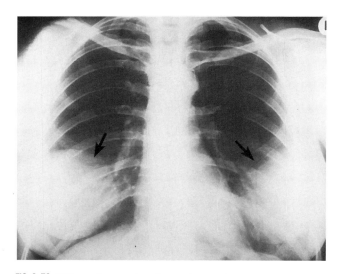

FIG. 8-73 Silicon breast implants (*arrows*).

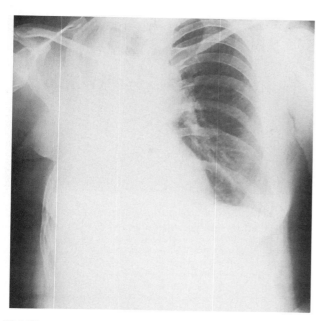

FIG. 8-74 Thoracoplasty.

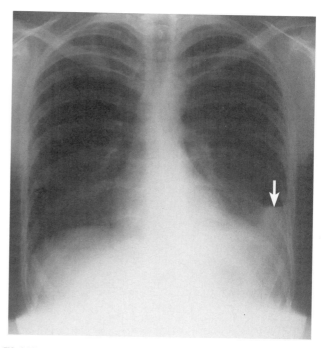

FIG. 8-75 Hydrothorax with an air-fluid meniscus level (*arrow*). The fluid occupies the left costophrenic sulcus.

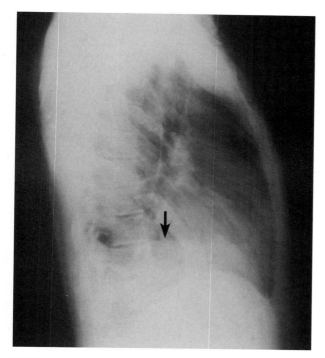

FIG. 8-76 Hydrothorax manifesting as an air-fluid meniscus level (*arrow*).

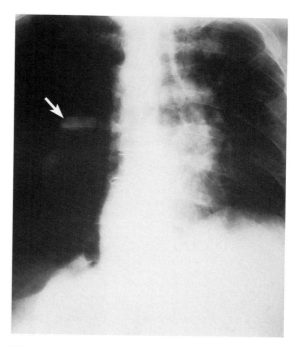

FIG. 8-77 Tension pneumothorax. Note the absence of bronchovascular markings in the periphery of the chest as a result of the entire lung collapsing toward the hilum (*arrow*). A contralateral shift of the mediastinum and its contents, including the trachea, has occurred, and the ipsilateral hemidiaphragm is markedly depressed.

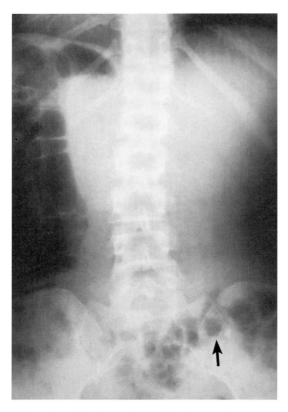

FIG. 8-78 Ptosis of the large bowel is observed (*arrow*). Redundancies of any part of the colon may also be seen incidentally as a normal roentgen variant.

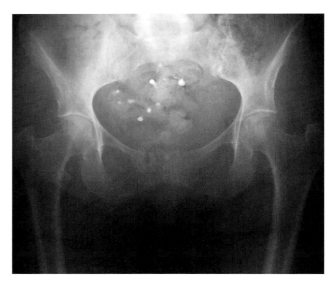

FIG. 8-79 Remnants of a barium sulfate enema examination are seen in small diverticulae in the sigmoid colon.

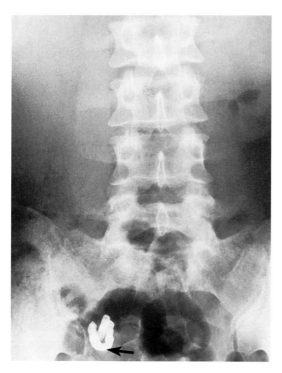

FIG. 8-80 Contrast medium is seen in the vermiform appendix (*arrow*).

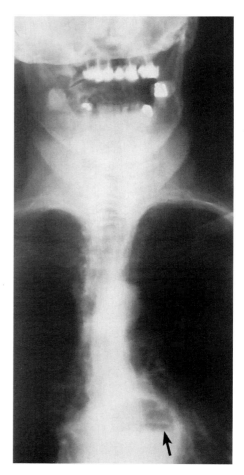

FIG. 8-81 Hiatal hernia. An air-fluid meniscus level (*arrow*) is superimposed on the cardiac silhouette. Gastric rugal folds are suggested in the roof of the hollow viscus.

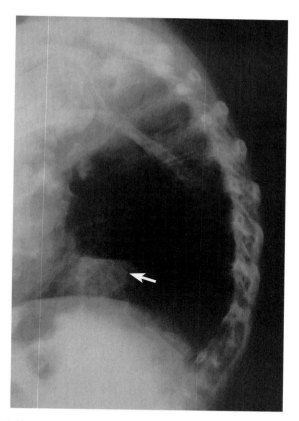

FIG. 8-82 Lateral view of a hiatal hernia (*arrow*) displaying the typical air-fluid meniscus sign in the middle mediastinum. This condition is most frequently observed in senior-aged women.

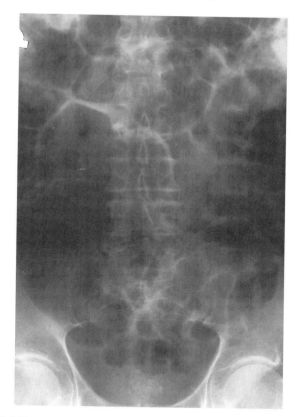

FIG. 8-83 Large bowel obstruction. Note the distention of the bowel walls by large quantities of gas.

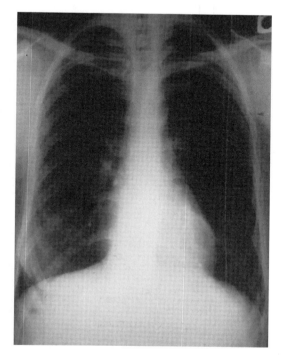

FIG. 8-84 The absence of a breast shadow indicates a mastectomy, which was necessary as a result of breast carcinoma.

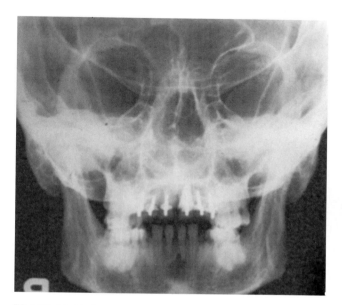

FIG. 8-85 Multiple dental implants.

SOFT TISSUE

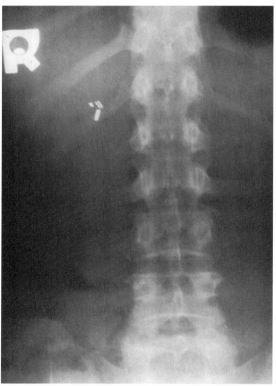

FIG. 8-86 Multiple surgical hemostatic clips in the right upper quadrant are suggestive of previous cholecystectomy.

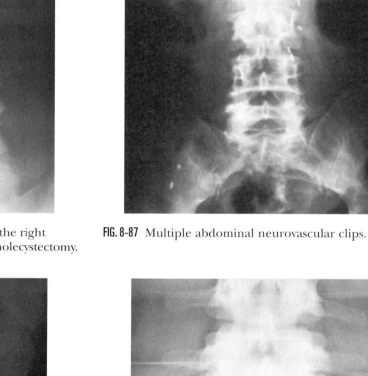

FIG. 8-87 Multiple abdominal neurovascular clips.

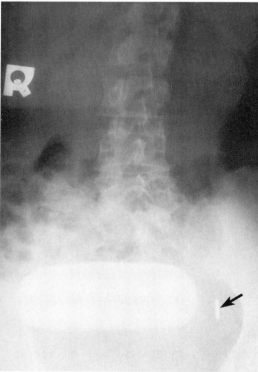

FIG. 8-88 Tubal ligation clip (*arrow*).

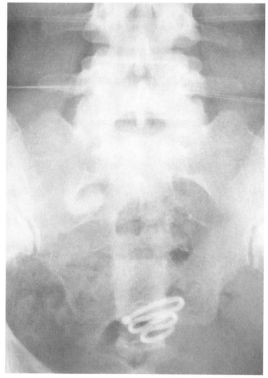

FIG. 8-89 Intrauterine contraceptive device: Lippe's loop.

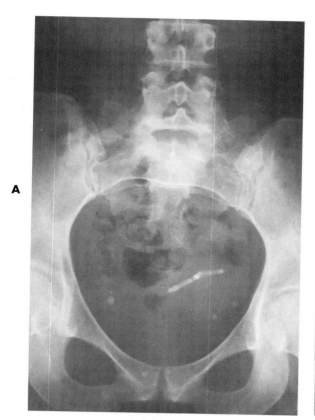

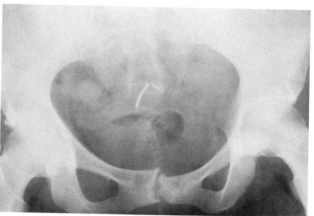

FIG. 8-90 **A** and **B,** Intrauterine contraceptive device: Copper T.

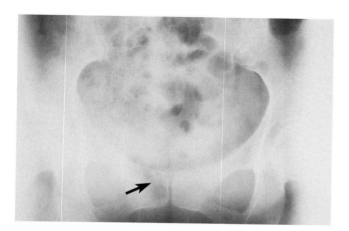

FIG. 8-91 "Tampon" sign (*arrow*) seen as a regular rectangular, radiolucent shadow.

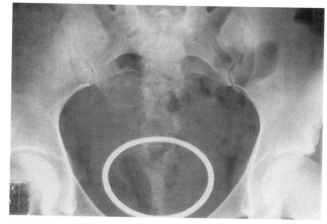

FIG. 8-92 This oval coiled spring is a contraceptive diaphragm.

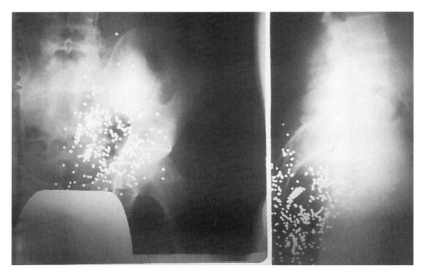

FIG. 8-93 Buckshot imbedded in the posterior pelvic musculature.

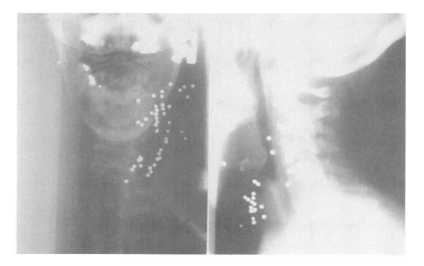

FIG. 8-94 Buckshot in soft tissues of the right anterior portion of the neck.

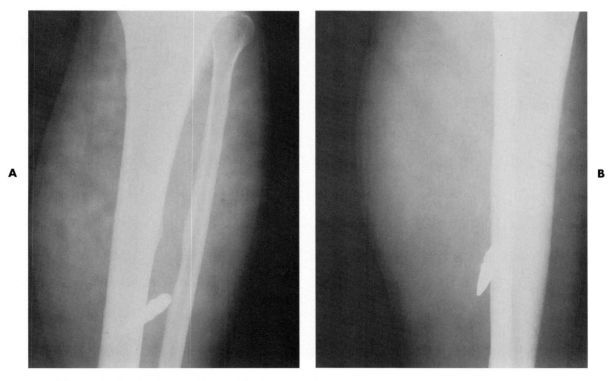

FIG. 8-95 A bullet is observed lodged in the posterior calf musculature. **A,** Anteroposterior. **B,** Lateral.

Scoliosis

Scoliosis is a term coined by the Greek physician Galen and is defined as any lateral deviation of the spine from the midsagittal plane (Figs. 9-1 and 9-2). An overview of the assessment of scoliotic considerations is presented in this chapter.

STRUCTURAL AND NONSTRUCTURAL SCOLIOSES

Structural

- ◆ Fixed lateral curve
- ◆ It does not correct on supine lateral, sidebending radiographs
  - Idiopathic: infantile, juvenile, adolescent
  - Neuromuscular (e.g., cerebral palsy, poliomyelitis, muscular dystrophy)
  - Congenital: wedge vertebra, hemivertebra
  - Neurofibromatosis
  - Tumor: osteoid osteoma
  - Infection: acute/chronic
  - Trauma: fracture, surgical (postlaminectomy)

Nonstructural

- ◆ The curve possesses no structural component and corrects or overcorrects on recumbent, sidebending radiographs.
  - Postural
  - Hysterical
  - Irritation of the nerve root: herniated nucleus pulposus
  - Inflammatory: appendicitis
  - Related to leg-length discrepancy
  - Related to regional hip contractures

MAJOR CURVE

- ◆ The largest curve, usually structural

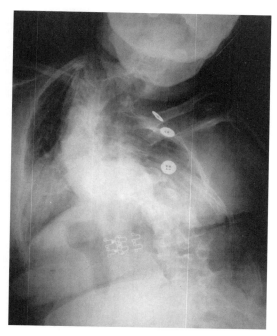

FIG. 9-1 Severe scoliosis. Note the nearly right angle formed by the spine at the curve's midportion.

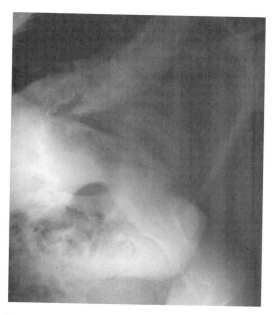

FIG. 9-2 Massive postural deformity accompanies this severe lumbar C-curve.

MINOR OR COMPENSATORY CURVE

- Located above or below the major curve
- Tends to maintain normal body alignment
- May be structural

Clinical Features

Structural

IDIOPATHIC

- Most common type
- Constitutes approximately 80% of scolioses
- Unknown etiology (possibly includes an inherited genetic defect)

Infantile

- The curve develops between birth and 3 years.
- The majority of curves resolve but rarely progress (usually characterized by a left convex thoracic curve in males).

Juvenile

- This includes children from 3 years of age to the onset of puberty (10 years of age).
- There is no gender predilection.

Adolescent

- Curvature develops in individuals when they are between 10 years of age and skeletal maturity (10 to 25 years).
- This is the most common form of idiopathic scoliosis.
- There is a female predominance of 9:1.
- This type may include rapid progression during the critical growth period of 12 to 16 years of age.
- Progression is unlikely after spinal growth ceases (denoted by Risser's sign).
- However, in adult life, the patient may acquire superimposed osteoarthritis resulting in increased curve and/or nerve entrapment.

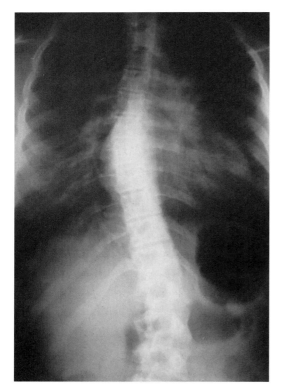

FIG. 9-3 This mild right thoracic convexity is characteristic of adolescent idiopathic scoliosis. (Courtesy Hartley Bressler, DC, MD, Toronto, Ontario.)

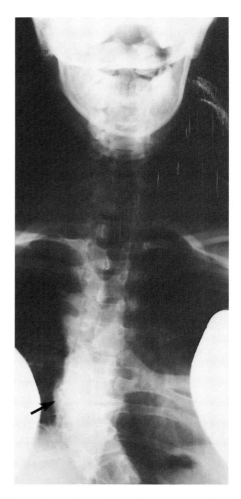

FIG. 9-4 T8 consists of a small wedge hemivertebra (*arrow*). In conjunction with multiple congenital block vertebrae (T4-T5, T6-T7, and T9-T10), a localized midthoracic convexity is formed. Also note the contralateral rib synostosis.

The most frequent pattern is a right thoracic convexity (Fig. 9-3). The patient may have permanent lateral wedging of vertebral bodies as a result of excessive compressive axial loading, resulting in impaired growth (Heuter-Volkman principle). The incidence of congenital heart disease is 10 times greater if the idiopathic curve exceeds 20 degrees.

Neuromuscular

Poliomyelitis

- Most common neuropathy with scoliosis
- Long C-curve extending from the sacrum to the lower cervical spine
- Convex to the side of unaffected musculature
- Possibility of severe intersegmental vertebral rotation
- Often rapid progression of angle between the ages of 12 and 16 years

Myopathic

- Infrequent; most common etiology, Duchenne muscular dystrophy
- Increased lordosis
- Rapidly progressive, severe

- Ultimately requires fusion by Harrington rods
- Virtual inevitability of scoliosis after patient confined to wheelchair

Congenital

- Anomalies of vertebrae and ribs possible
- Hemivertebrae, block vertebrae, spina bifida
- Rib deformities, fenestration, synostosis (Fig. 9-4)
- Typically a short C-curve
- Frequent association with genitourinary system anomalies

NEUROFIBROMATOSIS

- Congenital inherited disorder of neuroectodermal and mesodermal tissues
- Classic triad
  - Fibroma molluscum (elevated cutaneous tumors)
  - Café au lait pigmentation (coast of California margination)
  - Peripheral nerve neurofibromas
- Mild to severe scoliosis in 50% of patients
- Short angular deformities with vertebral body dysplasias
- Superimposed kyphosis
- Possible observation of enlarged intervertebral foraminae, posterior body scalloping, and "twisted ribbon" deformed ribs
- Tendency of scoliosis to advance, requiring surgical intervention to stabilize its progression

TUMOR

- Painful scoliosis, with lesion tending to be on the concave side of the curve

INFECTION

- One example: osteoma
- Possible promotion of scoliosis as a result of bony destruction and collapse (e.g., tuberculous spondylitis [Pott's disease])

TRAUMA

- Fracture of a lateral portion of a vertebral body possibly resulting in a permanent lateral spinal curvature

OTHER

- Degenerative joint disease with asymmetric advanced discopathy and facet arthrosis

COMPLICATIONS

- Cardiopulmonary
  - With severe scolioses, restricted rib cage excursion ultimately results in pulmonary hypertension and congestive heart failure.
  - This represents the single most common direct cause of death in the scoliotic patient.
  - Altered lung ventilation predisposes the patient to dyspnea and pulmonary infection.
- Degenerative joint disease
  - This occurs particularly in adults.
  - It is most pronounced on the concave side of the scoliotic curve.
  - Signs of osteoarthritis include decreased disc height, osteophytes, and intersegmental instability (Fig. 9-5).

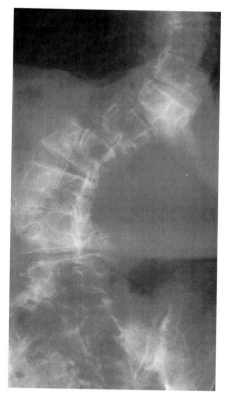

FIG. 9-5 This thoracolumbar S-curve in a 70-year-old woman demonstrates multiple levels of advanced degenerative disc disease, with laterolistheses at L4 and L1. (Courtesy Mrs. Freda Deltoff and Arnie Deltoff, DC, Toronto, Ontario.)

- This may lead to nerve root entrapment (e.g., lateral recess encroachment secondary to facet arthrosis).
- Progression of curve
  - This occurs particularly from 12 to 16 years, the time frame of the adolescent growth spurt.
  - The curve may rapidly increase by 1 degree per month.
- Joint dysfunction syndromes and fatigue
  - Altered biomechanical stresses, asymmetric joint kinematics, and muscular strain can produce significant pain and instability.
- Radiation exposure
  - The average increased risk of malignancy appears minimal.
  - There are long-term effects of repeated radiologic examinations (average of 22 studies during a 3-year period).

- Psychologic stress
  - The patient wears a brace.
- Skin irritations
  - These are secondary to long-term bracing.
- Surgical complications
  - Pseudoarthrosis
  - Instrumentation failure
  - Infection

X-RAY ASSESSMENT

- Important diagnostic modality
- Possible aid in determining etiology
- Evaluation of curve's site, magnitude, and flexibility
- Skeletal maturity determination
- Monitoring of curve progression and/or regression

Computed Tomography (CT) Evaluation

- CT aids in the description of the relationships of the rib hump, longitudinal axis rotation, lateral curve, and kyphosis-lordosis, with exceedingly small radiation doses.
- CT makes possible a direct measurement of the rotation of each vertebra.

- CT metrizamide myelography is an extremely important examination in congenital scoliosis with associated abnormalities such as dysraphisms.
- Magnetic resonance imaging (MRI) may provide information similar to that from CT without the hazard of radiation exposure.

MENSURATION

Cobb (Cobb-Lippman) Method

- This is the most accepted method.
- Construct a line along the superior border of the cephalad end vertebra (Figs. 9-6 and 9-7).
- Construct a line along the inferior border of the caudad end vertebra. (Use the tops or bottoms of the pedicles if the end plates are poorly visualized.)

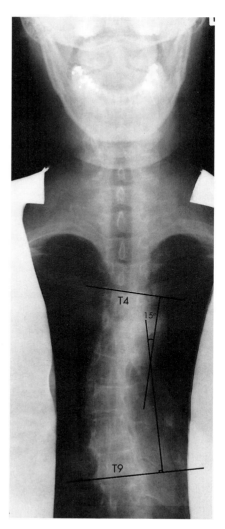

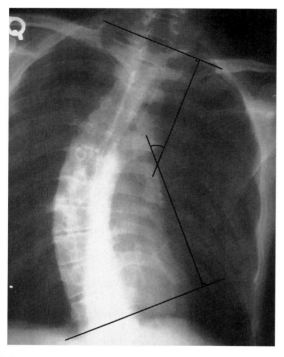

FIG. 9-6 The Cobb method of scoliosis measurement is demonstrated on this right thoracic convexity.

FIG. 9-7 A 15-degree right convexity is noted extending from T4 to T9. The Cobb method of mensuration is

- Construct a perpendicular line from each horizontal line.
- Measure the acute angle of intersection of the perpendiculars.

Risser-Ferguson Method

- Find the centers of the end and apical vertebral bodies (Figs. 9-8 and 9-9).
- Connect the centers of the superior and apical vertebrae.
- Connect the centers of the inferior and apical vertebrae.

- Measure the acute angle of the intersection of these two lines.

Rotation

- Rotation is related to the degree of external cosmetic deformity.
- The most accepted method of evaluation is the pedicle, or Nash-Moe, method.
- The movement of the pedicle is subjectively graded on the convex side of the curve between 0 and 4 (Figs. 9-10 and 9-11).

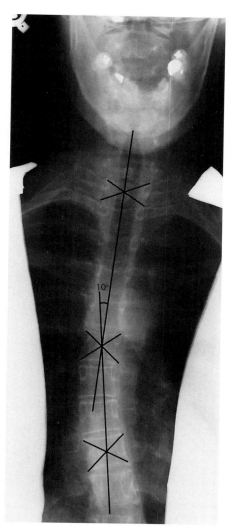

FIG. 9-8 A 10-degree right thoracic convexity in a 30-year-old woman is evaluated by the Risser-Ferguson method. (Courtesy Lisette Logan, MRT, Brampton, Ontario.)

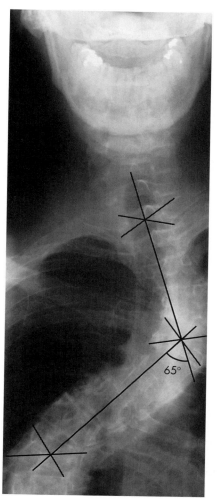

FIG. 9-9 The Risser-Ferguson method measures a 65-degree left thoracic convexity in this 40-year-old man. (Courtesy Robert Cannon, DC, Toronto, Ontario.)

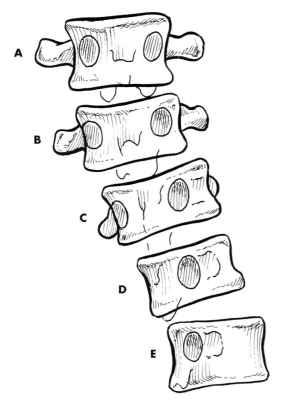

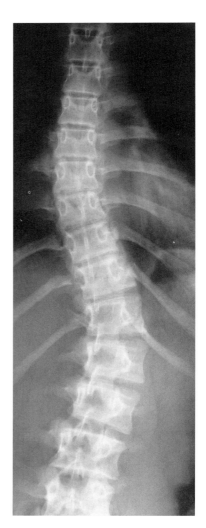

FIG. 9-10 The assessment of vertebral body rotation based on pedicle position, as viewed on an anteroposterior radiograph. **A,** Normal. **B,** Grade 1+. The convex-side pedicle is rotated slightly toward the midline. **C,** Grade 2+. The convex-side pedicle is rotated two thirds toward the midline; the concave-side pedicle is disappearing. **D,** Grade 3+. The convex-side pedicle is at the midline; the concave-side pedicle has disappeared. **E,** Grade 4+. The convex-side pedicle has rotated beyond the midline.

FIG. 9-11 Observe the multiple vertebral body rotation in the left thoracolumbar convexity in this 13-year-old girl. L1 demonstrates Grade 3+ rotation, T12 and L2 demonstrate Grade 2+ rotation, and T11 and L3 demonstrate Grade 1+ rotation. (Courtesy Lisette Logan, MRT, Brampton, Ontario.)

Flexibility

- *Flexibility* is defined as the degree of mobility in a scoliosis.
- A lack of flexibility is a contraindication to spinal fusion.
- The primary method of evaluation uses a supine lateral bending radiograph toward the convex side of the scoliosis.
- With the Cobb method, the degree of correction calculated is the measure of flexibility.

Skeletal Maturation

- Skeletal maturation is vital to the choice of therapy and determination of prognosis.
- Risser's sign is commonly used to assess the progression of skeletal maturity.

- Iliac apophysis usually appears laterally near the anterior superior iliac spine (ASIS) and progresses medially toward the posterior superior iliac spine (PSIS); this is referred to as *capping* (Fig. 9-12, *A* and *B*).
- Growth is graded as follows:
  - 1+ = 25%
  - 2+ = 50%
  - 3+ = 75%
  - 4+ = 100%
  - 5+ = apophysis fused to ilium
- Risser's sign becomes visualized at age 14 years in females and age 16 years in males.
- An additional year is required to reach Stage 4+.
- Stage 5+ occurs in 2 to 3 additional years.
- At 10 to 15 years of age, before iliac apophysis is visible, the scoliotic curve demonstrates its greatest potential rate of progression.
- After the iliac apophysis becomes evident, the curve progression slows, then eventually ceases following apophyseal fusion.

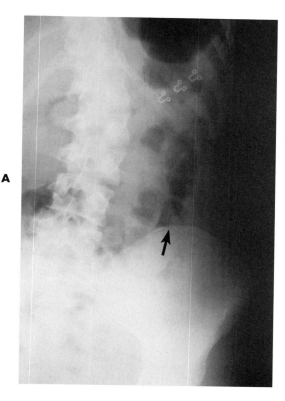

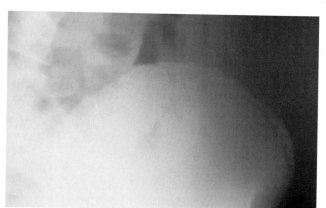

FIG. 9-12 Risser's sign. **A,** Observe the secondary growth center of the iliac apophysis (*arrow*) in this 18-year-old woman with a lumbar convexity. **B,** A close-up of the iliac crest, clearly demonstrating the unfused apophysis. (Courtesy Hartley Bressler, DC, MD, Toronto, Ontario.)

THERAPY SELECTION

- Therapy selection is based on the curve progression, effect on body function, and cosmetic appearance.
- Approximately 25% of curves exhibit some degree of progression.
- Indicators of likely progression are age, onset of menarche, and absent (0) or early (1+) Risser's sign.

Long-Term Monitoring

- Long-term monitoring includes an x-ray examination every 3 to 4 months until skeletal maturity is reached, as demonstrated by Stage 5+ Risser's sign.
- After brace removal, an annual x-ray examination is performed for 5 years. The patient is examined for any delayed tendency to curve progression. If curve progression is present, surgical stabilization may be indicated.

Surgery

- Relative indications
  - Determination whether underlying abnormality can be treated
  - Rapid progression in an immature spine
  - Curve greater than 40 degrees

POSTERIOR FUSION AND INSTRUMENTATION

Harrington rods

- This is the most widely used method of posterior fixation.
- It consists of distraction and compression devices.
- Distraction hooks located at each end of the rod are placed on the laminae of the vertebrae at either end of the concavity of the scoliosis.
- The compression rod is used on the convexity to supplement the Harrington distraction device.
- The average correction achieved is 30% to 55%.

Luque rods

- One Luque rod is positioned posteriorly along each side of the spine.
- Transverse forces are created by passing a wire under each lamina and then twisting the wire around its respective rod.

- Securing the spine at multiple points distributes the force across multiple levels, with resultant greater curve stability.
- Rods can also be contoured to maintain normal thoracic kyphosis and lumbar lordosis.

ANTERIOR FUSION AND INSTRUMENTATION

- Although posterior instrumentation and fusion is considered safest and is the most commonly used method for surgical correction of scoliosis, anterior fusion is generally recommended in the following conditions:
  - Paralytic lumbar and thoracolumbar scoliosis over 75 degrees with pelvic obliquity
  - Scoliosis with deficient posterior elements caused by myelomeningocele or extensive laminectomy
  - Scoliosis with spastic cerebral palsy
  - Idiopathic scoliosis over 80 degrees
  - Congenital scoliosis owing to hemivertebra or an unsegmented bar

Dwyer procedure

- This is the most commonly used method of internal fixation via anterior fusion.
- A staple is inserted into each vertebral body to be fused on the side of the convexity, and a screw passes transversely through a hole in the staple and into the center of the vertebral body. Each screw has a vertical opening in its head to allow passage of the cable.
- After it is slid through the opening in each screw, the cable is tightened to the desired tension and then crimped at each end to prevent slippage.
- This procedure allows dramatic correction of idiopathic scoliosis and more completely corrects the lateral deviation and rotation of the spine.

Zielke instrumentation

- A single screw is inserted transversely through the center of each vertebral body to be fused.
- Each screw is then locked onto a flexible stainless steel, threaded rod, which links all levels.
- This procedure has a greater ability to correct vertebral rotation, so it is generally preferred over Dwyer instrumentation when anterior internal fixation is the therapy of choice.

BIBLIOGRAPHY/SUGGESTED READINGS

Adams, Crawford J: *Outline of fractures,* ed 8, New York, 1983, Churchill Livingstone.

Adson AW: Cervical ribs: symptoms, differential diagnosis for section of the insertion of the scalenus anticus muscle, *J Coll Surg* 16:546, 1951.

Adson AW, Coffey JR: Cervical ribs, *Am Surg* 85:839, 1927.

Ardan GM et al: Assessment of scoliosis in children: low dose radiographic technique, *Br J Radiol* 53:146-147, 1980.

Aviolo LV: *Metabolic bone disease, vol I and II,* New York, 1977, Academic Press.

Bailey DK: The normal cervical spine in infants and children, *Radiology* 59:712, 1952.

Bailey RW, editor: *The cervical spine: the Cervical Spine Research Society,* Philadelphia, 1983, JB Lippincott.

Beckman CE, Hall V: Variability and scoliosis measurement from spinal roentgenograms, *Phys Ther* 59:764-765, 1979.

Berquist T: *MRI of the musculoskeletal system,* ed 3, Philadelphia, 1996, JB Lippincott.

Berquist TH: *Diagnostic imaging of the acutely injured patient,* Baltimore, 1985, Urban & Schwarzenberg.

Borkow SE, Kleiger B: Spondylolisthesis in newborn, *Clin Orthop* 81:71, 1971.

Brewer EJ, Giannini EH, Person DA: *Juvenile rheumatoid arthritis,* ed 2, Toronto, 1977, WB Saunders.

Brower AC: *Arthritis in black and white,* Philadelphia, 1988, WB Saunders.

Budin E, Spondheimer F: Lateral spread of the atlas without fracture, *Radiology* 87:1096, 1966.

Caillet R: *Scoliosis: diagnosis and management,* Philadelphia, 1975, FA Davis.

Carter CO, Evans K: Spina bifida and anencephalus in greater London, *J Med Genet* 13:343, 1973.

Cattal HS, Filtzer DL: Pseudosubluxation and other normal variations in the cervical spine in children, *J Bone Joint Surg* 47A:1295, 1965.

Chan SN, Seljeskog EL: *Spinal deformities and neurological dysfunction,* New York, 1978, Raven.

Chapman S, Nakielny R: *Aids to radiological differential diagnosis,* ed 3, London, 1995, Bailliere Tindall.

Chauman B: *The cervical spine: the Cervical Spine Research Society,* Philadelphia, 1983, JB Lippincott.

Conn HF, Conn RB: *Current Diagnosis,* Philadelphia, 1977, WB Saunders.

Connolly JF: *The management of fractures and dislocations, an atlas,* Toronto, 1980, WB Saunders.

Cowe P: Butterfly vertebrae, *Br J Radiol* 31:530, 1958.

Craignile TK: *Congenital anomalies of the spine in spinal disorders: diagnosis and treatment,* Philadelphia, 1977, Lea & Febiger.

Daffner RH: *Clinical radiology: the essentials,* Baltimore, 1993, Williams & Wilkins.

David Y: *Spinal injury,* New York, 1978, Appleton Century Crofts.

Debnan JW, Staple TW: Osseous metastases from cerebellar medulloblastoma, *Radiology* 107:363-365, 1973.

De Smet AA: *Radiology of spinal curvature,* St Louis, 1985, Mosby.

Dorland's illustrated medical dictionary, ed 26, Philadelphia, 1974, WB Saunders.

Dosch C Jr: *Radiology of the spine: trauma,* Berlin, 1985, Springer-Verlag.

Dyck D: Os odontoideum in children: neurological manifestation and surgical management, *Neurosurg* 2:93-98, 1978.

Eideken J, Hodes J: *Roentgen diagnosis of diseases of bone, vol I-II,* ed 3, Baltimore, 1981, Williams & Wilkins.

Eisenberg RL: *Atlas of signs in radiology,* Philadelphia, 1984, JB Lippincott.

Epstein BS: *The spine: a radiological text and atlas,* Philadelphia, 1976, Lea & Febiger.

Epstein BS: *The vertebral column: an atlas of tumor radiology,* Chicago, 1974, Year Book Medical Publishers.

Evants CM, Londsale D: Ossiculum terminale: an anomaly of the odontoid process: report of a case of atlanto-axial dislocation with cord compression, *Cleve Clin Q* 37:73, 1970.

Fielding JW, Griffin PP: Os odontoideum: an acquired lesion, *J Bone Joint Surg* 56A:187, 1974.

Fielding JW, Hensinger RN, Hawkins RJ: Os odontoideum, *J Bone Joint Surg* 62A:376, 1980.

Fischer FJ, Vandemark RE: Sagittal cleft (butterfly) vertebrae, *J Bone Joint Surg* 27:695, 1945.

Fornage B: *Musculoskeletal ultrasound,* New York, 1995, Churchill Livingstone.

Forrester DM, Brown JC, Nesson JW: *The radiology of joint disease,* Toronto, 1978, WB Saunders.

Francis KC, Hutter RVP: Neoplasms of the spine in the aged, *Clin Orthop* 26:54-66, 1963.

Freiberger R, Wilson PD Jr, Nicholas JA: Acquired absence of the odontoid process, *J Bone Joint Surg* 47A:1231, 1965.

Geber LH, Espinoza LR: *Psoriatic arthritis,* Toronto, 1985, Grune and Stratton.

Gehweiler JA, Osborne RL, Becker RF: *Radiology of vertebral trauma,* Philadelphia, 1980, WB Saunders.

George K, Rippstein J: A comparative study of the two popular methods of measuring scoliotic deformity of the spine, *J Bone Joint Surg* 6:809-818, 1961.

Gilbert GW et al: Epidural spinal cord compression from metastatic tumor: diagnosis and treatment, *Ann Neurol* 3:40-51, 1978.

Gilula LA, Yin Y: *Imaging of the wrist and hand,* Phildelphia, 1996, WB Saunders.

Glesson IO, Urist MR: Atlanto-axial dislocation with odontoid separation in rheumatoid arthritis, *Clin Orthop* 42:121, 1965.

Golding DN: *Rheumatic diseases,* ed 3, Chicago, 1978, John Wright and Sons.

Goldman et al: Osteitis deformans of the hip joint, *Am J Roentgenol* 128:601-606, 1977.

Gornall A: *Applied biochemistry of clinical disorders,* Toronto, 1980, Harper & Row.

Graham J, Harris WH: Paget's disease involving the hip joint, *J Bone Joint Surg* 53B:650-659, 1971.

Gray JF et al: Reduction of radiation exposure during radiography for scoliosis, *J Bone Joint Surg* 65:5-12, 1983.

Gray SW, Romain CB, Skandalakis JE: Congenital fusion of the cervical vertebrae, *Surg Gynecol Obstet* 118:373, 1964.

Greenfield GB: *Radiology of bone disease,* ed 3, Philadelphia, 1980, JB Lippincott.

Greenspan A: *Orthopedic radiology,* ed 2, Philadelphia, 1992, JB Lippincott.

Greenspan A, Montesano P: *Imaging of the spine in clinical practice,* London, 1993, Wolfe Publishing.

Griffiths HJ: *Basic bone radiology,* ed 2, New York, 1987, Appleton Century Croft.

Grilliot JR: Os odontoidum, *ACA J Chiro* 19:11, 1985.

Gwinn JL, Smith JL: Acquired and congenital absence of the odontoid process, *Am J Roentgenol* 88:424, 1962.

Hafen BQ, Karren KJ: *Prehospital emergency care and crisis intervention,* ed 2, Englewood, Colo, 1983, Morton.

Haller JO, Slovis TL: *Introduction to radiology in clinical pediatrics,* Chicago, 1984, Year Book Medical Publishers.

Halstead JA: *The laboratory in clinical medicine,* Philadelphia, 1976, WB Saunders.

Handy RC: *Paget's disease of bone, vol 1,* New York, 1981, Praeger.

Harris JH, Edeiken-Monroe B: *The radiology of acute cervical spine trauma,* ed 2, Baltimore, 1987, Williams & Wilkins.

Hawkins RJ, Fielding JW, Thompson WJ: Os odontoideum: congenital or acquired, *J Bone Joint Surg* 58A:413, 1976.

Helms CA: *Fundamentals of skeletal radiology,* Philadelphia, 1989, WB Saunders.

Hensigner RN, Fielding JW, Hawkins RJ: Congenital anomalies of the odontoid process, *Ortho Clin North Am* 9:901-912, 1978.

Hessler RM: *Management of common musculoskeletal disorders,* Philadelphia, 1983, Harper & Row.

Huvos A: *Bone tumors, diagnosis, treatment and prognosis,* Philadelphia, 1979, WB Saunders.

Jackson DW, Wiltse IL, Cirincione RJ: Spondylolysis in the female gymnast, *Clin Orthop* 117:68, 1976.

Jaffe HL: The classic Paget's disease of bone, *Clin Orthop* 127:4, 1977.

Jaffe HL: *Metabolic, degenerative and inflammatory diseases of bones and joints,* Philadelphia, 1972, Lea & Febiger.

James JIP: *Scoliosis,* Edinburgh, 1976, Churchill Livingstone.

Jarvis LJ: Involvement of the sacrum by recurrent carcinoma of the rectum, *Am J Roentgenol* 84:339, 1960.

Jeffreys E: *Disorders of the cervical spine,* New York, 1980, Butterworths.

Jehl J, Crummy P: *Essentials of radiologic surgery,* ed 6, 1993, JB Lippincott.

Jowsey J: *Metabolic disease of bone, vol 1,* Philadelphia, 1979, WB Saunders.

Katten J: *Trauma and non-trauma of the cervical spine,* New York, 1975, Charles C. Thomas.

Keats TH: *Atlas of normal roentgen variants,* ed 6, St Louis, 1996, Mosby.

Keim HA: *Scoliosis: Ciba Clin Symp* 30:1, 1978.

Kelley WN et al: *Textbook of rheumatology,* Toronto, 1985, WB Saunders.

Kozlowski K, Beighton P: *Gamut index of skeletal dysplasias,* Berlin, 1984, Springer-Verlag.

Krane SM: Paget's disease of bone, *Clin Orthop* 127:24, 1977.

Krishnamurthy GT et al: Distribution pattern of metastatic bone disease, *JAMA* 327:2504-2506, 1977.

Langenskiold A, Michelson JE: The pathogenesis of experimental progressive scoliosis, *Acta Orthop Scand Suppl* 59:26, 1962.

Lau LSW, DeCampo JF: *Notes on radiological diagnosis,* Artarmon, New South Wales, 1983, WB Saunders.

Lawrence D: *Advances in chiropractic, vol 3,* St Louis, 1996, Mosby.

Lester PN: *The essentials of roentgen interpretation,* ed 3, London, 1972, Harper & Row.

Lichtenstein L: *Diseases of bone and joints,* St Louis, 1975, Mosby.

Lutz J: Femoral fractures in Paget's disease, *Osteo Clin* 11:486-491, 1983.

MacEwen DG, Cowell HR: Familial incidence of idiopathic scoliosis and its implication in patient treatment, *J Bone Joint Surg* 52A:405, 1970.

MacRae JE: *Roentgenometrics in chiropractic,* Toronto, 1974, CMCC Press.

Manaster BJ: *Skeletal radiology,* Chicago, 1989, Year Book Medical Publishers.

Maroteaux D: *Bone diseases of children,* Philadelphia, 1979, JB Lippincott.

McCarty DJ: *Arthritis and allied conditions,* ed 10, Philadelphia, 1985, Lea & Febiger.

McRae DL, Barum AS: Occipitalization of the atlas, *Am J Roentgenol* 70:23, 1953.

Meisel AD, Bullough PG: *Atlas of osteoarthritis,* New York, 1984, Gower Medical Publishing.

Menelaus M: *The orthopedic management of spina bifida cystica,* ed 2, Edinburgh, 1980, Churchill Livingstone.

Merkow R, Lane J: Current concepts of Paget's disease of bone, *Clin Orthop* 15:4, 1984.

Meschan I: *Analysis of roentgen signs in general radiology, vol 1,* Philadelphia, 1973, WB Saunders.

Milgram J: Radiographical and pathological assessment of the activity of Paget's disease of bone, *Clin Orthop* 127:32, 1977.

Moe JH et al: *Scoliosis and other spinal deformities,* Philadelphia, 1978, WB Saunders.

Moore KL: *The developing human,* ed 2, Toronto, 1977, WB Saunders.

Mulvey RB: Peripheral bone metastases, *Am J Roentgenol* 91:155-200, 1964.

Murray RO: *The radiology of skeletal disorders, vol 1,* ed 2, New York, 1977, Churchill Livingstone.

Murray RO, Jacobsen HG: *Metastatic disease of the skeleton in the radiology of skeletal disorders,* ed 2, Edinburgh, 1977, Churchill Livingstone.

Nagashima C: Atlanto-axial dislocation due to agenesis of the os ondotoideum or odontoid, *J Neurosurg* 33:270, 1970.

Napoli LD et al: The incidence of osseous involvement in lung cancer with special reference to the development of osteoblastic changes, *Radiology* 108:17-21, 1973.

Nash CL, Moe JH: A study of vertebral rotation, *J Bone Joint Surg* 51:223-229, 1969.

Natasi AJ et al: Pain patterns associated with adolescent idiopathic scoliosis, *J Bone Joint Surg* 54A:199, 1972.

Newman PH: The etiology of spondylolisthesis, *J Bone Joint Surg* 45B:36-59, 1963.

Nicholson JT, Sherk HH: Anomalies of the occipitocervical articulation, *J Bone Joint Surg* 50A:295, 1968.

Ogden JA: *Skeletal injury in the child,* Philadelphia, 1982, Lea & Febiger.

Overton LM, Ghormley RK: Congenital fusion of the spine, *J Bone Joint Surg* 16:929, 1934.

Panush RS: *Principles of rheumatic diseases,* Toronto, 1982, John Wiley & Sons.

Passmore R: *A comparison to medical studies, vol III,* London, 1974, Blackwell Scientific Publications.

Paul LH, Juhl JH: *Essentials of roentgen interpretation,* ed 4, New York, 1981, Harper & Row.

Petersdorf RG et al: *Harrison's principles of internal medicine,* ed 10, New York, 1983, McGraw-Hill.

Phalen GS, Dickson JA: Spondylolisthesis and tight hamstrings, *J Bone Joint Surg* 43A:505-512, 1961.

Reeder M, Felson B: *Gamuts in radiology,* Cincinnati, 1975, Audiovisual Radiology of Cincinnati.

Resnick D: Osteomyelitis and septic arthritis of the hand following human bites, *J Skel Radiol* 14:263-266, 1985.

Resnick D, Niwayama G: *Diagnosis of bone and joint disorders,* Philadelphia, 1995, WB Saunders.

Riseborough EJ, Herndon JH: *Scoliosis and other deformities of the axial skeleton,* Boston, 1975, Little, Brown and Co.

Roback D: Topics in radiology, *JAMA* 245:9, March 1981.

Robbins SL, Angell MA, Kumar V: *Basic pathology,* Philadelphia, 1981, WB Saunders.

Romanus RH: *Pelvospondylitis ossificans,* Copenhagen, 1955, Year Book Medical Publishers.

Rothman RH, Simeone FA: *The spine, vol I,* Philadelphia, 1975, WB Saunders.

Rothman RH, Simeone FA: *The spine,* ed 2, New York, 1982, WB Saunders.

Ruge D, Wiltse LL: *Spinal disorders: diagnosis and treatment,* Philadelphia, 1977, Lea & Febiger.

Schaberg J, Gainor BJ: A profile of metastatic carcinoma of the spine, *Spine* 10:1, 1985.

Schultz EH Jr, Levy RW, Russo PE: Agenesis of the ondotoid process, *Radiology* 67:102, 1956.

Schmidek H: Neurologic and neurosurgical sequelae of Paget's diseases of bone, *Clin Orthop* 127:70, 1977.

Schmorl G, Junghanns H: *The human spine in health and disease,* ed 2, New York, 1971, Grune & Stratton.

Schumacher H: *Primer of the rheumatic diseases,* ed 10, New York, 1993, Arthritis Foundation.

Singer F, Mills B: The etiology of Paget's disease of bone, *Clin Orthop* 127:32, 1977.

Spjut H: *Tumors of bone and cartilage,* Washington DC, 1970, Armed Forces Institute of Pathology.

Sutton D: *Textbook of radiology,* ed 2, New York, 1975, Churchill Livingstone.

Taveras JM, Ferrucci JT: *Radiology: diagnosis-imaging-intervention,* Philadelphia, 1986, JB Lippincott.

Turek SI: *Orthopaedics, vol 2,* ed 4, Philadelphia, 1984, JB Lippincott.

Vaughan VC: *Textbook of pediatrics,* Philadelphia, 1979, WB Saunders.

Vernon H: *Upper cervical syndrome: chiropractic diagnosis and treatment,* Baltimore, 1989, Williams & Wilkins.

Von Torklus D, Rehle W: *The upper cervical spine,* New York, 1972, Grune & Stratton.

Wadia NH: Myelopathy complicating congenital atlanto-axial dislocation, *Brain* 90:449, 1967.

Weissman BNW, Sledge CB: *Orthopedic radiology,* Philadelphia, 1986, WB Saunders.

Wiltse LL, Newman PH, MacNab I: Classification of spondylolisthesis, *Clin Orthop* 117:23, 1976.

Wright V, Moll JM: *Seronegative polyarthritis,* New York, 1976, North-Holland Publishing.

Yochum T, Albers V: Cervical Paget's disease, *ACA J Chiro* 19:62, February 1982.

Yochum T, Rowe L: *Essentials of skeletal radiology,* ed 2, Baltimore, 1996, Williams & Wilkins.

Index